Neuropsychosocial Integration

Neuropsychosocial Integration

A Practical Approach to Discharging Trauma and Recovering the Authentic Self

Winniey E. Maduro, PhD

ROWMAN & LITTLEFIELD
Lanham • Boulder • New York • London

Published by Rowman & Littlefield
An imprint of The Rowman & Littlefield Publishing Group, Inc.
4501 Forbes Boulevard, Suite 200, Lanham, Maryland 20706
www.rowman.com

86-90 Paul Street, London EC2A 4NE

British Library Cataloguing in Publication Information available

Library of Congress Cataloging-in-Publication Data

Names: Maduro, Winniey E., author.
Title: Neuropsychosocial integration : a practical approach to discharging trauma and recovering the authentic self / Winniey E. Maduro, PhD.
Description: Lanham : Rowman & Littlefield, [2025] | Includes bibliographical references and index. | Summary: "This book explores manifestations of psychosocial trauma in the body and mind and offers practical interventions and resources for recovery and resilience"— Provided by publisher.
Identifiers: LCCN 2024023927 (print) | LCCN 2024023928 (ebook) | ISBN 9781538195840 (cloth) | ISBN 9781538195857 (paperback) | ISBN 9781538195864 (epub)
Subjects: LCSH: Psychic trauma—Treatment. | Post-traumatic stress disorder—Treatment.
Classification: LCC RC552.P67 M323 2025 (print) | LCC RC552.P67 (ebook) | DDC 616.85/21—dc23/eng/20240611
LC record available at https://lccn.loc.gov/2024023927
LC ebook record available at https://lccn.loc.gov/2024023928

To God
in whose wonderful image I am made and from whom I draw strength.

In gratitude to my ancestors
from whose struggles I draw inspiration.

Brief Contents

Foreword by William M. Singletary   xv

Preface: Authorship and Research Underpinning   xix

Acknowledgements   xxv

PART I: NEUROPSYCHOSOCIAL INTEGRATION IN RESEARCH   **1**

  1   Introduction to Neuropsychosocial Integration   3

PART II: NEUROPSYCHOSOCIAL (DIS)INTEGRATION IN CONTEXT   **15**

  2   Neuropsychosocial (Dis)Integration in Perspective   17

  3   Neuropsychosocial (Dis)Integration in the (In)Authentic Self   25

  4   Neuropsychosocial (Dis)Integration in the Dynamic Self   39

  5   Neuropsychosocial (Dis)Integration: Featuring Psychosocial Trauma   59

PART III: NEUROPSYCHOSOCIAL (DIS)INTEGRATION IN ANCESTRY   **73**

  6   Ances-Story in Neuropsychosocial (Dis)Integration   75

  7   Psychosocial Trauma as Legacy: Beginning in Early Life   91

  8   Psychosocial Trauma across Generations: In Practice   109

PART IV: NEUROPSYCHOSOCIAL INTEGRATION IN PROCESS   125

9 Neuropsychosocial Integration: Structures, Resources and Processes   127

10 Neuropsychosocial Integration: Aims and Steps   149

11 Neuropsychosocial Integration: Stages and Considerations   159

PART V: NEUROPSYCHOSOCIAL INTEGRATION IN THERAPY   167

12 Neurorelational Integration   169

13 Neuro-emotional Integration   185

14 Neuropsychological Integration   195

15 Neurosomatic Integration   209

PART VI: EMBRACING NEUROPSYCHOSOCIAL INTEGRATION IN WELL-BEING   223

16 A Survivor's Guide to Neuropsychosocial Integration   225

17 Beyond Psychosocial Trauma and Disintegration   235

Afterword   241

Neuropsychosocial Integration in Reflection   241

References   243

Subject Index   253

Name Index   265

About the Author   267

Contents

Foreword by William M. Singletary   xv

Preface: Authorship and Research Underpinning   xix

Acknowledgements   xxv

PART I: NEUROPSYCHOSOCIAL INTEGRATION IN RESEARCH   **1**

1   Introduction to Neuropsychosocial Integration   3
    The Neuropsychosocial of Our Native Need   6
    Adverse Lived Experiences in Context   8
    Structure of the Neuropsychosocial   10

PART II: NEUROPSYCHOSOCIAL (DIS)INTEGRATION IN CONTEXT   **15**

2   Neuropsychosocial (Dis)Integration in Perspective   17
    Neuropsychosocial (Dis)Integration in the Dance of Life   18
    Selfhood in Neuropsychosocial (Dis)Integration: Native SPEARS   20

3   Neuropsychosocial (Dis)Integration in the (In)Authentic Self   25
    Resilience in the Authentic Self: Resilience SPEAR   25
    The Authentic Self in Concept and Context   27
    Authenticity as a State of Self-Possession   30
    Automaticity in the (In)Authentic Self   31

4   Neuropsychosocial (Dis)Integration in the Dynamic Self   39
    The Self as Host of Life Stories: Survival and Pathological   40
    The Developing Self in the Absence of Pathology   43

The Functioning Self in a State of Pathology   48
The Protective Self Neurodynamics and Intelligence SPEARS   50
Metaphorical SPEARS for Neuropsychosocial Acrobatics   56

5   Neuropsychosocial (Dis)Integration: Featuring Psychosocial Trauma   59
    Automaticity in Neuropsychosocial Disintegration   59
    Disintegration in the Psyche and Soma   61
    Socioemotionality in Neuropsychosocial Disintegration   63
    Psychosocial Trauma in High Definition   68

**PART III: NEUROPSYCHOSOCIAL (DIS)INTEGRATION
IN ANCESTRY**   **73**

6   Ances-Story in Neuropsychosocial (Dis)Integration   75
    Transgenerational Trauma in Context   76
    The Neurobiological of Transgenerational Trauma   76

7   Psychosocial Trauma as Legacy: Beginning in Early Life   91
    The Neuropsychosocial of Transgenerational Trauma   91
    Social History of Psychosocial Stress: Beginning in Utero   94
    Psychosocial Stress in Adaptive Defences and Personality   99
        The Disposition to Engage Signals and Sources of Stress
            in Conflict: A Warrior Fight Response Pattern to
            Psychosocial Stress   99
        The Disposition to Dart Away from Signals and Sources
            of Stress: A Nomadic Flight Response Pattern to
            Psychosocial Stress   100
        The Disposition to Wander Aimlessly around Signals and
            Sources of Stress: A Nomadic Float Response Pattern to
            Psychosocial Stress   101
        The Disposition to Shape-Shift in the Face of Signals and
            Sources of Stress: A Settler Fold Response Pattern to
            Psychosocial Stress   102
        The Disposition to Submit to Despair in the Face of Signals
            and Sources of Stress: A Settler Furrow Response Pattern
            to Psychosocial Stress   104
    Spectrum of Autonomic Activation in Adaptive Defences   106

8   Psychosocial Trauma across Generations: In Practice   109
    Psychosocial Trauma in Intergenerational Family Life   110
        The Spirit of Family: Vector of Psychosocial Trauma   110
        The Spirit of Religiosity: Vector of Psychosocial Trauma   113
        The Spirit of Community: Vector of Psychosocial Trauma   114
        The Spirit of Education: Vector of Psychosocial Trauma   116

The Spirit of Ancestral Legacy: Vector of Psychosocial
 Trauma and Recovery 116
Legacy of Transgenerational Trauma in Destiny 119
Transgenerational Neuropsychosocial Disintegration 122

**PART IV: NEUROPSYCHOSOCIAL INTEGRATION
IN PROCESS** **125**

9 Neuropsychosocial Integration: Structures, Resources and Processes 127
 Neuropsychosocial Integration Essential Structures 127
  Social History in Neuropsychosocial Integration 127
  Social Psyche in Neuropsychosocial Integration 129
  Social Environment in Neuropsychosocial Integration 130
  Social Engagement Nerve in Neuropsychosocial Integration 130
 Neuropsychosocial Integration Essential Resources 134
  Integrous Empathy 135
  Embodied Mind-Heart-Soulfulness 136
  Psychosocial Integrity 138
 Neuropsychosocial Integration Fundamental Processes 141

10 Neuropsychosocial Integration: Aims and Steps 149
 Centering Authenticity in Neuropsychosocial Integration 149
 Essential Aims and Steps in Neuropsychosocial Integration 151
 Centering the Survivor for Neuropsychosocial Integration 154

11 Neuropsychosocial Integration: Stages and Considerations 159
 Neuropsychosocial Integration Core Stages 161
  Stage I 161
  Stage II 162
  Stage III 163
 Neuropsychosocial Integration Core Considerations 163

**PART V: NEUROPSYCHOSOCIAL INTEGRATION
IN THERAPY** **167**

12 Neurorelational Integration 169
 Neurorelational Well-Being 169
  Case Study: Misinterpreting and Mishandling Relational Trauma 170
 Neurorelational SPEAR 174
  Self-Compassion 175
  Presence 176
  Equanimity 177
  Altruism 179
  Resonance 180
 Neurorelational Therapy in Reflection 182

13 Neuro-emotional Integration 185
Neuro-emotional Well-Being 185
Neuro-emotional SPEAR 187
    Self-Regulation 187
    Positiveness 189
    Empathy 190
    Attunement 191
    Reflectiveness 192
Neuro-emotional Therapy in Reflection 193

14 Neuropsychological Integration 195
Neuropsychological Well-Being 195
Neuropsychological SPEAR 198
    Self-Esteem 200
    Purposefulness 201
    Enterprise 203
    Agency 203
    Righteousness 205
Neuropsychological Therapy in Reflection 206

15 Neurosomatic Integration 209
Neurosomatic Well-Being 209
Neurosomatic SPEAR 210
    Self-Sustenance 211
    Physicality 212
    Experiencing 215
    Anchorage 217
    Restfulness 218
Neurosomatic Therapy in Reflection 220

**PART VI: EMBRACING NEUROPSYCHOSOCIAL
INTEGRATION IN WELL-BEING** **223**

16 A Survivor's Guide to Neuropsychosocial Integration 225
Neuropsychosocial Integration as Purpose 225
Neuropsychosocial Integration: A Clinical Approach 228
Journaling Our Integration and Authentic Self-Discovery 232

17 Beyond Psychosocial Trauma and Disintegration 235
Post-traumatic Growth 235
Transgenerational Resilience 237

Afterword 241

Neuropsychosocial Integration in Reflection 241

References 243

Subject Index 253

Name Index 265

About the Author 267

Foreword

William M. Singletary

I consider it both an honour and a privilege to be asked to contribute the fore-word to Dr. Maduro's groundbreaking and inspiring book regarding trauma and recovery. This pioneering volume draws on her own personal under-standing, both familial and cultural, as well as her professional experience as a researcher and therapist in the area of trauma. Maduro begins with the consideration of an individual's adverse lived experiences, such as emotional, physical or sexual abuse due to psychosocial transgenerational trauma, and to collective/historical transgenerational trauma, such as that resulting from the Holocaust or the transatlantic slave trade. She considers both the epigenetic path from ancestors to child as well as the broader psychosocial path through behaviours, customary practices and traditions. Her integrative approach is most original and involves many perspectives, including psychoanalysis (Erikson, Bowlby and others) and Carl Rogers as well as the neurobiology of development under optimal circumstances, in contrast with the developmen-tal course under stress and adverse experiences. Her numerous perspectives include neuroplasticity and epigenetics, as well as mythology, spirituality and cultural healing practices. Dr. Maduro brings her unique viewpoint to bear on some of the most crucial issues of our time, including the physical and emo-tional effects of trauma and racism. Dr. Maduro's own life story is one of the hero's journey, in which she has use her own ultimately adaptive responses to traumatic experiences to achieve resilience and post-traumatic growth, which were required to make this remarkable contribution.

Here I will attempt to provide an extremely brief outline of my understand-ing of her work in order to prepare the reader to digest the feast she offers. For Maduro, there are two paths to survival in life, depending on whether or not one's primary experience is that of safety or of adversity and danger. First, the path of well-being and safety, including collective and social safety, involves a secure attachment to at least one caregiver, the capacity for basic trust and the development of caring relationships, which are all associated with an adaptive neurobiological and physiological response to stress that optimizes physical and emotional development and health. Predominantly experienced emotions include caring for others and feeling cared about, gratitude, the ability to forgive, the ability to process sadness and to mourn, as well as the ability to utilize a form of aggression the aim of which is not destructive but protective (Parens, 1979), and realistic hope in order to flexibly respond to life's challenges and grow and change over the lifespan. The second path, that of adversity, trauma and danger—including collective and social trauma and danger—involves the absence of a secure attachment to a caregiver and a basic mistrust which interferes with the development of caring relationships even with others who could or do care. These circumstances are all associated with pathological neurobiological and physiological responses to stress which interfere with physical and emotional development and health. For Maduro, under these conditions, the predominant emotions include loneliness, hatred, a desire for revenge instead of forgiveness, envy, greed, depression rather than processing sadness and mourning, a sense of stuckness and inflexibility, a strong resistance to accepting help and changing for the better, and ultimately despair.

For Maduro, healing involves neuroplastic changes and adaptive physiological regulation as well as adaptive psychological ways to manage stress. She includes the basic components of a healthy lifestyle, such as diet, physical exercise, stress reduction, spiritual practices and the maintenance and cultivation of positive relationships. In the context of treatment and the therapeutic relationship, Maduro feels that a person needs to be able to allow the therapist to help in order to heal and to develop personal resources. The capacities for acceptance, mindsight or the ability to look inward, and integration are critical. This necessitates a pattern of relating based on a secure attachment and the ability to form safe connections. The characteristics of altruism, courage, confidence, equanimity, positiveness and attunement need to be developed. As Maduro maintains, maladaptive ways to survive must be replaced by adaptive ones. Acceptance involves accepting oneself and one's life, including one's imperfections, vulnerabilities, hurts and losses. A pervasive sense of dissatisfaction with life can be changed to gratitude. Also, bitterness can be replaced by forgiveness and hatred by love. Healing requires developing the capacities for empathy and compassion for oneself and others, along with the cultivation of a feeling of well-being and a sense of meaning and purpose in life. One needs to acquire a sense of agency as well as enterprise and self-esteem. Furthermore, a feeling of righteousness and a sense of being able to sustain oneself and one's well-being need to develop along with a sense of groundedness.

Dr. Maduro concludes with the fact that the experience of psychosocial trauma is extremely common and that, while most people who engage in treatment because of psychosocial trauma benefit greatly, a substantial group of trauma survivors fail to benefit from therapy and continue to suffer. We must build on Dr. Maduro's work which highlights the psychosocial factors, both current and historical, involved in the creation of traumatic experience and ongoing suffering. We should be inspired by Dr. Maduro's work which illustrates the complexity of treatment of trauma and the multiplicity of factors that need to be considered. We have much to learn regarding the treatment of individuals who are stuck in suffering from their maladaptive responses to traumatic experience. The refusal to accept the vulnerability felt in allowing someone to help us forms the cornerstone of such intractable conflict. We feel defenceless when we give up our protective stance of hostility and omnipotence. Thus, we reject the positive experience of caring about and being cared for by others who can help us become able to experience positivity, goodness and strength within ourselves and purpose and joy in life (Singletary, 2024).

Understanding the historical and psychosocial factors involved in the genesis of traumatic suffering should lead us to accept our responsibility and obligation not only to develop new and more effective treatments for survivors but also to enlarge our efforts towards the primary prevention of traumatic experiences in early childhood, such as child abuse and neglect (Olds, 2019). In addition, effective early intervention and treatment for young children who are already experiencing emotional and behavioural disturbances secondary to trauma need to be more widely available (Korom et al., 2024). Finally, programs for disadvantaged children which significantly improve developmental outcomes for disadvantaged children in terms of education, health and employment could have a major positive impact on society (Heckman et al., 2013). Dr. Maduro's inspiring work shines a light on the path forwards and brings much realistic hope for the future.

REFERENCES

Heckman, J., Pinto, R., & Savelyev, P. (2013). Understanding the mechanisms through which an influential early childhood program boosted adult outcomes. *American Economic Review, 103*(6), 2052–86.

Korom, M., Valadez, E. A., Tottenham, N., Dozier, M., & Spielberg, J. M. (2024). Preliminary examination of the effects of an early parenting intervention on amygdala-orbitofrontal cortex resting-state functional connectivity among high-risk children: A randomized clinical trial. *Development and Psychopathology*, 1–9. https://doi.org/10.1017/s0954579423001669

Olds, D. L. (2019). Can home visitation improve the health of women and children at environmental risk? In D. E. Rogers & E. Ginsberg (Eds.), *Improving the life chances of children at risk* (pp. 79–103). Routledge.

Parens, H. (1979). *The development of aggression in early childhood.* Jason Aronson.

Parens, H. (2012). Attachment, aggression, and the prevention of malignant prejudice. *Psychoanalytic Inquiry, 32*(2), 171–85.

Singletary, W. (2024). Resolving rapprochement challenges: The process of metabolizing love-fueling development, therapeutic growth, reparation, and healing. *Psychoanalytic Study of the Child, 77*, 225–50.

Preface

Authorship and Research Underpinning

On completing my doctorate at the University of Manchester, which explored implications of psychosocial resources for life outcomes among Caribbeans as an internally diverse but historically disadvantaged group, I began exploring the possibility that persistent intergenerational disadvantages in essential domains of success in ordinary life—mainly within the contexts of family, community, education, health and enterprise—may have a neurobiological underpinning. Hence, I began my career as a research psychologist and an academic by focussing on the neurobiology of the psychosocial, with special interest in trauma and neuro-(mal)adaptations. I recognise this can be interpreted in any number of ways, so it is helpful to specify that my research is guided by the neuroscience of human development, psychosocial processes and the impact of adversity on well-being, my approach being an integrative one that brings into focus without prejudice the somatic, emotional, psychological and social manifestations of adverse life events (ALEs) that give rise to trauma. An ALE can be a palpable wounding that can exist freely and be discernible or be tangled and tricky to parse. This definition bears a special import because not so long ago in clinical science what qualified as trauma needed to be physical, like a broken limb. Neuro-atypicality, likewise, involved peculiar life events about which there was little clinical insight, except among analysts for whom neuro-atypical features were manifestations of neuroses and personality disorders.

Not exactly an exciting backstory, but one in the light of which exposing trauma as much more than has ever been recognised seems remarkable. More precisely, prolonged suffering in settings and traditions in which we are socialised is a reliable origin not only of neuro-adaptations that explain neuro-atypicality but also of trauma and neuropsychosocial disintegration that respond well to neuropsychosocial therapy. By this conceptualisation, it is possible that you begin to see yourself and people around you as trauma troughs in need of therapy, as a fairly normal response to trauma work. To guide you in qualifying or quantifying this response, you might find my ALEs assessment questionnaire helpful (table 0.1).

The ALEs questionnaire divides into two lots. Nine questions make up Lot I and are interested in childhood at the point at which all neurobiological structures are developed, even if not fully matured. These questions derive from Vincent Felitti's seminal work on childhood adversities, with which we shall become familiar in chapter 1. What is important to know here is that, in a sample of eighty-seven respondents—across five world regions—whose ALEs were analysed for the purpose of this preface, an excess of three *yes* responses pointed to an early life exposed to significant psychosocial stress and a life trajectory that bore a significant risk for protracted suffering, which the survivor may be able to alter with healing connection, nurturing relationships and reorganisation of their life story. An excess of three *myself* answers in Lot II suggested adversities experienced throughout the life cycle inform maladaptive and high-risk behaviours that correlated with severe disadvantages, disabilities and suicidal attempts at a point in life. For the whole sample (N), a total of 539 ALEs gave a mean value of six, among which 349 and a mean value of eight corresponded to a life lived with considerations and adjustments for a special need, disability or health condition affecting daily life.

The intricacies of the neuropsychosocial mean that it is not necessarily easy to ascribe specific adverse health outcomes to any specific ALE. However, we can infer causation from correlation, by the strength of the correlation and consistency across different people groups. And when we do that, an overall score exceeding three *yes* and three *myself* responses, in other words a score higher than six, points to poor overall health and normalised hardship. This translates to historical sufferings and symptoms of ALEs that may or may not respond to neuropsychosocial therapy and more healthful life choices. For instance, an ALEs score of 8 or higher across the two lots correlated with acquired disabilities, diseases and dependency on psychotropic intervention. A score of 12 that included the loss of a father in childhood, whether through abandonment or premature death, correlated with unrelenting poverty and suicidality, in addition to a nearly 500 percent increased likelihood of severe disease and disability, which reflect—in the words of the Canadian physician Gabor Maté—'an entire life lived, one that arises from a web of circumstances, relationships, events, and experiences' (2023, p. 9), which bears enormous import for our individual and collective well-being.

The questionnaire in this sense is an invaluable information-gathering and analytic tool with which we can begin to unravel this web, for it undertakes to open us up to origins and trajectories of ALEs that give rise to psychosocial

Table 0.1 Adverse Lived Experiences Assessment Questionnaire

Lot I			
1 Before your sixteenth birthday, did a parent or other adult in your household often swear at you, insult you, put you down or humiliate you?	Yes	No	Maybe
2 Before your sixteenth birthday, did a parent or other adult in your household often hit or beat you? Or act in ways that made you feel afraid you might be physically hurt?	Yes	No	Maybe
3 Before your sixteenth birthday, were your parents or other principal caregiver often unable to take care of you because they were sleeping excessively, too drunk or too strung out on drugs?	Yes	No	Maybe
4 Before your sixteenth birthday, did you often feel that your family did not love you enough or did not treat you like you were important or good enough?	Yes	No	Maybe
5 Before your sixteenth birthday, did you often feel you did not have enough to eat and had no one to provide enough for you to wear, stay clean or keep warm?	Yes	No	Maybe
6 Before your sixteenth birthday, did you often feel that your family members did not care for each other or support each other enough?	Yes	No	Maybe
7 Before your sixteenth birthday, was a biological parent ever lost to you through adoption, abandonment, death, disease, divorce or other reason?	Yes	No	Maybe
8 Before your sixteenth birthday, were you left for any extended period of time by one or both of your biological parents?	Yes	No	Maybe
9 Before your sixteenth birthday, were you directly exposed to sexual activity (including sexually stimulating touching and conversations, voyeurism or exposure to pornography)?	Yes	No	Maybe
Lot II			
10 At any time in your life, have you or anyone close to you suffered with a severe disease, taken medication for a chronic illness or had to be hospitalised for a major surgical intervention?	Myself	Family Member	Friend

11 At any time in your life, have you or anyone close to you attempted suicide, self-mutilated or self-hurt (including deliberately cutting, burning, striking, ripping off or breaking parts of your own body)?	Myself	Family Member	Friend
12 At any time in your life, have you or anyone close to you often felt alone, lonely, isolated, abandoned or unable to build close and trusting relationships?	Myself	Family Member	Friend
13 At any time in your life, have you or anyone close to you suffered from drug-misuse addiction (including alcohol, nicotine, cannabis or synthetic vape)?	Myself	Family Member	Friend
14 At any time in your life, have you or anyone close to you suffered from domestic violence?	Myself	Family Member	Friend
15 At any time in your life, have you or anyone close to you been affected by a premature death (suicide, homicide, disease, accidental death)?	Myself	Family Member	Friend
16 At any time in your life, have you or anyone close to you suffered abuse or forced exit from a revered collective space (such as a school, religion or community) and needed help from family welfare, refugee, exile or human rights services?	Myself	Family Member	Friend
17 At any time in your life, have you or anyone close to you suffered with homelessness (not having a safe place to sleep and self-care for any length of time)?	Myself	Family Member	Friend
18 At any time in your life, have you or anyone close to you suffered imprisonment (not including short stays in police custody related to civil protests)?	Myself	Family Member	Friend
19 At any time in your life, have you or anyone close to you needed to be hospitalised or medicated for a severe psychiatric condition (such as schizophrenia, eating disorders, depression, alcoholism, anxiety, etc.)?	Myself	Family Member	Friend
20 At any time in your life, have you or anyone close to you submitted to a mental healthcare practitioner or counselling therapist (voluntary or involuntary)?	Myself	Family Member	Friend
21 At any time in your life, have you or anyone close to you ever required adjustments or consideration for a special need, disability or health condition that affects your daily life?	Myself	Family Member	Friend

trauma and attendant pathologies that afflict most of us in some way. Our goal is then to use the information we glean to predict the behaviour resulting from ALEs and trauma in our body and mind. This proved to be particularly helpful throughout the COVID-19 global health crisis, when I developed it with the help of my psychotherapy students, who were desperate to help their clients to cope with multitudes of stressors in experimental virtual clinics—experimental in the sense that the scale on which they were delivering psychotherapy virtually was unprecedented in our history. Since then, I have had responses from respondents in five continents and used the findings, still yet to be officially published, to assess patterns of psychosocial trauma and evaluate accessible therapy for people who come to the task of ordinary life with traumas that cause them at times unimaginable suffering. Hence, this research fills an urgent need for creative healthcare but also addresses a historical gap in access to evidence-based psychosomatic therapies. I'd say this is a decent contribution to the field, one that extends as well to supervising postgraduate research.

And now, to this book.

Table 0.2 Adverse Lived Experiences: Insight from the Data

All People	Number	Disability/Severe Health Issue in Daily Life	
Sample (N)	87	N (s)	46
ALEs	398	ALEs	348.5
Mean	**6**	**Mean**	**8**
Sex	**Number**	**Arbitrary Racialised Identity**	
Male	21	Black	24
Female	24	White	16
Nonbinary	1	Brown (non-Black/White)	4
Unspecified	0	Unspecified	2
Total	**46**		**46**
Region	**Number**	**Disability/Adverse Health Issue in Daily Life**	
North America and Canada	3	Acquired Disability	20%
Caribbean	12	Mood Disorder	10%
Asia and Australasia	13	Hyper/Hypotension	10%
Europe and Great Britain	9	Arthritis	10%
Africa	9	Anxiety Disorder	6%
Total	**46**	Sleep Disorder	6%
		Total	**62%**

Acknowledgements

With gratitude and inner warmth, I write these acknowledgements for the people without whom this book would not have been possible, as well as the people for whom it is written. In the first tribe is my octogenarian grandmother Catherine E. Andrew née Carbon. At age eighty-eight, she is fully present, our talks still very much animated with the intense curiosity of my five-year-old self, whose safety screening she exceeded with little difficulty and from then allowed herself to become my safe person. Our organic and untiring talks—infused with wisdom, truthfulness and caution—were a source of my interest in matters of the body, mind and spirit. But also, equally important, the ancestral stories I honour and feel fortunate to share. So interest and honour had their seeds planted early in our relationship of resonance. This, I would say, allowed my vulnerable child-self to come into ordinary life, which I consider a gift from the gods. For it is to our relationship that I credit not only the personality I continue to refine but also my bringing this book to life with its offering of faith in neuroscience and the individual's capacity—in spite of unimaginable suffering—to actualise authentic self-expression and lead a life that is fulfilling.

The life stories of my mother, Lily; sisters, Amina, Carina, Erica and Giovanni; brothers, Jerry and Edwin Jr.; and many others among my relatives have been inspiring. To my aunts Shona, Agatha, Marietta, Diane, Monette, Delores and Vivian and my uncles Antoine, Lewis, Samuel and Sam, thank you for sharing your lives with me and entertaining my spirit of inquiry. It is my hope that, where I have called on your experience, I have done justice to your courage, dignity and strength. To Shem, Micah, Kenyan, Nancy, Marvin, Sheena, Kevin, Alexandre, Germain, Tanasha, Vanessa, Valentine, Veron, Earl, Nixon, Joakim and all your posterity, I am glad to have you as cousins; you are stronger than you know. To my friends and peers who have encouraged me on this adventure in exploring, learning and writing about the neuropsychosocial, I also extend my gratitude. Heather, William, Wilworth, Mario, Zulkhuu, Illiriana, Magdalena and Sakina, I love you!

Now that I've spoken of my first tribe, I feel obligated to speak of the other—the people for whom this book is written. Here I owe gratitude to the participants in my research and therapeutic experiments, many of whom were survivors of adverse life events that troubled their ancestry and lives. The cumulative as well as unique wounds left by such events, as hallmarks of experiences lived, presented themselves without prejudice in haunting memories and otherwise continuous suffering from which they actively sought relief. I consider it a privilege to have been entrusted with alliance on their journey to find relief, to be well and to lead a life filled with purpose and satisfaction. Without their faith, commitment and strengths, this work would not be what it is, so it is also for them. Composites of their lives that do not betray confidentiality or privacy have allowed me to answer their questions about where and how to find information about the 'things' we address in our therapeutic meetings. 'Things' that are indelibly complex but decipherable with education. Which brings me to my ultimate audience: the curious demographics—including my students—who find value in my lectures and research on neurobiology of the psychosocial, psychosocial [mal]adaptations, resources, trauma and trauma-informed integrative therapy. *Neuropsychosocial Integration* is written for you, to enrich your perspective on heritable traumas that impact the body, mind and soul, and to turn to for guidance in a practical approach to discharging the chaotic energy of psychosocial trauma and recovering authenticity in the self.

Winniey E. Maduro
Sale, Cheshire, December 2023

Part I

NEUROPSYCHOSOCIAL INTEGRATION IN RESEARCH

Chapter 1

Introduction to Neuropsychosocial Integration

The neuropsychosocial arises when somatic, emotional, psychological and social rhythms of life converge. Rhythms are energy pulses that merge into waves, energy waves that arise in and transcend our body and mind in search of resonance in our social orbit. Sufficient resonance is the feedback that we are not alone, we are part of something social that holds us, and being held, as we shall learn in this book, is important for our well-being, as it is for our very survival.

As I understand it, these waves debut at conception when the zygote begins the task of becoming an autonomous sentient. Before autonomy, however, comes the attachment relationship through which the developing child receives sustenance and information about the world. This relationship is first physical, involving a neural cord that binds mother and child until its severance at birth, long before the infant can self-sustain or appreciate survival away from the mother's body and its familiar rhythms, to which she is attuned and through which she learns her native needs will be met. As an experienced mother from the Ashanti tribe (an Akan people) of Ghana once told me, the mother's body is the 'baby's natural home, the baby knows it, and loves it'. Ancient cultures and social worlds honour this implicit 'knowing and love' by holding babies in their home, safely swathed along the curves of their mother's back, waist or bosom. As the baby vibes to the rhythms of resonance emanating from the mother's heart, lungs and veins, she learns, is reassured and grows. Learning, assurance and growth, it turns out, depend on rhythms of resonance and our profound rhythmicity. And when there is insufficient resonance with our caregiver or we fail to get feedback in our social orbit that our rhythms are welcomed in a cogent synchrony, in other words, when our rhythms are met with dissonance or disturbance, so too will be our capacity to grow, rest and experience and respond to life events with flexibility.

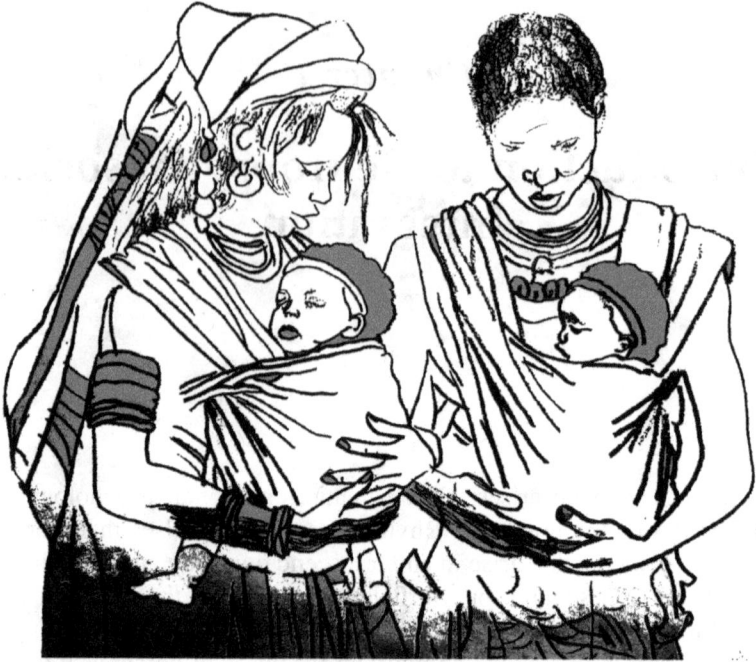

Figure 1.1. Baby Wearing. An ancient cultural practice that promotes secure attachment, intelligence and growth. In ancient warrior-settler-nomadic cultures, young children were offered what is now recognised as an optimal parenting environment. This was a social world in which babies, for as long as they needed, were held both rhythmically and physically. Practically wrapped into the deep curves of their mother's back, waist or bosom where—as they vibed to the rhythms of her heart, lungs and veins—they were kept warm, comforted and safe and learned that they could trust caregivers to fulfil their needs—the first psychosocial developmental prerequisite for secure attachment, intelligence and growth. *Figure courtesy of Dagmar Roelfsema.*

The American neuropsychologist James Prescott at the Institute of Child Health and Human Development in Bethesda, Maryland, was on to something ancient when he undertook to analyse hundreds of cultures and to notice that the less violent ones—with less domestic violence—emphasise holding babies both physically and rhythmically (Prescott, 1975). For disturbance in the small child's bodily rhythm, a surge in the chaotic energy of sadness that needs to be expressed, for instance, is a violent psychosomatic event to which her cry reflex will respond, as she has little capacity to respond with cognitive flexibility, say when she is hungry, cold or both, to mindfully suppress the pangs of hunger or to delay a petition for warmth until mother returns from gathering groundnuts for dinner.

Evidently, these life events intersect the biological and psychosocial, both of which stoke the child's emotions and psychology that she cannot yet reconcile, for emotional and psychological reconciliations are outputs of complex executive functions that develop in tandem with neural maturation and social-relational input over time. The psychosocial, in this regard, involves a continuous developmental course that spans the entire life cycle—from infancy to the elderly years. Its progression was first explored by the German American child psychoanalyst Erik Erikson (1998) in his classic work *The Life Cycle Completed*, in which he wrote convincingly of eight discernible stages in terms of core virtues—namely, hope, will, purpose, competence, fidelity, love, care and wisdom.

In context, the virtue of hope emerges in infancy in relationships with caregivers, wherein the infant learns to trust that existential needs, such as being fed and held, will be met and that the child will be trusted to express these needs. Will or willpower, Erikson argued, emerges in toddlerhood, between the twelfth and twenty-fourth months of life, when we learn we can do things freely with our body and for our own self, such as control our bowels and protect and dress our body with warm and pretty clothes of our choosing. This is the need for autonomy, in the absence of which self-doubt can take root. The virtue of purpose emerges between the ages of three and six in early childhood to drive initiatives like organising, building and creating things that bring joy and satisfaction. The paper roses and butterflies the five-year-olds I often work with create in their own time and give to me at a given opportunity is an expression of this need. In the absence of its fulfilment, the chaotic energy of guilt sets in. In middle childhood, between ages seven and ten, the need for competence emerges to promote industriousness, say in school or sports. In the absence of its fulfilment, a sense of inferiority easily takes root. In adolescence, between ages of eleven and nineteen, fidelity shapes identity in social relationships and averts confusion about who we are, our status among our peers and what we can and cannot achieve. In early adulthood, between ages twenty and forty-four, the need for romantic love promotes intimacy and protects us from aloneness and genealogical obliteration. In middle adulthood, between ages forty-five and sixty-four, our impulse to care in a way that promotes our generativity emerges to protect us from the suffering of stagnation—our need to make life meaningful emerging to prepare us for the final lap in the life cycle. This takes place beyond the age of sixty-five, when our accumulated wisdom promotes our integrity and protects us from the despair that having lived a meaningless life potentiates.

Evidently, these stages of psychosocial development speak to the emergence of native needs that mesh with the demands of society, a meshing that gives rise to challenges and conflicts to which we are liable to respond in either of two ways—adaptively or maladaptively. I shall discuss these different ways of responding to life events throughout the chapters as they relate to specific needs at the different stages in the life cycle, beginning in early childhood.

THE NEUROPSYCHOSOCIAL OF OUR NATIVE NEED

At this stage, we can be convinced that the genesis of every aspect of our development throughout our life cycle lies in impulses that emerge from a surge of free energy. According to the British psychiatrist Jeremy Holme (2020, p. 35), free-flowing energy ensures the nervous system has enough fuel to resist disorder and maintain homeostasis—a fancy word for stability. In a homeostatic state, our more discernible rhythmic systems—examples of which include our heart rate, blink rate and respiratory rate—are steady, continuous and synchronous. Truly a reflection of a coherent orderliness on the inside, psychosomatically speaking. And the nervous system achieves this by binding free energy into stable states of 'action' in service of its survival and 'rest' in service of its renewal and resilience. Naturally, action relies on sensory input, while rest facilitates the reduction of internal chaos that gives rise to disorder and the establishment of integration. Derived from the Latin word *integrare*, which translates as 'to make whole', integration speaks to the unification of body and mind, creating an authentic self through synchronized nervous system and psychological and social processes.

In the first stage of our psychosocial development, in early infancy, our impulse to trust our caregiver with whom we are in resonance and from whom we learn about responding to life events is driven by free-flowing energy that binds and integrates when this impulse is met with action from our trustworthy caregiver. This happens when we are hungry and our caregiver provides nourishing food to quell our hunger, our bowels are full and our caregiver provides a safe means for defecation, we are afraid and our caregiver provides reliable comfort and reassurance that we are safe. This is our introduction to the charge-and-discharge cycle, which begins with a tension that creates a surge in energy and ends with a release of this tension and a return to homeostasis. More important, however, is that our caregiver is acting to ensure we appreciate what is nourishing and what is harmful, and by extension how to play to fulfil our needs in the gritty sandbox of life with the tender, innocent and vulnerable lamb but not the rabid predatory lion. Where this developmental challenge fails, say because our caregiver cannot act or effectually respond to our need to trust in service of our safety, we are liable to experience a flood of unbounded energy—fuelling rhythmic disturbance that will establish itself in our body and mind as an absence of a secure base (Ainsworth, 1979). Energetically speaking, this is the surge of energy and need for information about our survival at this stage freezing at their local address in the nervous system, and these will stay there until intentionally differentiated and contextualised, or discharged, in a word. According to the lore of psychosocial development, throughout the life cycle, this disturbance will echo the wanting of trust left unfulfilled in early life. The ensuing vacancy giving rise to maladaptive perceptions, beliefs and behaviours that prevail, especially within relationships, and will also curtail curiosity and exploration in the realms of the physical, emotional, psychological and social. This suffering, hindering the ability to prune complexity, discern a good life and figure out how to fulfil needs, is one the adverse life experiences (ALEs) relational questions (see preface) seek to unveil and validate. Curiosity and fear—both native instincts that drive our impulses—will proffer their input as we develop into our personality. Curiosity will impel us to explore our environment, to reach out and discover, while fear will curtail this impulse and push us towards our default stress response—our pattern of response to ALEs that installs itself in our nervous system (Adolphs, 2013). The absence of a co-regulating caregiver to help us bind and contextualise the energy that fuels our fear could mean we retain it in our body and mind—where it will certainly stoke some kind of disturbance—and it never gets discharged from our nervous system, which depends on co-regulation, before we can learn self-regulation.

This comes together tidily as our native need for somato-psycho-emotional attunement and relational security, a need with which we come to the task of life and will suffer terribly when it is unfulfilled. The neuropsychosocial is both structural and functional in enabling us to fulfil this need, but this all depends on whether it is integrated or disintegrated. We shall get to the definitions of these concepts and attendant states in subsequent chapters. Here I want to focus, first, on how this need influences our life outcomes and, second, on childhood experience and the early stages of childhood development, when the fulfilling of this need is critical in ways we continue to learn about. For, as it turns out, 'The first seven years of life are crucial, but the first three are the nub of it. Get those first three years right, and parents can relax. In getting them wrong, however, parents are liable to engage in remedial parenting throughout their entire career' (Dr. Gabor Maté on London Real, January 2019), a poignant claim with which Maté punctuated his talk with investigative journalist Brian Rose on London Real in January 2019. The conversation that followed was nothing short of fascinating, but the substance was not new in that it echoed empirical wisdom. For instance, the eighteenth-century French philosopher Jean-Jacques Rousseau's (1712–1778) observation that life events in early childhood establish behaviours in adulthood. Perhaps drawing on Rousseau's observation, the nineteenth-century Russian biosocial psychologist Lev Vygotsky (1896–1934) also emphasised in his seminal work the role of the social and cultural in early life in how we respond to such events throughout our life cycle (Vygotsky, 1978). In the twentieth century, the American psychologist Urie Bronfenbrenner (1917–2005) developed this idea further and led a school of thought that emphasised the import of complex relationships we enter in early life and within which we learn and grow. For it is within complex relationships that we learn about how our body and mind serve our needs, in ways that range from virtuous self-regulation to harmfully hiding our wounds and suppressing our authentic self, according to the American clinician Vincent Felitti, from whose work the widely known concept of 'adverse childhood experience' derives.

ADVERSE LIVED EXPERIENCES IN CONTEXT

In 1985, Felitti was running an obesity clinic in San Diego, California, when a twenty-eight-year-old nurse's aide entered the program. In fifty-one weeks, her weight went from 408 to 132 pounds, but when Felitti saw her again a few months later, she had regained an extraordinary amount of weight—more than he thought was biologically possible. What had happened? Sexual interest from a male coworker had triggered her to overeat again, even at night when she had trouble staying asleep. The woman revealed to Felitti that growing up her grandfather had sexually abused her, and she now finds sexual interest frightening. Her coworker's suggestion had, almost literally, flipped a switch in her. Felitti investigated further and found that among the 286 obese patients with whom he conducted interviews, most of them had experienced sexual abuse in childhood. Their excessive eating soothed the fear, anxiety and depression triggered by memories of the abuse. Their morbidly large bodies, he would also discover, acted as a shield against unwanted sexual interest and helped them to cope with life events in adulthood, including the life-threatening cardiopathy, diabetes and hypertension they often suffered with.

This finding prefaced further research Felitti (Felitti et al., 1998) convened a team to undertake with over thirteen thousand mostly white, middle-class and college-educated Americans to determine the extent to which household dysfunction and exposure to emotional, physical and sexual abuse in childhood affected their lives, brought them suffering in adulthood and predicted premature death. These events clustered around physical abandonment, insults, neglect, sexual abuse, violence, substance misuse, severe disease, loss of caregivers and separation from an attachment figure. A scoring system awarded one point for each yes answer. This meant if the interviewee answered yes to parental separation, parental addictions and sexual abuse, they had an ACE score of 3, which would reflect the experience of roughly two-thirds of us in childhood.

This observation comes with my confidence in my own findings surrounding ALEs that give rise to woundedness in the body, mind and spirit. Left untreated, this woundedness embeds in the nervous system and expresses itself in emotions, thought processes, behaviours and somatic symptoms. Taken together, this is a trauma that cleaves the soma and the psyche in ways that are discernible and even tractable for many survivors who seek reintegration. A part of this book, thus, is about surfacing and discharging the chaotic energies that fuel this trauma through therapeutic reworking of life stories that bring respite to what ails and insight into what fulfils, which is important to me.

I have interrogated my body and mind to find that my curiosity surrounding trauma and the broader interest from which it stems—both personally and professionally—is prefixed by my history with a brain injury sustained from being struck by a cyclist at the age of eleven and events of adversity throughout my ancestry and my own life that have caused me to suffer. However, according to my neurologist, as well as my own sense of how I am functioning, I seem to have recovered well from these events and have experienced post-traumatic growth, as opposed to depletion or afflictions redolent of traumatic stress and wounds.

This seemingly little trouble with which I have emerged from my volley of adversities—both lived and inherited—is an experience I feel lucky to share, considering the chronically adverse lives and sufferings I am often confronted with in my research and therapeutic practice. My loving-kind grandmother would say it's my blessing. However perceived, my life experiences have left me with a deep yearning to understand how my nervous system—and the nervous systems of others—manages to self-repair and recover from assaults. Not purely for my private sake, but so that I can be of help to others who might benefit from that process. The possibility that there is utility in my experience for how we do therapy is also a faithful visitor to my mind, and I am curious about that too.

Therapy, much like neuropsychosocial integration, is a nuanced concept, and I recognise it could mean different things, and perhaps everything, to those who reap its benefits. In principle, it is subjected to interpretation and, for my purpose, must be understood as that safe space where the trauma survivor shows up vulnerable and disintegrated and the attuned and integrated therapist brings a restorative presence to establish a relationship of resonance. Disintegration—counterintuitively—is about preservation of life. The body and mind coming apart to keep us alive after we have been exposed to adversity. The designation *survivor* in this sense implies an event of adversity has been lived and some impact remains—unprocessed at an address—in the body and mind. In other words, as far as nature is concerned, a significant event or lack thereof occurred in the course of life, resulting in a trauma that may or may not be perceived. This trauma, nonetheless, has the potential to cause profound and enduring disintegration in the nervous system, fragmentation in the self and disease in the body (van der Kolk, 2015). In the therapeutic space, the goal is to confront these consequences and help the survivor to discharge the chaotic energy that sustains their trauma. This is to promote neuropsychosocial integration and the flow of energy that affirms well-being over the chaotic energy that fuels maladaptive defences that leave the survivor feeling stuck, unsatisfied or unsafe in their body, mind and relationships—so, not with drugs, gadgets, images or even compassionate inquiry alone, but by developing and deploying metaphorical SPEARS to alter the trajectory of their adverse life, beginning with their impulses, their genetics and the psychosocial that express at the level of neurons, the building blocks of the nervous system, and that undertake necessary and complex roles in the experience of life. Naturally, this implicates the big brain and spinal cord, which together form the central nervous system.

STRUCTURE OF THE NEUROPSYCHOSOCIAL

The brain is an extraordinary organ that depends on a remarkable network of nerves—led by the spinal cord—to provide it with a constant flow of information from within the body and the world that it undertakes to interpret and orient in service of our survival. It is also through this network that it sends its interpretations and reactions that then cascade to target nerves and muscles in the peripheral nervous system (PNS). *Peripheral* implies on the edge of something core, more central. However, within the context of neuropsychology, the PNS is recognised as a core division in its own right of an extensive nervous system.

Much like the spinal cord, which continues from the brainstem down to the lower back, the PNS consists of a network of nerves that allows us to react to life and stimulation in our environment. This includes the nerves lying outside the brain and the spine. These nerves are further divided into somatic and autonomic nerves, and autonomic nerves are divided further into enteric, sympathetic and parasympathetic nerves. The functions of these different systems of nerves and how they interrelate will become clearer as I explore manifestations of adverse lived experiences, psychosocial trauma, well-being and post-traumatic growth. It is enough to say here that we cannot afford to overlook the interconnectedness among these nerves, for it is at the helm of how we are put together and function as relational sentients. However, this may be overshadowed throughout the chapters by a pointed emphasis on the activities of the central and autonomic nerves, the nerves that innervate voluntary action, perception, bodily state regulation and executive functions that are vital for survival and with which we shall necessarily become familiar.

Voluntary action is what we do that is afforded by nerve cells throughout our body, but we do it volitionally. Say I want to hug my grandmother, which I found myself wanting to do more and more throughout the COVID-19 pandemic, and I reach out with my arms—at times virtually—and I hug her. This is a volitional action. Similarly, if a strange hand touches me in the dark and I screech or flinch, this would be volitional, but it is an emotional reaction too. It comes from an emotional memory that is encoded in my nervous system—perhaps from my own experience or from an inherited reaction to strangers' touch in the dark. Anyone with the 'stranger danger' acculturation from childhood might relate.

These actions—driven by the central and autonomic nerves—are adaptations we can use to orient our body and mind. And, in addition to alerting us to danger, invoking a sense of safety is arguably the most natural reason for which we might do that. I say arguably because volitions that are informed by emotional memories can betray consciousness that promotes distance between affect and action. Consider, for a moment, that vocalisation functions independently of somatic states. An example from my early enculturation is the saying that 'sticks and stones can break my bones but words can't hurt me'. However we might like this to be true, and I am glad to share that it isn't, the autonomic nerves do not distinguish between suffering that is inflicted by stones and suffering that is inflicted by words, or even malicious silence, upon the body and mind.

Before neuroimaging technology and biofeedback permitted us to observe and measure this event in vivo, we learned from Freud that words have magical powers, and life and death are truly in the power of the tongue. Thus, words can bring the greatest happiness but also the deepest despair. This truth, we also know, is because vocal expressions, including tones, mutters and spoken words, are interpreted in the nervous system in much the same way as action—in this case, volitional action that involves use of the mouth, larynx and diaphragm.

At this level of familiarity with the neuroscience of voluntary action, of what it might involve at least, the next core survival function with which we shall necessarily become familiar is that of perception. First is that, unlike voluntary action, perception is involuntary. It is what we appreciate about the way we feel and function. This may be translated to how we make sense of what is going on inside of our own body and mind, in the bodies and minds of other sentients we interact with, and what we do with the information. Needless to say, much of this processing is subconscious. For instance, my heart rate, blood pressure and body temperature as well as those of my partner are actively interpreted in my brain as safe or unsafe, though I may not be conscious of this. If I'm asked, I could make an educated guess. But that is because I am a neuroscientist and I have an idea—a reliable cognitive schema—of what heart rate, blood pressure and body temperature should be under normal conditions. Alas, I cannot be as confident with the less reliable of perceptions that extend to our natural senses—of hearing, smell, taste, vision, balance—and position in the world, for such perceptions derive from information about how we are, who we are, where we are and what we can and cannot become. This is a large amount of information that will be processed by our sensory nerves and filtered in the half second before the most salient reaches our consciousness—with its very little capacity for information (Norretranders, 1999). Perceptions of these events, however, can be brought to consciousness with some effort, even if unreliable.

The third core function of the central and autonomic nerves is the regulation of physiological states in relation to the external environment to promote synchrony in energy surges that inform the quality of neural connection with the rest of our body and mind. This is the essence of homeostasis, wherein the body is within safe and stable functional limits. Ensuring, for instance, we have enough oxygen, blood and energy, as well as regulated rhythms— the rhythms of our breath, blood flow, heartbeat and sleep that stay the same throughout the life cycle as we go from childhood to adolescence, adulthood and older age, from being provided for to providing for others and creating legacies and traditions to pass on to posterity.

This is a safe thought with which to turn to executive functions, the ultimate of our autonomic-nerve-driven activities. There are different descriptors that are scattered in the neuroscience literature, such as *cognition, perception* and *reason*, none exactly perfect. My preference is *cognition*, and for my purpose, *cerebral-cognitive* and *cognitive functions* are also appropriate. These include activities like thinking, feeling, use of language to express our needs and use of memory to stay safe. How we self-relate, interrelate with others and survive the gritty sandbox of life are also among the activities this function facilitates.

By merging neuroscience, psychosomatic insights and ancestral wisdom, we are offered an integrative prism to appreciate these uniquely human capacities we all have a birthright to. Additionally, this merging functions to expose us to a more comprehensive approach in making sense of psychosocial trauma and recognising that this type of trauma is fuelled by a chaotic energy that is liable to respond to therapeutic intervention. And, with this understanding, we could confront traumatic memories stored in our body and mind—outside of our awareness—and safely bring such memories to awareness, to be contextualised and reoriented in a neural sense. Importantly, however, the goal is not to extinguish such memories, for we must consider our traumas—in much the same way as our survival—as components of our life story that should not be forgotten, erased or redacted in the way the act of extinguishing assumes. Rather, what we want is healthful ways to cope with ALEs and resilient capacities to recover when traumas embed in our body and mind and disturb our life. We want unbounded energies that sustain traumas discharged, so that they do not inhibit our well-being and resilience. That would mean enjoying life free from maladaptive trauma-based responses that imprint at the neural level with their very own epigenetic, neurobiological and psychosocial signatures.

I perceive this expedition as one towards neuropsychosocial integration, which begins with survivors of ALE coming to a therapeutic relationship in a state of vulnerability that is characterised by deleterious loss. This may be a loss of self, loss of purpose or loss of safety, which, incidentally, is also in itself an adverse experience that can upset the survivor's body and mind like any boo-boo—in other words, embedding itself in the nervous system as a psychosocial trauma and attendant neuropsychosocial disintegration. However, loss can also shape us in wonderful ways if we know how to let it, as we become aware of how we can live fulfilling lives, make good sense of our experiences and learn to direct healing energy to our thoughts and perception in ways that are life promoting. This is consistent with the sense in neuropsychology that the psyche is best understood in the light of the neurobiology that informs it and the social contexts within which it develops and expresses itself. Social context is about relationships in which resources and resourcefulness are cultivated to meet fundamental needs of safety. As such, resourceful social relationships are important not only in meeting our needs for food and warmth but also in the pursuance and sustenance of well-being in our body and mind.

Integration, thus, is an undertaking to sustain well-being relationally, but one no doubt fraught with risks, in much the same way as the therapeutic relationship bears the risk of mirroring important relationships in the survivor's life that are sources of suffering. The aim, nonetheless, is to appreciate that cultivating authenticity in the self and building resilient capacities in the body and mind are undertakings along which the survivor will change, and so too will the nature of their relationships, including with themselves and the social world. Some such changes will inevitably be easier than others. One might consider, for example, the cultivation of self-compassion and healthy relational boundaries, which can feel less frightening than the more radical and emotionally challenging tasks of severing family connections, losing friends or retiring lifestyle tenets that sustain traumatic wounds and contribute to neuropsychosocial disintegration.

This brings me back to the idea that neuropsychosocial integration necessarily centres meaningful and nourishing relationships, and throughout the coming chapters, I draw on lived experiences and observations to explore this centeredness. One might imagine this involves biographies and quasi-ethnographies, and this is true. Beginning in part II, I introduce survivors' experiences moving through life in a state of disintegration stoked by unmet psychosocial needs and protected by maladaptive defences, including the native need for somato-psycho-emotional attunement and relational safety, which incidentally derives my acronym *SPEARS*, echoing the word for an ancient tool used to secure food and safety, but which can cause injury if we fail to protect it or use it appropriately.

These native SPEARS, much like the others spears we shall learn about throughout the chapters, is among the psychosocial resources that are vulnerable to maladaptive defences. Many of such defences, we shall learn, are attached to psychosocial traumas. Their structures, which include both biological and psychosocial components, are explored within a sociohistorical context in part III. The focus, however, is on utility and the persistence of psychosocial trauma and adaptive responses across generations. In part IV, I draw on polyvagal theory to explore nervous system states in neuropsychosocial disintegration and integration. This includes a pointed exploration of key aims, steps and processes in neuropsychosocial integration. Part V follows with considerations for cultivating psychosocial resources and application of relational, emotional, somatic and psychological SPEARS in the therapeutic space. Finally, in part VI, I review implications of neuropsychosocial integration for general health and well-being, innate intelligences, psychosocial resources and resilient capacities.

In a pragmatic sense, think of these as a mixed bag of SPEARS survivors utilise along the journey from disintegration to integration. Or, more precisely, essential tools survivors deploy to discover and restore authenticity in themselves and to settle any tenuous inauthenticity in its rightful context. I am especially satisfied that some insights I drew upon as I explore this journey derived from my experience of having descended into my own body, mind and ancestry to restore and nurture authenticity in myself. And that I have arisen with an impulse to nurture authenticity in the selves of others I work with, care about and feel inclined to keep safe.

Part II

NEUROPSYCHOSOCIAL (DIS)INTEGRATION IN CONTEXT

Chapter 2

Neuropsychosocial (Dis)Integration in Perspective

Neuropsychosocial integration is essentially an exploration of life as a dynamic, purposeful and relational experience. This is a notion of life that takes me home to the Caribbean, where life—as in the wider Americas—is experienced largely in relationships loosely strewn together by relatives who are available at any given time to share in the gift of presence and connection. A suitable backdrop, I would say, for my incursion into the until-now-still-obscure terrain of neuropsychosocial (dis)integration. One against which I want to introduce the lived experience of a gentleman, whom I shall call Alex, who was born and raised in the Turks and Caicos Islands. Alex's life story includes the experience of deep woundedness and a related drive to self-heal. Throughout this book, I will have a lot to say about relatedness. Here it suffices to say that we experience relational woundedness and the impulse to heal in our bodies, minds and spirits and, by design, are equipped to heal our woundings as and when they occur. This includes wounds we experience and those we might inherit from our forebears. These are all ours to heal from, with resources we have available to us, inside us and in our ancestral legacy.

For Alex, this task began with a specific and inflexible purpose: to break patterns of income insecurity and fatherlessness that existed for as long as he could remember in his extended lineage. As he told me of this purpose, I sensed his profound drive to act in its service, which directed his energies and led him to a career in hoteliering and a married life in which he felt safe enough to father three children. Until disrupted by a near fatal road accident and subsequent decline in his marriage, this was a relatively decent life that, incidentally, also represented an important achievement for him. One may consider these events life-altering, adverse lived experiences (ALEs), or even psychosocial stressors, that would initiate a series of life changes that led Alex to Britain. However, at the age of thirty-eight and five years into this

17

novel life in Britain, in a fairly secure job, he was suffering. Suffering from a sense of immense loss and stuckness in a world that felt mostly alien and difficult to navigate.

NEUROPSYCHOSOCIAL (DIS)INTEGRATION IN THE DANCE OF LIFE

Alex felt besieged by incessant negative moods and insufficient resourcefulness to apply himself fully in his family, at work and in tasks of ordinary life. He recounts having had his 'life blown up many times, but nothing ever like this'. Under the conditions of the global health crisis we have come to know as the COVID-19 pandemic, Alex's symptoms were exacerbated by the unnaturalness of 'social distancing' the world's population was forced to practise. Of not being able to get together with family, friends and helpers we normally depend on to help us navigate or overcome the challenges of ordinary life. Which, based on the global accelerated rates of psychopathologies during the pandemic (Newlove-Delgado et al., 2021), appeared to drive survivors into an existence in the canal of fear—a place of high anxiety and aloneness that eroded general well-being and social engagement systems and, for Alex, this included his important relationships with himself, his loved ones and the socially distant but otherwise well-intentioned psychotherapist whom he was referred to for help.

After a few sessions in 'socially distanced' therapy, Alex discharged himself and began self-medicating with alcohol and isolation within the walls of his small apartment. When I asked him why he had discharged himself prematurely from the therapeutic relationship, he was remarkably resolute in his response: 'The therapist doesn't know what she is doing. I am telling her that I am having difficulties doing basic [daily] tasks, [and] she is giving me tasks to do. She is not getting it' (Alex, Greater Manchester, England, 2022).

There is no shortage of assumptions we can draw from this short excerpt in terms of what might be happening for Alex. For one, we could almost immediately appreciate the injury to his safe relationship with his children, within which he experiences intimacy and commitment to love. The bounded energy of this need acts to oppose the unbounded chaotic energy of aloneness and isolation that can surge when our hope for a nourishing social life and intimacy with our loved ones is eroded. It is in this state we are inclined to doubt that the social world can 'hold' us and we can in some way survive isolation from our loves and intimate relationships. This need—we learned in chapter 1—shows up for fulfilment between the ages of eighteen and forty—the sixth of the eight stages of our psychosocial development, a la Erikson. This points us in the direction of a psychosocial problem, as opposed to, say, one of resourcefulness. For we could also appreciate that Alex was not incapable of carrying out tasks in his daily life, as he clearly demonstrated resourcefulness, even with little, if any, psychosocial resources and support.

Beyond assumptions, it turned out that Alex's stuckness was more about his inability to act to protect what gave meaning to his life, and that involved his ability to be available as a father to his children and to provide for his family, both of which were stifled under the rigid conditions of the pandemic. His truncated ability to meet these needs, which was manifestly a consequence of his inability to influence the conditions of life under COVID-19, exposed in him a vulnerability to which he reacted with what amounts to psychosocial paralysis and a furrow into the depth of despair. To use the language of emotion, this was a state of helplessness, wherein he felt unable to influence environmental events that were reshaping his life and causing him to suffer. As I shall explore in part III, this furrow response to ALE hopelessness presents with a discernible neurobiology and behavioural expression. Equally important is that the vulnerability from which it derives is a carefully guarded component of the 'it' the therapist failed to 'get'. An 'it' that bares utility for Alex's well-being and must be appropriately acknowledged and engaged in his experience of life.

This 'It' incorporates both the inherited and acquired stories with which we come to the task of ordinary life, what I shall call our psychosocial legacy. The word *legacy* in itself is quite telling, coming from the Latin verb *legare*, which translates in English to what we inherit, acquire and leave behind when we transition to the afterlife. We can, therefore, think of psychosocial legacy as the collection of experiences and instructions, which include beliefs, values and wisdom, we inherit from our ancestors, as well as those we acquire in our lifetime and will pass on to future generations. Importantly, this also includes our disposition to respond to life events in either an adaptive or a maladaptive way, which we learned in chapter 1 is a construct of our psychosocial development that we cannot afford to exclude or overlook in the bigger story of how and why we exist. Naturally, this kind of legacy will be of different value to different people, but my sense is that it is an important ally in our experience of life. One that shows up reliably in my own reflections and work within academic and nonacademic contexts, including with survivors of ALEs. Its utility, I have discovered, is fairly practical in the sense that it involves agency and value we can rely on and attach to our purpose.

We have agency when we can act or move to help ourselves. Agency, thus, is that feeling of independence and resourcefulness trust in our self and abilities gives rise to when we are held relationally. In our resonant relationships, that is, with competent and reliable caregivers, such as a parent, lover, teacher, mentor or therapist. Much like trust, in the absence of which distrust takes root, agency is a native need that shows up for validation and integration in the course of our psychosocial development between the eighteenth and thirty-sixth month of life. This is the second and third stages of our psychosocial development, wherein we are driven by will and purpose and learn to take initiative—to do, move and act—in order to protect ourselves from unpleasant sensations like shame, doubt and guilt. When the familial relationship within which we ought to achieve this is vacant, perverse or unpredictable, we experience tension, and our agency may fail to develop. In a psychological sense, this is the incapacity to act or move competently to achieve what we want and bring us what we need, and to maintain a degree of influence over our life outcomes (Bandura, 2006).

The chaotic energies of shame, doubt and guilt that sustain this state take command of the body and mind when agency is vacant or eroded, so survivors might present with inactiveness or indifference in the face of ALEs. They cannot seem to move or act to help themselves, or all attempts fail. However, as we shall learn in part V, with the help of predictable input from nourishing relationships and development of psychosocial resourcefulness, survivors can learn to differentiate what comes from within themselves and what comes from others, and they can rework their life story to promote agency and free themselves from the hold of shame, doubt and guilt.

This differentiation will initiate for them a sense of selfhood and agency that can encourage them to open up and engage with the social world in ways that are not fuelled by the energy of shame and doubt, which cautions against engagement and mobilises our defences—encouraged to act, in a word, like a sovereign curator and sufficiently resourced choreographer in the dance of life. This type of agency, however, with its vulnerability to shame and doubt, is inclined to shield itself and may not be easily apparent to the uninitiated. In fact, expressions of psychosocial agency naturally favour relational intimacy. This is the native sense that we are heart-centred sentients. As one of my mentors put it wisely, it is like 'I heart you and you heart me', which underlies our existence as relational beings; existence necessarily involves being 'in relationship'.

SELFHOOD IN NEUROPSYCHOSOCIAL (DIS)INTEGRATION: NATIVE SPEARS

This was no different between Alex and me. I came to know him through our work for a British medical regulator, an institution in which we were a handful of non-white faces in a conspicuously white workforce, so 'it was easy for us to find ourselves', he once observed. He was acquainted with my research on Caribbeans' experience in Britain (Maduro, 2018). Our experience as Caribbeans was a common theme in our conversations, and we often talked warmly about how we navigate the relational spaces in which we find ourselves, spaces in which we act in a variety of roles, bearing identities such as colleague, associate and even friend. These spaces, ironically, also qualify as ones in which we are not encouraged to attend to our quiet yearnings, hopes, fears and agency. As such, we never felt sufficiently safe to expose the parts of ourselves that are intelligent, sovereign and motivated to build a good life, or to experience the greater goods in life. Here I am introducing tangentially the idea that we come to the task of ordinary life with our self as a collection of parts that serve us in different ways.

The self being a complex phenomenon that can transcend comprehension (Jung, 2016) and whose parts, or subselves, promote our survival but can also conflict with our native and adaptive defences. And this is especially true for those parts we are not encouraged or invited to expose in the course of our ordinary life, but which embody true competency, esteem and purpose. Those that are truly authentic and, in suppression or obscurity, give rise to dysregulations and deficits in our nervous system, our psychology and the way we present our body in the social world, embedding in our life as a psychosocial trauma and attendant neuropsychosocial disintegration. In early life, this can mean that authenticity and self-esteem fail to develop or, where fragile, altogether vacate the self. In his exploration of optimal self-esteem, the social psychologist Michael Kernis (2009) described authenticity as the 'unobstructed operation of one's true, or core, self in one's daily enterprise'. In the absence of this resilient true self, survivors are prone to struggle with feelings of inauthenticity, emptiness and unwholesomeness, to which they could well respond by imitating another organism's self, adopting a false self or rejecting and allowing to be destroyed physiological features—natural sex and sexual organs, for example—that inform the self, in a way that undermines well-being.

Authenticity that encourages survivors to pursue wellness is therefore a feature of neuropsychosocial integration. This is because, in addition to promoting a resilient true self and inner capacities, cultivating authenticity in the self is also about recovery from loss. Loss can be current and ongoing, but it could also be ancient, occurring in a distant ancestry. In that case, the pursuit of wellness is also about discovering who we might be in the absence of both past and ongoing losses that evoke despair and compel us to hide, rebuke or destroy who we truly are, our authentic self.

On this journey of self-discovery, our native SPEAR is indispensable, in that it functions to establish our somatic, psychological, emotional and relational attunement and safety that are important for our sense of self and our future.

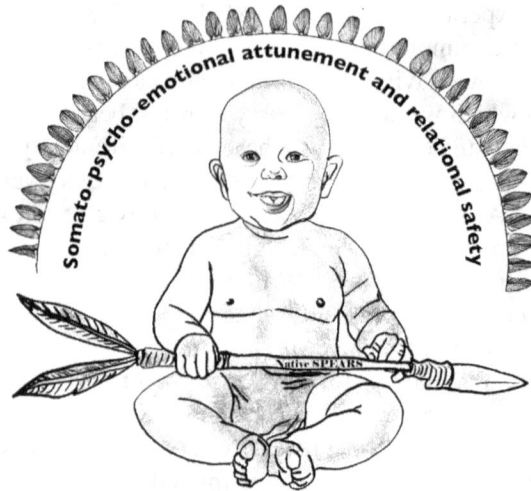

Figure 2.1. Safety Embodied—Native SPEARS (Somatic Safety, Psychological Integrity, Emotional Attunement, Relational Satisfaction and Self-Authenticity). We come to the task of life with the need to feel safe in our body, in our mind and in our social environment. This is our need for somato-psycho-emotional attunement and relational safety. *Figure courtesy of Dagmar Roelfsema.*

In chapter 1, we learned that attunement happens when the rhythms originating in our bodies and mind are undisturbed and validated in our social world. In somato-psycho-emotional attunement and relational safety, these rhythms merge into an energic synchrony that informs our sense of self. Ultimately, this is our most resilient identity, a need that emerges in the fifth stage of our psychosocial development. Between the ages of twelve and eighteen, when we are energised to reflect on our experiences, confront the expectations in our families and community, and develop aspirations that are value laden. This is, in a word, the undertaking to assert our true self. However, in the absence of a resilient true self that we are proud to assert, confusion about who we are—our name, sex, gender—and what we can and cannot achieve abounds, fuelled by the chaotic energy that impels us to neglect or injure our body, mind and self more generally. It is in this state that survivors are most liable to self-destruct and attack or alter the body in which they live and suffer with harmful objects—blades, drugs, needles and so on. This is the experience question 11 in the ALEs questionnaire seeks to surface for exploration, asking for information surrounding survivors' attachment to self-destructiveness, self-mutilation or self-injury, which includes suicidality, cutting, burning, striking, ripping off or breaking parts of their body.

I am compelled to pause, to rest here, as I am mindful of the negative resonance, or perhaps dissonance, in this observation. Particularly of its power to induce an inhibitory emotional state as a perfectly organic reaction. This conversation, however, continues in subsequent chapters, wherein I revisit the authentic self and its embodiment of competency, esteem and purpose, alongside its vulnerability to psychosocial trauma and neuropsychosocial disintegration that transcends generations. One could think of this conversation as a nod to intrapersonal, interpersonal and intergenerational relations that—we shall learn—invite compassion, presence and altruism to promote neuropsychosocial integration. Relationality, thus, is not merely a native need. It represents a metaphorical quiver of neuropsychosocial well-being SPEARS that serve us as we engage in the delicate dance of life and, even whilst exposing us to injury, orient to our adaptive needs, including our need for healing when we are wounded and resilience to sustain our well-being. Much like a terrific tango through which we can be savagely wounded but also derive flexibility, strength and well-being. It is my hope to have conveyed by the end of this book that this must involve cultivating and orienting resourcefulness to attend to our wounds, pains and vulnerabilities, and taking charge of experiences that shape our life. In a word, we must be resourced in the dance of life to navigate neuropsychosocial integration and disintegration that express at the level of the self.

Chapter 3

Neuropsychosocial (Dis)Integration in the (In)Authentic Self

The previous chapter introduced the self as a vessel for virtuous competency, purpose and authenticity, but also one within which these virtues can be badly lacking. This configuration is central to our understanding of integration and disintegration in the self, and as such, its exploration continues here, drawing insight from scholarly literature that emphasises the importance of authenticity as a psychosocial resource and an aspirational trait. As a psycho-social resource, for instance, authenticity honours vulnerability in the self in the same way as natural strengths and yearnings, say, for safety, operate in the body and mind. For the psychoanalyst Alice Miller (2008), this human need is primal in the drama of being a child, and each stage of the life cycle informs adaptive ways of surviving adversity, pursuing fulfilment in nourishing relationships and delighting in sophistication, all of which curve back to the need for a resilient true self and a sense of safety in the body and mind. This makes authenticity a good subject with which to begin my exploration.

RESILIENCE IN THE AUTHENTIC SELF: RESILIENCE SPEAR

At the level of the individual, resilience is the sense that 'I am safe in the world; I am cared for, cherished and sufficiently resourced internally and externally', not only to cope with adversity but, crucially, to lead a fulfilled life and grow in spite of adversity. Beyond this sense, resilience includes the capacity to learn in service of the needs for safety and growth and, ultimately, to apply learning to promote safety. Resilient safety is the wholesome state of somatic safety, psychological integrity, emotional attunement, relational sat-isfaction and self-authenticity. These are fundamental needs of the whole self,

Resilience embodied
Metaphorical spears

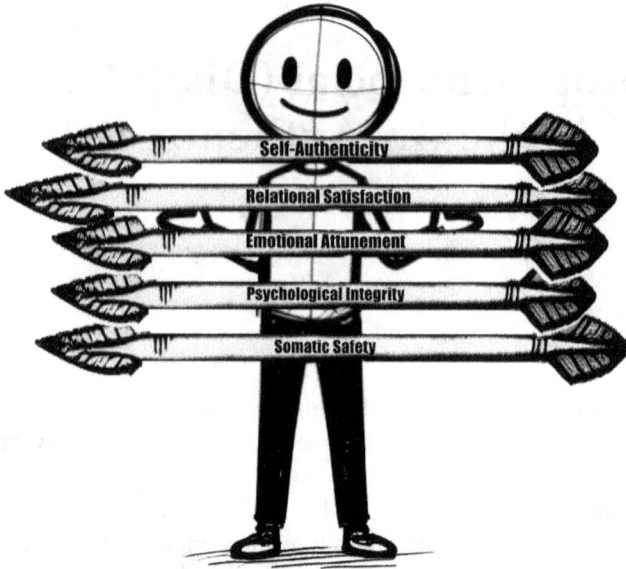

Figure 3.1. Resilience Embodied—SPEARS. *Figure courtesy of Dagmar Roelfsema.*

and, remarkably, when ordered, as illustrated in figure 3.1, they derive the acronym SPEAR. We might think of this as a quiver of resilience SPEARs.

- Our soma, the Greek word for 'body', keeps a record of how we experience the social world in its memory system (Rothschild, 2000). *Somatic safety* is a task of our autonomic nerves, which are responsible for signalling whether we feel safe or unsafe, moving us to engage in social interactions with positive energy and prosocial intentions.
- Upward from somatic safety is *psychological integrity*, our need for our mind to be free from false input in its experience of the world, and our thoughts to be congruent with reality and authenticity in our self.
- *Emotional attunement* reflects our deeper subcortical connections, undertaking to honour and bring regulation to the demands of our emotional state and that of other sentients we relate with (Goleman, 2003).
- *Relational satisfaction*, in the simplest of sense, is that sensation of nourishment we derive from our relationships.
- *Self-authenticity*, synonymous with 'rightness' or 'being upright', is our native morality mandate, to have a resilient moral compass that directs our behaviour in the world and our relationship with the laws of nature.

This quiver of SPEARs points me to social interaction that necessarily reinforces resilient capacities in our body and mind, and this extends to authenticity in our self. Interaction serves not only as a mechanism through which we develop contacts we rely on for resources in times of need, especially when we are wounded, but also for learning the rules of play and achieving our goals. In addition to the basic rules of survival that guide us, this is essentially about the need to influence our outcomes and keep at bay the chaotic energy of guilt. For it is at this stage in our psychosocial development—the third stage—that our need for 'calling shots' presents itself, so that we can learn to decide, take initiative and develop ambition. Our resilience SPEARs function to ensure we are equipped for this stage and to respond to the demands on us with courage and flexibility.

These SPEARs are not neurobiological features of the body and mind we can observe but useful metaphors for essential tools with which to move through life. They take us far back in time, to the time of our ancestors who lived in small groups of up to fifty individuals. The spear—physical, pliable and pointy—was essential for fulfilling their needs for food and safety. Notably, it was used to hunt for and gather food from the land and keep enemies away. Naturally, among these ancient ancestors, there were those who were aggressive, peaceful or curious, enduring dispositions that seem to have influenced patterns in contemporary personalities explored by the Welsh psychotherapist Terrance Watts (2000) in his important work on self-discovery. I shall explore these personalities in some depth in chapter 7. It suffices here to say that they inform authenticity in a self that is equipped not only for safety but also to benefit from the conception of authenticity as a progressive trait.

THE AUTHENTIC SELF IN CONCEPT AND CONTEXT

The influential psychologist Carl Rogers's insight in *On Becoming a Person* (1977) establishes a connection between authenticity and progression, as observed in both individuals and groups, enabling hypothetical and practical exploration of authenticity as a progressive trait. The hypothetical proposition is that authenticity fosters a virtuous concept of the self, that is, a self that does not accelerate towards a distorted identity, such as an identity suffused by a sense of unworthiness, inferiority or even superiority. A self that avoids such distortions is, in a word, integrous.

In a practical sense, the whole self, enthused with authenticity, is vulnerable in a way that does not evoke despair in the mind or paralyses in the body or lead to premature death. According to this characterisation, the self is actualised to affirm life and resilience as central aspects of the human condition, as the social psychologist Abraham Maslow (2011) explored in his seminal work on our core motivations and needs. Beginning with our basic needs for food, warmth and getting our genes and ways of surviving adversity into the next generation. These needs span the entire life cycle in much the same way as our psychosocial needs. As these needs are fulfilled, we open up to the more sophisticated needs for esteem, morality and relational intimacy. In neuropsychosocial integration, this is the sense that we are self-directed, but, within the bounds of nourishing relationships, we are important and, ultimately, virtuous. The practical tools, our SPEARS, with which we can fulfil these needs, Maslow—for reasons unknown—left for us to design. This is my task in part V.

So far this is a rather simplistic way of understanding human needs and the role of the self in fulfilling these needs, for we are indelibly complex and conflictual organisms. Take our selfish instinct to survive as individuals, which encompasses resilient emotional attachment, self-autonomy and predation that originates in our ancient neural substructures. It is safe to think of these forces as primordial, even reptilian. Many of the selfish urges these forces promote are ones we share with the most ancient reptile, the tuatara. This includes self-destructiveness and conspecific predation, also known as cannibalism, as seen in more contemporarily evolved reptiles that 'eat their own tails' or unempathically prey on their offspring or others of their species (Cloudsley-Thompson, 1999). This is as destructive as one can get, but nonetheless it is a truth about us that compels us to consider our needs and how they are categorised. Perhaps they should be hierarchically ordered, as with Maslow, and at the apex, the authentic person is fully self-accepting, unconditionally pro-life and living righteously in congruence with reality. Congruence, in this sense, is about reactions to life that embody core capacities and motivations to

- appropriately contextualise and integrate lived experiences;
- honour universal wisdom, moral boundaries and the sacredness of life; and
- engage in appropriate and vulnerable expression of the whole self.

Appropriately contextualising and integrating our experiences is contingent on our ability to accurately evaluate our environment and act in ways that reflect organic processes in our body and mind. Our big brain and its network of nerves facilitate these processes, which begin with sensory stimulation and end with interpretations and reactions in our mind. More on this in part IV.

The second capacity—to honour moral boundaries, universal truths and the sanctity of life—involves reconciling our core needs with those of others in our social orbit. This calls for innate intelligence, which I shall explore in the next chapter. Here it suffices to say that this involves our ability to recognise what is going on in our body and mind and to tune into the bodies and minds of other sentients.

This latter ability—to tune into the nervous system of autonomous sentients and perceive emotional and other nonverbal cues—is what we call empathy. It is native to limbic and cerebral creatures, like ourselves, and is among the more sophisticated executive functions we develop to enable us to more effectively self-regulate and co-regulate as we participate in the delicate dance of life.

I described this dance earlier as terrific and tango-like, tango being a folk dance native to the deprived Río de la Plata area that straddles the border between Argentina and Uruguay. In a metaphorical sense, this area is a good representation of the limitations and stuckness with which survivors of historical traumas move through life. Nonetheless, it offers hope with the story of the evolution of the tango, which integrates influences from Afro-Latin *candombe*, habanera and milonga in a celebration of the wonders of interpersonal relationships that are complex, conflictual and demanding of resilient boundaries to keep our selves safe.

The aggressive yet carefully crafted moves, sensualness and interdependence of the tango speak to a defensive yet cautious agency in us. The guardian of this agency is our own 'private dragon' whose purpose is to keep us safe, and it is meant to be engaged to protect life and defend integrity. The literature inclines us to consider this task one with which our adaptive defence system is charged, manifesting itself as a valiant but bindable energy that is equipped with an autonomous 'fire'. This is the instinct of anger, bravery and justice that can be deployed freely to ward off a valid threat, protect kin, settle disputes and recover from assaults on the body and mind. Another way to think of this fire is as a flexible aggression that responds to discipline when we can access and temper its neural circuit. An ancient clump of neural cells known as the ventromedial hypothalamus that hides itself deep within the social-emotional brain system, from where it regulates our impulse to deploy violence in service of self-preservation and survival, which incidentally also includes sex (Hashikawa et al., 2017). By this awareness, we are able to validate our 'private dragon'—its tendencies and competencies which we can harness in different situations—as well as keep it disciplined and uninterested in spewing its fire in unexpected ways and unwanted places, especially not on the path towards integration and authentic self-actualisation.

Lastly, the third feature of congruence—the capacity to perceive accurately and engage in appropriate and vulnerable expression of the whole self—is to show up as we are naturally. By which I mean with all of our wounds as well as our need for SPEARS, and the expression of this need with interpersonal and intrapersonal compassion. Compassion is a psychosocial resource at the heart of neuropsychosocial integration, which I explore in some depth in chapter 12.

AUTHENTICITY AS A STATE OF SELF-POSSESSION

Taken all together, the core features of congruence offer up authenticity as a possession through which the authentic self acts to stay safe and fulfilled. We could think of this as a culture that requires cultivation and nurturance of a divine wisdom with which the authentic person steers life to a state of relative security that is sustained by truth. This kind of wisdom is also unique in that it embraces losses, pains, anxieties and even despair that vulnerability can evoke.

In the absence of congruence, thus, vulnerability is liable to oppose truthfulness, which poses a problem for authenticity in a self in which they must coexist. This is a need that presents itself in the eighth stage of our psychosocial development, when the healing energy of wisdom and integrity must battle the chaotic energy of falsehood and pretence. The British psychoanalyst Donald Winnicott (1984, 12) introduced the concepts of the 'true self' and 'false self' in an inverse relationship to speak about this battle. This relationship can be interpreted in any number of ways, but Winnicott nonetheless holds firmly that the authentic self is not corrupted by falsity. The life that the authentic person leads, in other words, is one that is true, and it is in denying this aspect of the self that we are liable to show up to the task of ordinary life dis-integrated, disordered and inauthentic.

This leads me to think of the inauthentic self as an existential threat, in that it can render survivors impaired in the face of life challenges for which they must show up wholesome and competent. Consider, for instance, the challenge to provide enough food, warmth and security for one's family. Another may be to face the challenge of a global health crisis. For many, the list of such challenges feels endless. My conviction, nonetheless, is that where life challenges invoke adaptive but inadequate defences, as opposed to resilient capacities to self-rescue and self-preserve, the survivor is at risk of further peril.

This vulnerability surfaces in various contexts throughout the chapters. Here it is in a pernicious manifestation wherein it betrays the authentic self. The self that accurately interrogates relational environments to detect cues of safety as well as cues of hostility and moves us to respond appropriately and adapt in our body and mind. More precisely, in service of our survival and well-being, the authentic self that encourages adaptation in the ways we present ourselves, how we carry ourselves, how we think of ourselves and how we relate. For it is in this service that its vulnerability to betrayal lies.

Where it can be unwelcomed, unrewarded or feel threatened in any other way and yield to an inauthentic configuration, even switching place with the inauthentic self in varying social-emotional contexts. Thereby, surrendering authenticity. Even when what we are reacting to is superficial, but nonetheless stoking our protective dragon or rattling its circuitry. *Circuitry* simply refers to neural substructures that connect chemically or energetically to fulfil biological functions. Our native defence circuitry, within which our protective dragon acts, is better understood because of its involvement with defences, aggression and trauma.

AUTOMATICITY IN THE (IN)AUTHENTIC SELF

Until now, I have treated neural substructures, circuitries and processes as autonomous and unconnected in the nervous system. They are, in fact, to a degree autonomous but not unconnected in the nervous system that provides the self with the information it needs and uses. This relationship begins with the neural cells. The magnificent neurons that—among many competencies—use complex appendages to exchange energic signals—also known as action potentials, firing, impulses and spikes—across tiny neural gaps called synaptic clefts.

These signals are transported by neurochemicals—neurotransmitters that are contained in vesicles in the synapses—and the intended synapse on the other end of the cleft can receive them because of a notable energy charge difference inside and outside both the sending and receiving neurons. The synaptic cleft, for instance, is ordinarily a heavily charged and busy environment, whereas the energy level of a neuron at rest is about negative 70 millivolts, roughly 0.03 percent of the power of a UK main socket. The inside of a neuron, in other words, is 70 mV less than the outside. When an urge or demand to take action arises, say in response to a curiosity originating in the mind, specific neurons experience a surge in energy, making signals more likely to occur, even involuntarily, and this happens very quickly, within milliseconds.

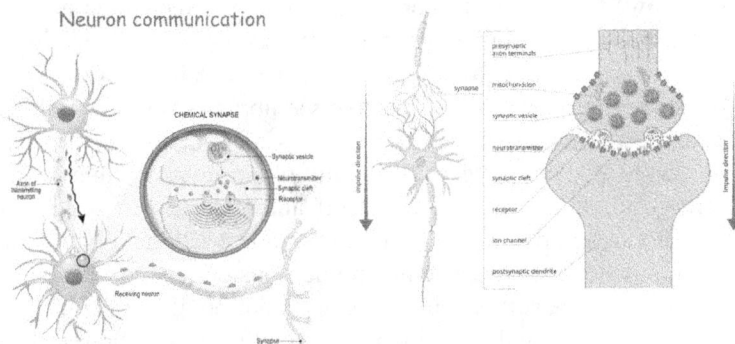

Figure 3.2. The Magnificent Neuron. *Image © ttsz / iStock / Getty Images and Olha Pohrebniak / iStock / Getty Images*

Neurons, like the body and mind they communicate to govern, are incredibly self-protective. Protection is a task they undertake with great flexibility, considering their complexity and vulnerability to trauma. For instance, neurons can transfer charged molecules across their membrane to the synaptic cleft in an effort to rapidly adjust their energy level and avoid being overwhelmed. Obviously, this only applies to molecules tiny enough to cross the sheaths of their membrane, like the hydrogen protons and sodium, potassium, calcium, and chloride ions that are naturally energising and easily moved. You may recognise these as nutrients and minerals we get from foods. Their increased levels in neurons reflect in neural vigourosity. The inverse too is true. Their levels deplete as they are used, and the neurons return to a state of rest.

We can appreciate that neurons achieve this masterful control of their activities by swiftly opening and closing channels—tiny holes—in their membrane, a fancy name for the protective sheath that surrounds the neuron. But they also have a specialised transport system that move content in and out of their body to preserve stability, or even to avoid being overwhelmed by molecules flowing inward during channel openings. Incidentally, these channels are also integrated in receptors on appendages called dendrites that bind to molecules deposited in the synapse. By these openings, proton and ion molecules also exit through respective channels, releasing inner content to mitigate the risk of being overwhelmed and neuronal descent into anarchy. Obviously, neuronal activities are more intricate and complex than shuttling molecules and exchanging and regulating signals, but this is a tidy way to begin to understand how they maintain health and functionality, as well as allay vulnerability to trauma.

When molecules bind to neuronal receptors, they excite, inhibit or neutralise neuronal activity, affecting whether the neuronal energy is bounded or increased and allowed to flow freely. Neuroimaging technology, such as EEG and fMRI, which lay bare neural activities under conditions of stress and stasis, has allowed researchers to observe these phenomena and how energy waves in the brain synchronise and reinforce each other, giving rise to big signals that are strong enough to activate our native defence circuitry. These signals, so strong, permeate the protective membrane of our central nervous system to trigger reactions in our heart, lungs and veins and, in effect, the rhythm of our heart rate, oxygen intake and blood flow. By this set up, our native defence circuitry can activate itself automatically in service of our survival, without cognitive input—such as thoughts, rationality and mindfulness. And this is possible because its autonomous circuits are located in the brainstem, from where survival instincts and core bodily functions, such as deep rest, wakefulness and movement, are regulated. The brainstem is the most ancient of the four organising structures of the central nervous system, the other three being the superior midbrain, neocortex and inferior spine.

Separate from the peripheral nerves, these structures are protected by multiple layers of tissue collectively known as meninges, from *meninx*, the ancient Greek word for 'membrane'. Reminiscent of a deadly insect, I recall becoming acquainted as a child with this peculiar term, which made me think of some deadly insect. I heard it long before I had learned the words *nervous system*, for it was associated with death in people, who, however unfortunately, had become exposed to harmful microbes. This was the lethal disease known as meningitis, characterised by inflammation of the meninges.

Essentially, the meninges membrane consists of an inner layer called the pia mater, an outer layer called the dura mater, and a middle layer filled with fluid called the arachnoid. The term *arachnoid* implies complexity and sophistication, much like the dwelling of arachnids, or spiders. Together, these layers ensure that neurons in the brain and spine are actively protected and not easily breached by harmful microbes. It is also important to note that the neural substructures couched within the borders of the meninges are protected further by endothelial cells that fend off microbes in the bloodstream that could disturb neural activities. Figure 3.3 shows some of these substructures in the midbrain, from where their neurons extend and connect in networks. Neurons' bodies and dendrites make up the outer cortex, which can be identified as deep greyish matter on functional resonant images of the

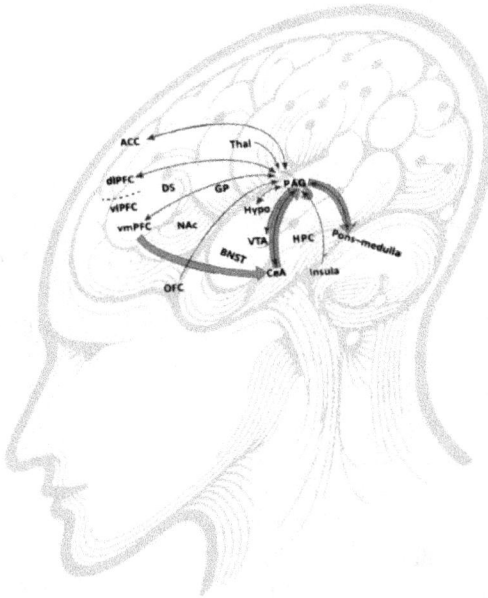

Figure 3.3. Neural Substructures and Circuitries in the Midbrain. *Figure courtesy of Dagmar Roelfsema.*

brain. Their connective appendages, called axons, are swathed in an insulat-
ing myelin, a proteinous fatty white sheath, and folded beneath the cortex.

The periaqueductal gray (PAG), for instance, plays a crucial role in regulating pain and response to danger. In these tasks, its neurons project to other
neural substructures in established safety networks. Disintegration in these
networks, thus, may alert to its presence via chronic pain and maladaptive
response to danger. Other important neural substructures involved with this
autonomous process include the hypothalamus, which works to keep the
body within safe physiological limits; the thalamus that regulates consciousness and alertness; the hippocampus that plays a role in learning and recall
memory formation; the amygdala that regulates emotional states and informs
adaptive defences; and the insula that plays a vital role in sensorimotor and
complex social-emotional functions. Interconnection in the socioemotional
limbic system—between the neocortex and brainstem—allows these substructures to inform perceptions.

We think of perceptions as the output of the mind, implying that the limbic
system has a mind of its own. If the amygdala detects vulnerability, say to
shame, the thalamus will dutifully pass on this information to the neocortex,
which will provide context, assuming the cortical lobes are unimpaired. The
amygdala and thalamus, in this sequence, are acting intelligently in the service of survival, naturally with input from the hippocampus, hypothalamus
and periaqueductal gray.

It will become clearer in subsequent chapters that this system of intelligence is instructed by neuromodulators to work continuously in service
of life and safety, much like a fire alarm scanning for smoke. Thus, outside
of our awareness, it monitors our environment for threats—large and small,
real and imagined. This could be events linked in memory to bad outcomes,
events that are unfamiliar, unpleasant relationships we want to avoid or even
imagined terror. In all these situations and others where we might feel vulnerable or unsafe, this integrated system of intelligence directs our behaviour—
sometimes at our peril. At peril because it can be short-circuited or hijacked,
thereby creating the conditions for neuropsychosocial disintegration that lead
even incredibly smart people to concede authenticity and to self-sacrifice.

In bringing this all together, I am compelled to share a story about a brilliant Ayurvedic doctor with whom I once had the joy to work. I'll call him
Dr. Amjeet. Like every one of us, he came to the task of life with himself as
a collection of parts, which included being an intelligent naturopathic doctor,
a selfless father of two children, an insulin-dependent diabetic who managed
his health with a natural diet and a member of a family of well-being practitioners in India. All this is to say that Dr. Amjeet was not naïve in his approach
to life. Yet, in response to enduring disapproval, insults and odd demands
from his employer, he was disposed to fold into a toady version of himself.

An incident I can share is that of a manager's proposal to have Dr. Amjeet's young children come to work with him to help package items for service users. In response, Dr. Amjeet, without expressing objection, offered to carry out the task himself. The socioemotional message conveyed was 'in order to keep his children safe, he submits to suffering'. This apparent need to be needed, as implied by the role of keeping vulnerable children safe and securing the future, is one that emerges at the seventh stage of our psychosocial development, according to Erikson, between the ages of forty and sixty-five, when the impulse to generate can express itself in sacrificial undertakings to give to family, community and society. This impulse could also express itself in undertakings to succeed in a meaningful task or career in order to ward off the chaotic energy of stagnation and unusefulness.

From a neuropsychosocial perspective, this kind of suffering is one that the spirit of parental love, acting to fulfil the evolutionary biological imperative to protect posterity, can mitigate. Psychosocially, too, this is about submission to a part of the self that is equipped for the pain of stagnation and unusefulness. I cannot say with certainty whether this was Dr. Amjeet's native or adaptive response to adversity. He had not had a chance to take my adverse lived experiences (ALEs) assessment, which would tell me about historical events of adversity that informed his reaction to life events. His apparent servility, however, pointed to a native disposition, beneath which a servile socioemotional impulse promotes a fold to numb his sense of suffering, whilst allowing him to protect his children from exploitation and provide an income for his family. Both of these would triumph over an impulse to engage his 'protective dragon' to reshape or relinquish the injurious relationship and the workplace in which he suffered, where, incidentally, he was not encouraged to apply himself to resolve the complex health problems—the arthritis, gut dysbiosis and impotency, for example—of which his patients complained.

The temptation to view this kind of self-sacrifice as virtuous or altruistic is also palpable. Altruism, we shall learn in part V, is rooted in the instinct, which we call compassion, to alleviate suffering. This kind of self-sacrifice, however, lacks the virtue of compassion. In its own unique way, it is as harmful as Alex's self-abandonment in chapter 2. In fact, until Dr. Amjeet's fold had rendered him dispensable and he was freed from his professional duties, he felt compelled to appease his disapproving employer in an effort to feel secure in himself.

Dr. Amjeet's attachment to this effort, though, stoked in him a fear of being judged unworthy—say, of respect, reward for his competencies or even job security—that held him stuck in a state of loss. This autonomic state, in which his inauthentic self, in a position of dominance, demanded concession, was bad for him, as is common with concessions that involve self-sacrifice demanded by the inauthentic self. The conceder feels compelled to neglect their own loss and pain whilst promoting and fulfilling the needs of others. Here loss includes negative consequences that one can acquire or inherit, and which are attached to conditions that one has little to no control over. An example would be an inherited ethnic penalty, where the individual is denied opportunities or faces undeserved contempt due to an ascribed or inherited ethnicity. In the face of such injustice, self-sacrificial concession—as in over-extending one's self or quieting one's yearning—can serve a desperate need for inner peace. And this is possible because such concessions in service of peace are autonomously invited in response to psychic tensions and pains, a phenomenon identified in the interpersonal neurobiology literature as fawn-ing (Walker, 2013).

More precisely, fawning behaviours—as in acting to appease an antago-nist—mitigate injury momentarily. For Dr. Amjeet, this injury was largely emotional, being made to feel ashamed, incompetent and unimportant. But injury can be physical, as in being beaten, or psychological, as in being dehumanised and disenfranchised. Whatever the source of the injury, the neurobiology of fawning, much like that of any self-protective state, engages the autonomic nerves in ways that signal the immune system to begin repair in the body and mind. As such, fawning as a default self-defence adapta-tion may give rise to autoimmunity, in order to enable the immune system to detect and repair neuronal impotence, damage or depletion as it occurs. Similar to a chronically frightened person who goes through life in a state of hypervigilance for cues of danger, these neurons will be hypersensitive to cues of injury rather than cues of safety, leading to hyperreactivity. This could then result in a fragile state of hyper-hypo activation that undermines the survivor's ability to stay safe (see part IV).

For the survivor, the foremost question—from a frightened inner voice—is 'What do I need to be or do so that I don't get hurt?' The output is likely to be a combination of self-serving and self-sacrificing cognition and behav-iour. Think of servility in the abused child, passivity in the battered spouse or subservience in oppressed people groups, all of whom are stuck between the instinct to stay unhurt and the need for care and resonance in relationship.

The compulsion to please others in people who come to the task of life with relational traumas that are complex and compounding also comes to mind. This stuckness in itself is also complex, especially when it invokes and sustains a toxic liaison between the autonomous defence impulse and the attachment impulse. When activated at the same time, these two survival instincts give rise to the volatile neurobiology of a traumatic wound that cuts the survivor off from inner sensations through which to express the need for nourishing relationships that are germane to emotional and social intelligence.

It would not be inappropriate to think of this adaptive response to ALEs and attendant traumas in the same way as any self-sacrificing tendencies that are rooted in injurious early life relationships and—in the absence of remedial intervention—may block the authentic self from developing (Walker, 2013). Even if only for this reason, self-sacrificing, of which self-folding and fold-fawning are examples, is a feature of psychosocial trauma that establishes the conditions for neuropsychosocial disintegration with which I am concerned. An auxiliary task will be to declare it an expression of an inauthentic self that can be invoked and sustained by the instinct to survive. However, not unlike inauthenticity, self-sacrificing is inimical to survivors' long-term well-being and, as such, it is maladaptive in its consequence.

Part III considers this maladaptation and its features within the context of intergenerational survival, as they were appropriate for my enslaved ancestors and socioeconomically disadvantaged forebears. Foremost is to appreciate that maladaptive impulses manifesting in the self bear wisdom as well as consequences for well-being that are handed down across generations. And these consequences, too, constitute psychosocial legacies that we cannot afford to ignore.

Recall from chapter 2 the 'it' that Alex's therapist failed to 'get' and the implications for his experience in therapy. My lived experience, along with insight from the literature on black identities and white therapies (Charura & Lago, 2021), informs me that this is plausible because it was not a legacy the therapist was disposed to acknowledge and honour. Not necessarily because of hardiness or prejudice on her part, but more that it was the kind of legacy she was unlikely to have been exposed to in her psychoeducation, conventional psychotherapy or practice of psychodynamics, which emphasise cognitive analysis and brain-based therapy for the here and now (Charura & Lago, 2021). It is in the light of these conjectures that I am led to believe the root of this travesty lay in a lack of empathic attunement, a key component of our native and resilience SPEARs. This is essentially a deficit in ability to establish a therapeutic relationship within which distress that comes into focus is naturally validated, regulated and reflected on, and new meaning emerges in the reworking of a life story within which it is contextualised, free of chaotic energy. But, more importantly, it is also a deficit in the ability to connect and resonate with another sentient and, in Alex's case, in a way that gets to legacies of maladaptive impulses and inauthenticity that give rise to disintegration in the dynamic self, to which I shall now turn.

Chapter 4

Neuropsychosocial (Dis)Integration in the Dynamic Self

That the self can assimilate both adaptive and maladaptive impulses as its own speaks to its dynamism, fluidity and resilience, even when it is inauthentic or its dynamism leaves it vulnerable to contradiction and pathology. Here I am rather pessimistic about the self, but this is important, for this is the story of the inauthentic self. In fact, the *Oxford English Dictionary* defines *inauthentic* as 'lacking sincerity' and 'not genuinely belonging to a style or period'. To put this in other words, inauthenticity in the self is an adaptation that is unbounded, and the inauthentic self is one that is inadequately or inappropriately adapted for the environment or situation in which it presents. This suggests that the inauthentic self is not only liable to travel in time and across space, but also to influence environments in which it is novel, to reflect the one in which it developed.

This adaptability speaks to profound wisdom in the inauthentic self, its disposition to preserve survival in the face of adversity, even though with little regard for authenticity. In this role, the inauthentic self acts as a guardian of experiences the nervous system cannot yet process safely. The reasons for this can be varied and complex but ordinarily include neurobiological limitations and psychosocial inquietudes. Bearing this in mind, another of my discoveries—both in practise and in the scholarly literature—is that experiences the inauthentic self is disposed to protect often include deep secrets, repressed miseries and quiet yearnings that would be unsafe in exposure, for the good reason that exposure invites judgements that imperil the need for relational security.

The inauthentic self, working to keep us safe from this kind of peril, is nothing short of noble, although its suppression of authenticity in this service cannot be overlooked and is in fact centred in traditions in which the self is perceived as a host of stories that are implicated in survival as well as pathologies. Welcome to the self as a host of life stories with implications for survival and pathologies!

THE SELF AS HOST OF LIFE STORIES:
SURVIVAL AND PATHOLOGICAL

I think of life stories as memories that bear two important profiles—the first is neurobiological, and the other is sociohistorical. Memories, in other words, are complex biosocial implants, the mechanics of which are beyond the scope of this book. We can, however, satisfy ourselves with the broad categories of negative and positive. Negative memories are associated with adverse life events that give rise to trauma and, as such, can be aptly labelled as traumatic memories.

Overwhelming sensations by which traumatic memories are characterised are mostly stored in the body, where there is storage space in a physical sense. Beginning in childhood, the chaotic energies of relational traumas with caregivers, for instance, that do not complete the charge-and-discharge cycle and embed in the nervous system can feature in bodily aches and irritations that are primitive but far more accurate than cognition and emotion that distract from real danger in the environment. More abstractly, the self hosts these memories in its subselves. And, collectively, the subselves constitute the mind and body, or psyche and soma.

In the psyche, memories are records of emotional and cognitive changes that occur in response to stimulation. Think of these as emotions and thoughts arising from an actual or perceived lived experience. In the soma, however, memories are chemical and physical changes in biological tissues that are expressed in behaviour, sensations and physiological disturbance. Hence, one might perceive memories—where negative, traumatic and embedded in the nervous system—as vulnerabilities that give rise to psychosomatic pathologies.

Pathologies that defy the psyche's and the soma's native resolve and power to self-heal. This includes healing from a state of neuropsychosocial dis-integration that I argue is achievable with active therapy that involves a reworking of life stories and freeing the self from the claws of chaos, beginning with the idea that the state of wellness, as is that of pathology, is influenced by varying configurations of who we are, how we are and what we can and cannot become. This is our whole self, which challenges us to reconcile its varied configurations.

Historical insights surrounding the psyche, especially in psychodynamics, have taught us this is not a simple task. Any attempt inevitably comes up against defences in a powerful part of the psyche and invariably the self. These are repressed, to use the Freudian term. I remain convinced, nonetheless, that the psyche, as is the self, is dynamic, and in ascribing mutable descriptors such as adaptive, maladaptive, authentic and inauthentic to the self, I affirm this to be true.

In fact, I perceive the self as malleable and multipart, which aligns with the school of thought that frames the self as an expression of distinct identities with which we move through life and which we use to make sense of our experiences and expressions. I think of these identities, however undisclosed, as consolidating around three core subselves—namely, a primal-instinctive, social-emotional and cerebral-cognitive.

I am concerned, foremost, with authenticity, which I believe is native to the primal-instinctive self. This is not by any means an original idea, for psychoanalysts have long argued that a crude component of the self offers up authenticity in the purest of sense, an instinct that presents at birth equipped with reflexes to support a drive to survive. This drive, however, it is said, is vulnerable to a latent death instinct that mobilises towards destruction, including self-destruction (Freud, 2003). At the surface level, this theory appears wholly inadequate to address the nuanced and complex interplay between neurobiology, psychology and social forces that shape the self. Yet it retains credibility that has utility for the psychology of well-being and has evolved since its unveiling in the nineteenth century to guide scholarship surrounding the psychogenesis of wellness and pathology.

Empirical insights surrounding emotions derived from the seminal work of the American psychologist Paul Ekman (2003), for instance, have suggested that the survival and death instincts of which psychoanalysts speak relate to equally powerful instincts to maximise positive and comforting emotions and minimise negative and upsetting ones. This encourages me to think of emotions as agents of a relatively sophisticated social-emotional self as well as neurobiological programs for instincts that derive from the instinctive self.

Thus, positive and comforting emotions move us to engage in activities that promote our survival, as in the preservation of life, but also in activities that promote somatic safety, psychological integrity, emotional attunement and relational satisfaction. The resilience SPEARS, which we learned about in chapter 3, that are essential for well-being. By this assumption, our SPEARS and emotions appear to coalesce and move us to behave in ways that are good for us, but they can also move us in ways that are not good for us. To focus first on the good, consider the positive and comforting emotions of kindness, gratitude and love that derive from the spirit of altruism.

Kindness moves us to care for the more vulnerable of our kind, which is also in service of our bid for social security. We also care in order that we will be cared for, too, should the need arises. Gratitude can move us to invest generously in relationships that offer attunement, appreciation and care. And love moves us to engage in coupling from which we can derive the pleasures of intimacy as well as the gifts of procreation and posterity and the nurturing of our children, to be available to them and supplement their growth.

These axioms are among my favourites to share in my talks on emotions, often prefixed with the biological fact that we do not have neuronal receptors we can ascribed to any particular emotion, but we can measure the neuro-chemistry of dopamine fuelling the pleasure we derive from kindness, sero-tonin fuelling gratitude and oxytocin fuelling love. Emotions, therefore, are the output of neurochemical reactions. And although we do not have neuronal receptors for kindness, gratitude or love, our nervous system knows when we are not getting enough and expresses this in the tiny synaptic clefts between neural cells, where the neurons converse and signal for action.

I think of love, for instance, as this incredible emotion we can access when we are vulnerable. By vulnerable, I mean when we open up ourselves to love, to be loved and to fall into the depth of emotional pain. It is the state in which Alex experienced a more fulfilling life, within the context of a marriage through which he fathered children and was sufficiently resourced to meet his family's material needs. It is also the state in which Amjeet lived and self-sacrificed to provide for his family and keep his vulnerable children safe. This kind of love moves us to honesty and openness in our bid for inner harmony, but it can equality bring us disharmony and death. My point is that emotions bear significance for the sense of safety and fulfilment around which we are inclined to organise our life.

I have noted neurochemistry, but, more discernibly, we experience the benefits of emotions through our moods, curiosities and motivations, or lack thereof. These are psychosomatic responses we are disposed to recognise. One may find, for instance, that kindness evokes hopefulness, gratitude evokes contentment and love leads to happiness. Although happiness—a positive state—can derive from negative emotions too. Earlier, I alluded to emotions being used in ways that are not good for us, even if we are in a prosocial state that dopamine rewards with feel-good sensations. This could be true with, for instance, Schadenfreude, that depletive emotion through which one derives delight, perhaps even ecstasy, from others' suffering. Preceding this sensa-tion, however, may in fact be some other deleterious emotions. Take envy and jealousy one can feel towards a nemesis, a friend or one's own children. Envy reveals itself in intense sensations of unfulfillment and destructive behaviours that accompany wanting what the other—the target of the envy—has. This could be anything from that person's spouse to their virtues. As such, it is experienced as a threat to self-esteem. Jealousy, likewise, involves a perceived threat to self-esteem, but unlike envy it reveals itself in active fear of loss. This could be fear of losing a desired relationship or a perceived opportunity, which gives rise to emotional pain and attendant toxicity—a depletive emotional state, in other words, that is included in the mixed bag of psychosomatic states we can experience at varying levels of intensity, which also correspond with motivation to express or to suppress them.

Disturbance in this system betokens pathology. In fact, every negative emotion outlined in the *Diagnostic and Statistical Manual of Mental Disorders (DSM)* and the International Classification of Diseases (ICD) is associated with a distinct pathology and attendant symptoms. Envy and jealousy are examples of depletive emotions that evoke anger and sadness, and chronic anger and sadness are associated with emotional and behavioural disorders.

For far more troubling examples, consider chronic fear, disgust and hopelessness associated with premature death. At an extreme deviation, these negative emotions overwhelm the instinct to survive adversity and preserve life. Think of the anorexic person who perceives food as disgusting and starves to death. Disgust, in a word, can trump the will to live. Likewise, hopelessness can invoke the neurobiology of suicide. And fear, which is arguably the most studied of our emotions, can eclipse sexual urges and inhibit the pro-life instinct to procreate.

Considering our biological imperative to stay alive, procreate and safeguard posterity, emotional states that beget genealogical destruction, such as with suicide and filicide, are anathema in the story of human survival, especially where these emotional states, examples of which include disgust, fear and shame, incite the deadliness of unbounded disturbance in our social-emotional self or the predatory urges we share with the ancient reptile that hide in our instinctive self. Within the safe bounds of his acclaimed docudrama *Murdered by My Father*, the British dramatist Vinay Patel offers a palpable insight into this deadliness. Its incidence in reality, however, is far from drama or escapable, as we could readily learn from the widely mediatised life and death of seventeen-year-old Shafilea Ahmed in Britain; the Shafia sisters, Zainab, Sahar and Geeti, in Canada; and the Saeed sisters, Amina and Sara, in the United States. Young women who were slain by their families in apparent 'honour' killings that speak to the universality of an unforgiving death instinct, which appears to prioritise itself over the instinct to preserve life and posterity. In a word, this is a feature of a pathological self—whether social-emotional or instinctive—that emotes and behaves in ways that lead to its own demise as well as that of its genealogy.

THE DEVELOPING SELF IN THE
ABSENCE OF PATHOLOGY

Now that we are acquainted with both positive and negative manifestations of emotions in the whole self as a host of life stories, it is safe to say that it is in the absence of pathology that the instinctive self—debuting in infancy—is mobilised to survive and is preoccupied with tension that can be resolved by satisfying survival needs. Aloneness and hunger that invariably evoke acute fear and despair, for instance, can be resolved with attention and sustenance, and the cry and suckle reflexes support these needs without regard for consequence.

Again, in the absence of pathology, whether so deriving from emotion or instinct, sensitivity to consequence in the young child co-develops with self-awareness and identities that are separate and different from those of caregivers. Consider, for a moment, the crude identities of boychild, girlchild, grandchild and slavechild, which are distinct from those of mama, dada, grandma, and master. These identities, one may argue, are consequential in that they evince the psychosocial, which is what is constructed when the psyche meets and adapts to society.

Specifically, the psychosocial develops from interaction between the nervous system and society, which, incidentally, is created by the psyche. Here, we have a bidirectional flow between psyche and society, synched in a delicate tango, creating, shaping and reshaping each other whilst memories are installed in the nervous system to promote survival behaviour. All this is to say that the nervous system, as is society—the environment in which we learn about ourselves and what we can and cannot become—is an active co-creator of the psychosocial. The psychosocial, in this sense, sanctions behaviour as acceptable or unacceptable and, in so doing, links behaviour with emotion, so that emotions can function as biological agents that move us to act in service of our survival as well as social agents that help us to interpret our experiences.

Recall the examples of love, which moves us to protect our loved ones and relate in ways that favour well-being; that of fear, which warns us against injurious intimacy and moves us to avoid contact in service of self-protection; or even that of shame, which reflects insult to our honour and incites us to act in service of its restoration. Much of these processes occur at a subcerebral-subconscious level. Manifesting somatically, for instance, in our heart by lowering its rate when we feel loved; in our gut by invoking a churn when we feel vulnerable; and in our limbs, facilitating the numbness and paralysis we experience when we are terrified.

Invariably, the intensity of these emotions and the psychophysiology they invoke vary depending on the chemistry the neurons release or do not release in response to how we are experiencing our world, that is, whatever we are sensing, doing or thinking. My focus on emotions in the nervous system thus emphasises the absolute magnificence of neurons. Among functions, for instance, neurons bear responsibility for storing the energy used in the nervous system, host memories, and, above all, they are building blocks of the nervous system itself. The many billions in this latter role are necessarily involved in how life is experienced through emotions as well as through action and present themselves structurally suited for their tasks.

Basic Neuron Types

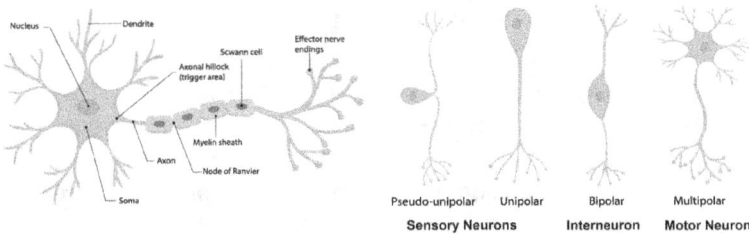

Figure 4.1. Three Types of Neurons. Neurons are highly specialized for the processing and transmission of cellular signals. Based on their roles in the nervous system, they can be divided into three classes: sensory neurons, motor neurons and interneurons.

This speaks to a complexity—both in structure and functions—that defines neurons, in addition to the unique features by which they can be categorised. Those that take information to the brain for perception and sensory processing can be identified by their relatively long receptor dendrites and short axons through which they communicate. Those that innervate muscles throughout the autonomic nervous system to summon movement are appropriately called motor neurons.

In the opening preface, I talked about my need to hug my loving-kind grandmother during the COVID-19 pandemic. Imagine this need originating with an emotional sensation, say a fear of losing my grandmother to disease and a corresponding yearning for connection and closeness to her. Its actualisation, however, will begin in my social-emotional brain with a signal that travels through my instinctive brain, down my spinal chain and along its meandering way into a physical embrace involving leaned-in bodies, interlocking necks and curled arms. These voluntary movements are made possible by the motor neurons, distinguished by their fairly short dendrites and long axons that can extend up to a metre in length.

But the motor neurons receive instruction from the other categories of neurons, most directly from interneurons that relay information between sensory and motor neurons using relatively short dendrites and axons that vary in length. In my example, these interneurons would also act to ensure that affirmation of the hug and its corresponding sensations of attunement, comfort and love travel back to my emotional brain.

These emotionally nourishing sensations engulfing my body, mind and spirit are jewels of psychosocial fulfilment we can experience, in spite of terrible suffering we might also be experiencing in other areas of life, all enlivened by neurochemistry, involving, for instance, the earlier cited dopamine, serotonin and oxytocin, as well as other neurochemicals. By this role, neurochemicals, as are their circuitries, are necessarily active or inactive in the eventuation of any given psychosomatic state. And, like our breath, they are endowed with incredible powers, versatility and abundance.

Consider, for instance, that the eighty billion neurons in the brain alone use two of the most versatile and abundant neurochemicals—gamma-amino-butyric acid (GABA) and glutamate—to achieve either of two outcomes, to inhibit or excite us. GABA, on the one hand, is the primary neurochemical present in our inhibitory states, such as hunger, depression, numbness and somnolence. And, glutamate, on the other hand, is the primary neurochemical present in our excitatory inner states, examples of which include the kindness, gratitude and love I have already mentioned, but there is also happiness, hopefulness, desire and others.

Just as with any emotion we can feel, these states are modulated in the synapses and bloodstreams. Neurochemicals classed as neurotransmitters, of which dopamine, serotonin, GABA and glutamate are examples, act in the synaptic cleft and differ in versatility from those classed as hormones, which travel around the body in the blood but are no less involved in the specific ways our mind, bod, and nervous system work. They are all, in a word, psychosomatic agents that inform how we are put together, present ourselves, think and behave. Earlier, I gave the examples of GABA and glutamate that inhibit or promote neural activities that reflect in our expression of emotions. The task of inducing these effects in the synaptic cleft where neurons interact and exchange signals for action is naturally quick and short lived, following a precise science. Tidiness is important for good communication. Hence, the tighter and more tidily kept the synaptic cleft, the more effective neuronal communication will be modulated by chemistry. The opposite is true where synapses are blocked or synaptic clefts are congested, spacy or both.

This science, at the heart of how we function as humans, extends to input from endocrine hormones that, in much the same way as neurotransmitters, act to modulate nervous system activities and, crucially, regulate essential bodily functions—ranging from procreation to stress response. Hormones are the output of endocrine glands, of which we have eight, namely, the hypothalamus, pineal, pituitary, thyroid, thymus, adrenals, pancreas, ovaries, and testes—from where they secrete into the bloodstream.

However, unlike neurotransmitters, the effects of hormones in the body are characteristically reactive and long lasting in carrying out a variety of tasks. My best example is cortisol, perhaps the body's most versatile hormone, which is crucial for our survival and, as such, is among my favourite neurochemicals, if I were to choose. It is produced by the adrenal glands from atop the kidneys, and it bears responsibility, among competencies, for regulating stress in the body and mind and modulating potential for injury with its anti-inflammatory properties.

The term *stress* is held to have been first used in this sense by the influential Hungarian endocrinologist Hans Selye, who defined it as 'the non-specific response of the body to demand for change' (1978). This is a fairly simplistic definition of stress that—short of nuance—betrays stress's complex and diverse presentations, both the good ones and the not so good ones. For instance, there is the virtuous hormetic stress we invoke when we are fasting or exercising to strengthen our body and mind and to build neural reserves, so stress can be essentially beneficial in that it promotes well-being (Kouda & Iki, 2010). There is the baseline level of stress we need to wake up in the morning, keep ourselves safe, build resilient capacities in our body and mind, and shield psychosomatic vulnerabilities that are associated with an ill-set baseline, one informed by abnormal levels of cortisol and consequent toxicity in the body. A chronically low level of cortisol, for instance, may lead to clinically disruptive hypocortisolaemia, or hypercortisolaemia in the case of a chronically high level.

Relative to baseline and virtuous stresses, there is the mundane jaws-clenching stress of ordinary life. Think of getting a toddler to tidy a toy box, being stuck in gridlock traffic or the acute stress of being hit, infected or injuring a limb. The cumulative burden of this stress is better known in the scholarly literature as allostatic load (Guidi et al., 2021). *Allostatic* from the Greek *állos* and *stasis*, means a varying stable burden, which speaks to the body's ability to adjust steady-state conditions based on input from environmental stressors.

And, ultimately, there is distress (Selye, 1974), which encompasses the traumatic stress of being alienated, battered, enslaved, invalidated, sexually violated, neglected, or harmfully stereotyped as well as persistent insecurities about food, health, money, housing or environmental disaster. Because of the universality of these ALEs, traumatic stress is a global health emergency we cannot afford to ignore. For my purpose, it is at the centre of neuropsychosocial disintegration, and as this chapters progress, there will be insights into its manifestation in the body and mind, especially in a state of chronicity when it functions to dysregulate native defence systems, impair neurons, stymie neuroplasticity and procure degeneration in circuitries that connect different parts of the nervous system. With this in mind, cortisol—as deeply as it is involved in the experience of life—is seen as holding properties that can be both good and bad in attending to its tasks. Which it does without prejudice, even whilst the different types of stress it modulates compete for urgency.

With reference to urgency, we might consider cortisol's role as a glucocorticoid through which it regulates glucose levels in the body. As cortisol level increases, the nervous system converts glucose into energy that the body can use in its functions. A chronically high bodily demand for energy, however, can translate to a chronically high level of cortisol and excess glucose in the bloodstream, more than we need or can use.

THE FUNCTIONING SELF IN A STATE OF PATHOLOGY

A chronically activated nervous system saturated in cortisol and glucose establishes among other vulnerabilities the prediabetic condition of hyperglycaemia, what my elders would refer to colloquially as 'sweet peepee' or 'the sugar' and attempt to remedy by restricting their intake of carbohydrates and other sugars.

Something they would say about diabetes is that it is like 'snuffing the sweetness out of life', which happens to be true in a literal sense for many patients whose treatment for the disease includes restriction of sugar intake. It is a precarious neurobiological state to which the endocrine system, and other defence systems, are alerted in order to counteract the threat to well-being. The word *precarious* is meant to emphasise that—in the absence of intervention—excess blood glucose begets severe adverse health events. At the level of the nervous system, there is the toxicity to neurons, which could lead to the debilitating disease of neuropathy and premature death. To mitigate this vulnerability, the pancreatic glands below the liver, in the body's cavity, are primed to release insulin to direct excess glucose into storage, storage being adipose tissues, from where this glucose could be later drawn for energy and metabolisation of stress. This is an incredibly intelligent system that is supplied with autonomic nerves—to operate autonomously—and the body should be able to handle its processes with little trouble. However, high levels of cortisol that increase bodily glucose and insulin levels can lead to chronic disturbances and maladies in the body and the mind.

Take insulin resistance, a condition in which adipose tissues—also known as fat cells—do not respond well to insulin, typically because the insulin receptacles on the cells are stretched out of shape and cannot easily bind to glucose molecules in the blood. The pancreas may then respond in one of two ways. By secreting more insulin to help glucose into the cells, which could lead to insulin buildup and hyperinsulinemia. Or by ceasing secretion of insulin upon receiving signals of an excess in the bloodstream. More insulin is not needed, in other words. This may be a virtuous intervention, until it leads to insulin deficiency, or hyperinsulinemia.

In either case, insulin dysregulation and its connection to abnormal cortisol and glucose levels in the blood will contribute to the development of dysautonomia, a fancy term for dysregulation in the autonomic nervous system that gives rise to a range of symptoms. For instance, chronically dysregulated sympathetic nerves could lead to complaints of intrusive thoughts about traumatic events at inapposite times, difficulty with sleep and restfulness, inexplicable tension in muscles, and difficulty focusing the mind on complex or abstract tasks. Chronically dysregulated parasympathetic nerves, in a similar vein, could lead to complaints of persistent tiredness, cravings, hopelessness, depression, worthlessness, shamefulness, difficulty with memory, and autoimmunity that is associated with neurodegeneration. I shall explore some of these symptoms in some depth throughout the chapters that follow. Here it suffices to appreciate that dysautonomia manifests in a range of discernible psychosomatic maladies.

At the somatic level, I have mentioned diabetes, but other common incidents such as chronic fatigue, hypertension and obesity that wreak havoc on the body over time we may not associate with the psyche but are indeed psychosomatic, as we shall learn. In the big brain alone, the consequences are especially catastrophic when toxic levels of cortisol that give rise to dysautonomia impair the cerebral structures involved in perception, learning and memory retention, thus increasing the risk for neuropsychiatric maladies (Echouffo-Tcheugui et al., 2018), such as Alzheimer's, schizophrenia and forms of dementia that are associated with the middle-age and geriatric years. This gets trickier in the psyche, especially with subclinical dis-ease. Hyphenated *dis-ease* in itself infers internal disturbance that ranges in intensity and expression.

My point, however, is that the neurochemistry of traumatic stress has a lasting impact on well-being, impairing psychosomatic defence systems such as survival instincts and memory. At a clinical level, dysregulation in survival neurochemistry and the attendant dysautonomia also have implications for psychosocial functioning. Consider cognitive impairment, a neural disturbance wherein survival neurochemicals suppress or restrict executive processes and systems in the brain. This may be brought on by trauma that prevents images, sounds and words from being processed and combined into semantic memory, that is, what things mean. This disturbance may also inhibit information from being sequenced and imprinted for recall in the hippocampus—the site of our working memory circuit—or may even corrupt patterns of experiences and behaviour that consolidate into habits, what we call emotional and procedural memories.

When these neural disturbances bereave executive input, the body is liable to deploy cortisol, not simply to procure inflammatory molecules to mitigate injury but also to increase the potential for somatic memories to be laid down. This is the body using its native intelligence to facilitate its survival even whilst cognitive and emotional functions are compromised. One could think of this intelligence as an anthropological legacy—an adaptive intelligence, a somatic intelligence, or both—and it is among the distinct human capacities the English psychologist Charles Spearman (2005) unveiled in his seminal work *The Abilities of Man*. These capacities, it is clear, orient toward safeguarding the life within the body, independently of cognitive input.

This adaptation, however, keeps the body in a defensive state, wherein, faced with stress and negative emotions, survival neurochemicals come to the rescue. Take embarrassment, isolation or imprisonment, which activate our stress response circuitry and incline us to fight or flee stressors. Adrenaline secreted to muscles in our arms is to serve us in a fight, noradrenaline to muscles in our legs is to serve us in fleeing, and cortisol that converts glucose into energy is to sustain us. It may also occur that our fight-or-flight impulse is inhibited, say when GABA inhibits our motor neurons, causing us to freeze in a state of unreactivity or immobility.

The American somatic psychologist Peter Levine (1997) describes this counterintuitive survival response as an ancient reaction to imminent danger, originating in neural substructures in the instinctive brainstem, where pain modulation begins with opioid-like endocrines—namely, endorphins, enkephalins and dynorphins. The literature tells us too that neuronal signals for these endogenous opioids come from the prosocial periaqueductal grey (see figure 3.3), and, in addition to analgesia, they hold euphoric properties, which helps to explain why some people 'enjoy' pain. But in a chronic state, this cannot be good, for, as I mentioned earlier, the effects of endocrines in the body and mind are typically long lasting and disposed to invoke bodily and mental states that are hostile to our native and resilience SPEARS, the neurochemistry that promotes these needs, and the protective self.

THE PROTECTIVE SELF NEURODYNAMICS AND INTELLIGENCE SPEARS

The protective self keeps us safe in the face of adversity, although fending off adversity is not its favourite job. In fact, the protective self relies on information and resources from other parts of the whole self to fulfil its role. As such, it inclines naturally towards prosocial behaviours that are nourishing and resourcing, more so than adversities that deplete it, taking its cues from the more ancient neuron (see figure 3.2), whose natural state is one of flexibility, constant change and adaptability as it processes input from internal and external environments.

Recall that environmental input is processed in neural networks within which individual neurons behave in much the same way as individual people do, in terms of connections in families, communities and the wider society that confer resources and promote capacity to weather adversity and to grow. Without these resilient connections, we are disposed to feel bereft of resourcefulness and purpose, a state of being we became acquainted with in chapter 2 in meeting Alex, who felt cut off from his family during the COVID-19 pandemic and found himself in the depth of despair. A place wherein, starved of connection, life bears a certain purposelessness that kills the self figuratively or inclines one to die literally. It is in this similar way that, without connections, neurons are starved of purpose, perceive themselves as unuseful and die in a process called apoptosis. Conversely, the better their connections with other neurons in a diversity of circuitries, the more flexible, adaptive and growth inclined they are.

This is the spirit of neurodynamics, the natural state of flexibility, adaptability and growth that characterises neural systems, making each one resilient in its own right. In particular, the complex neurochemistry that rewards sensations of fulfilment, which are germane to a fulfilling life, allows us to appreciate this more fully. Earlier, I talked about serotonin, dopamine and oxytocin, three of our better known prosocial neurochemicals. Serotonin is vital for restfulness, sociality and emotional stability; dopamine is vital for motivation, memory and pleasure; and oxytocin is vital for emotional attunement and relationships that are nourishing and rewarding, even if superficially. Hence, the neuronal syntheses of these chemicals are crucial as the social-emotional self develops—debuting in early life to incubate deep memories, socialisation and attachments, and to regulate expressions of biologically programmed behaviours that are not the result of socialisation—the

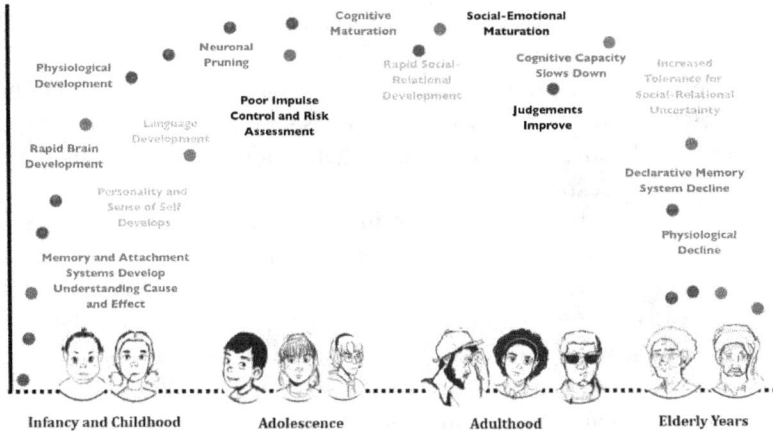

Figure 4.2. Natural Competencies and Instincts throughout the Life Cycle. From infancy to old age, the life cycle encompasses eight psychosocial developmental stages throughout which natural competencies and instincts emerge for validation and fulfilment. The idea is that individuals go through a sequence of developmental stages within the contexts of family, community and society, and every stage not only relies on previous stages but also prepares for the next stage. At each stage, conflicts emerge and mark significant milestones in psychosocial development. *Art courtesy of Jesse James.*

brute instincts we share with ancient reptiles, for instance. For us, in the early stage of our development, our social-emotional self, guided by native intelligence, carries out this task with crude physicality, getting better in time as it submits to virtues and ideals the cerebral-cognitive self promotes. Thus, this course begins with instincts and develops throughout the life cycle.

My experience working with young children in preschools, adolescents in secondary schools, college students, middle-age professionals and senior citizens in residential homes acquainted me with these instincts across the life cycle. In the three-year-old child, for instance, who bites and strikes playmates but delights in play and sharing toys at age five, as she completes the third stage of her psychosocial development, through which she discovers her capacity for initiative, enterprise and guilt and learns to assert control over her impulses and environment. This capacity, however, will continue to mature as her social-emotional self develops and promotes the need for intimacy that can be achieved with friendliness and in friendships, and the capacity to regulate emotions in service of that need. The adolescent child's ability to relate is now mediated by more mature memory systems, the ability to understand cause and effect, and the use of complex language and social cues.

This represents the cerebral-cognitive, the ultimate part of the protective self to mature and establish its connections in neural networks until around age twenty-five. Among its tasks, the cerebral-cognitive promotes socialisation and prosocial behaviour in service of achievement and well-being, in spite of the ever-present risks of trauma and disintegration. The impulse to achieve, which asserts itself at the fourth stage of our psychosocial development, is especially active in this part of the protective self, motivating the pursuit of external accomplishments—say in family, community or industry—that we can reflect upon with pride. As such, it fosters a sense of well-being, particularly in the senior years when pride in achievement buffers against feelings of despair.

I have defined well-being as a state in which our native needs for secure psycho-emotional attunement and relational safety are promoted by resilient somatic harmony, psychological integrity, emotional attunement, relational fulfilment and self-authenticity. These are two metaphorical SPEARS our neurobiology appears to select for by chemically rewarding prosocial behaviours that promote the relationships within which we develop them. The integration of the cerebral-cognitive into the whole self serves this developmental need and is therefore an imperative upon which the protective self depends to be guided in its tasks. In carrying out its tasks, however, the protective self relies on somatic, psychological, emotional, adaptive, reflective and social intelligences, the initials of which also spell SPEARS. Accordingly, we might consider these intelligences as a set of SPEARS with which we are equipped for the task of life.

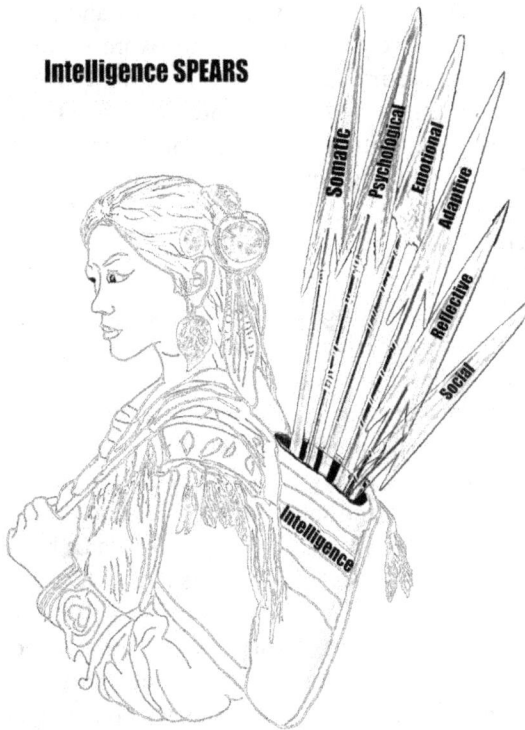

Figure 4.3. Intelligence Embodied—SPEARS. *Figure courtesy of Dagmar Roelfsema.*

- *Somatic intelligence*, much of which derives from our genetics-loaded cells, is the key to unlocking the wisdom of our body and ancestral memory, the complete set of instincts and response patterns that are responsible for our ancestors' survival and which they passed on to us. To support our body's remarkable capacity to survive adversity, heal itself and achieve somatic harmony by drawing upon its resources to promote integrity, restore stability in the nervous system and prepare the protective self for learning, growth and resilience. Somatic intelligence, thus, ensures we are sensing, protective bodies, and, importantly, our protective self has agency over inner workings that move us to inflict pain upon bodies, including our own and those of our loved ones. As the American scholar Antonio Damasio put it, 'we are feeling machines that think' (2021), ascribing priority to the body in the system that generates survival behaviour over the cerebral structures that centre the mind. This is a priority we begin to exhibit from around the fifth month in gestation, when we can use our developing body to express sensations, such as contentment and distress (Verny & Kelly, 1982). By the time we are born, we will have fully developed capacities to suckle, startle, cry, grasp, fence with our limbs and step with support—all of which are ways we use our body to express our needs. By these capacities alone, somatic intelligence is primal, and in promoting somatic harmony, one of its salient features is interoception. From the Latin root words *inter* and *capere*, 'within' and 'get', interoceptions are messages our protective self gets from within our body and can use to keep us safe as well as to reestablish somatic integrity when such is lost. This is the wisdom of the body, the knowledge and capacities it possesses that can be parlayed in service of well-being.

- *Psychological intelligence* necessarily promotes psychological integrity in the protective self. The American Psychological Association (2018) defines this intelligence as the human capacity to derive information, learn from experience, think, reason and correctly utilise the mind to regulate the body, guide behaviour and predict consequences of actions and inactions. Psychological intelligence thus governs flexibility in mental processes that curves towards integration and safety in the body and mind, even if not necessarily away from injury. This basic law, which dates back to Spearman's insight in *The Ability of Man* (2005), impels the protective self to establish safe conditions for survival with the tools of the mind—our thoughts and logics, for instance. For it is by doing this that we are encouraged to stay mindful of hypocrisies that undermine true safety, particularly in the families and communities that form the societies we create. And also undertake to honour our agency over the inner workings that move us to violate bodies and minds, which is arguably what sets us apart among emotionally intelligent sentients.

- The *emotional intelligence* that underpins emotional attunement speaks to the human capacity to turn both inwards into the self and outwards into other sentient selves with empathic flexibility that promotes growth and safety. Throughout this book, I have explored different expressions of this capacity, as they are important for understanding neuropsychosocial disintegration and integration. Ultimately, the sense is that emotions drive us. The word *emotion* itself, translated from the Latin verb *motere*, suggests 'a tendency to act is implicit in every emotion' (Goleman, 1996, p. 6). For our protective self, this intelligent tendency encompasses the capacity to cultivate and regulate inner states that move us to act in the service of our survival, foremost, and then well-being as a more evolved motivation. This is central to anchoring our nervous system in a state of receptivity and openness, as opposed to one of rigidity and reactivity that betrays the imperative in our body and mind to adapt in the service of life.

- *Adaptive intelligence* consolidates somatic, psychological and emotional intelligences in our biological and behavioural adaptability as we interact with our environment. For our protective self, this is the capacity to 'learn from the environment' and 'reason about the environment' in order to 'make sense' of the demands environmental changes impose upon us and adapt to those changes with biological wisdom and creative and practical behaviours (Sternberg, 2021). Biological wisdom features in instincts, sensations, vivid mental images and dreams that use ancestral memory patterns, rather than logical thoughts, to inform reactions and responses to life events. As such, in undertaking its important tasks, the protective self benefits from ancestry in adjusting the body and mind to survive in the environment, changing the environment to accommodate the body and mind, and discovering or constructing new environments if needed, driven, presumably, by instincts to self-preserve in the face of adversity that potentiate our extinction, whether that of our entire species, our gene pool or our individual self. Instincts are sensitive to biological as well as sociocultural factors. So these include not only how tall we grow, the amount of melanin our skin contains and the shape of our eyes, but also how the foods we eat, clothes we wear, intonations in our voice and ways we relate shape or select our environments. Perceptibly, this flies in the face of human activity that insults the natural environment our existence depends upon. Consider, for instance, how we exploit our planet in ways that exacerbate global climate change, the effects of which are resulting in deaths through extraordinary environmental events, such as rising heat and increased hurricanes, snowstorms and typhoons. Adaptive intelligence enables us to upregulate our capacity to survive such hostile life events whilst promoting behaviours that create more habitable conditions for future generations. The obverse would be the definition of maladaptive.

• *Reflective intelligence* speaks to our capacity to cultivate wisdom from our historical experiences and congruous discoveries in order to deepen our knowing of our self and project into the future with confidence (Perkins, 1996). It is through this capacity that we derive hindsight and insight we can use to self-monitor and cultivate valid foresight about how our life story unfolds, a role the protective self undertakes to ensure we are perceiving clearly, choosing wisely and acting with moral judgment in the service of our growth and resilience (Graham, 2018). For it is this intelligence that underpins our capacity for self-awareness and authenticity. Self-awareness, like authenticity, invites us to consider not only what we are experiencing, say poverty, isolation or inutility, but also how we are experiencing in our body and mind, say in our head as an ache and confusion, in our chest cavity as a constriction and broken heartedness, in our gut as a wrench and collapse of intuition or in our legs as an impulse to escape and be far away from a perceived stressor. This kind of reflection brings context to our experience of life events, which is important for integration in our body and mind.

- *Social intelligence* speaks to our capacity to cultivate interpersonal relationships that shape our life experiences and outcomes in ways that fulfil
our need for relational satisfaction. It is what enables our protective self to
foster nourishing connections in our social orbit by accurately 'reading'
social cues and acting accordingly (Goleman, 2007). By this intelligence,
our protective self is disposed to engage with our social environment in
ways that promote our well-being and reflect our relational successes,
more so than our failures, say, in friendships, romantic opportunities and
family life. For, in cultivating social intelligence, our protective self is
equipped to open us up to discover and experience the nourishing power
of psychosocial resources—such as cooperation, altruism and compassion—within the context of safe relationships. Social relationships within
which we learn to function as prosocial organisms to protect ourselves
against social dis-ease and gain capital that serves us in times of need,
which is always.

METAPHORICAL SPEARS FOR
NEUROPSYCHOSOCIAL ACROBATICS

Tied all together, our native intelligences constitute a third set of metaphorical SPEARS with which we can move through life and promote our integration and well-being, the essential needs with which the protective self is
concerned. As such, it is safe to say that the protective self relies on these
native intelligences insofar as they promote our essential needs, including our
need to protect the relationships within which our needs are fulfilled and to
honour the social rules that govern these relationships, such as those set by
families and faiths. This cannot be a simple task, for it involves reconciling
demands of our crude instinct with those of cultured norms, mainly in institu-
tions of socialisation, such as in the family, schools and religion. This makes
better sense when one considers that a SPEARS-less and unregulated social-
emotional self can produce malady in the host as well as in others when it
expresses itself, for instance, in roguish personalities and chaotic relationships that are inimical to well-being. Consider a roguish social-emotional self
embodying selfish traits that render the host unlikeable, or conceitedness in a
roguish cerebral-cognitive self that renders the host intolerable. At the level
of the individual, these traits are the kind that might have landed our ancestors
in social isolation and imminent danger. Being unlikeable and intolerable are
socially unappealing and incompatible with our native needs for emotional
attunement and relational satisfaction, which is to say that our natural state
is one that resists neural dysregulation, binds chaotic energy and anchors in
homeostasis.

Given that unsatisfied needs effect distress in the body and mind, in response to which the social-emotional self is liable to engage adaptive defences, it is helpful to explore this process—even if only to get a sense of how adaptive defences serve us. I shall begin this task with the idea of identifying and metaphorically tai chi–ing sensations across the nervous system in what amounts to neuro-acrobatics. The art of tai chi is an apt metaphor that speaks to engaging the body and mind gently and naturally with movements that are soft, spiralling and continuous, as opposed to those of more offensive arts, such as karate and tae kwon do, where movements are hard, fast and focused on dominating or defeating a threat.

The goal in neuro-acrobatics, as in tai chi, is to use metaphorical SPEARS to protect the whole self—containing soma and psyche—from injury. In response to ALEs, this may involve organising defences at levels of consciousness that are distinct but connected, generating cognition and action that favour immediate safety, and consigning distractions, including disruptive memories and painful sensations, to the unconscious until they can be safely surfaced and discharged of their unbounded energy. Throughout the chapters, I use the terms *cerebral-cortical conscious*, *subcortical subconscious* and *instinctive unconscious* to infer these distinct levels of neural processing, terms I drew from the scholarly literature to support my organisation of experiences and adaptive defences at distinct levels of security in the nervous system, much like data in a secure volt. In a concrete sense, experiences and defences that are readily available—such as thoughts and feelings—are organised at a cerebral-cortical conscious level. Experiences and defences that can be retrieved with effort, say by connecting life stories, are at a subcortical subconscious level. The instinctive unconscious retains all that dwells in our soma and psyche but of which we may be unaware. This includes the bulk of eleven million bits of experiences and memories careering towards our nervous system every given second for processing (Wilson, 2002).

An observation that is both convenient and interesting is that these distinct levels of consciousness correspond with the brain structures discussed in chapter 3. That is, the conscious is housed in the cerebral cortex, which is the most recently evolved part of the brain and is responsible for higher executive functions, like reasoning and complex problem-solving. In neuropsychology, as in information theory, the capacity of consciousness—which is not particularly extensive if measured in bits, the unit of measurement for information—is better understood than the origin of consciousness in itself. This tells us our precortical ancestors survived with little consciousness or cognitive information and relied much more on their subconsciousness.

The subconscious—occurring below the level of the conscious—begins with the limbic midbrain, which hosts emotional regulations and stress response signals among its tasks. This includes feelings, preferences and impulses surrounding life events we may not have ourselves experienced but of which we hold emotional memories, perhaps acquired vicariously or inherited ancestrally. It is not uncommon to find that the exercise of collecting and connecting our life stories surfaces these events—at times spontaneously—to allow meaning making and reflection to occur.

Lastly, in the lower subconscious, in the remoteness of the self, the relatively vast unconscious exists. Some of its activities are aptly mediated by neural substructures in the brainstem, which connects superior substructures and activities to the rest of the body and regulates autonomic processes at the level of the unconscious. These include instincts and memories that inform adaptive defences, even when neural activities in the conscious and upper subconscious are suppressed, albeit with consequences, notably that of disintegration, a mind-body state wherein native intelligences are whelmed by traumatic wounds that lead people to act against their authentic selves, environment and well-being, which I shall explore next.

Chapter 5

Neuropsychosocial (Dis)Integration

Featuring Psychosocial Trauma

The previous chapters sensitised us to the nervous system in its role shaping the selves with which we show up to the task of life and the idea that trauma wounds the protective self and inhibit its native intelligences. In this chapter we are encouraged to think of this wounding as a measure of neuropsychosocial disintegration that affects survivors somatically, emotionally, psychologically and relationally, and which they cannot resolve on their own. It is a psychosomatic state to which they will adapt as the nervous system undertakes to retain its eminence in directing their experiences and defences in service of their survival. This adaptability, Thomas Hübl (2020) humbly leads us to recognise, sustains the nervous system as the caretaker of our humanness. Organising from the brain and spine, it is like a vast library that keeps a record of the whole of our history and adaptations, including every tradition our ancestors crafted and every developmental adjustment we have made to get us to where we are—undertaking this task with automaticity that does not prejudice disintegration.

AUTOMATICITY IN
NEUROPSYCHOSOCIAL DISINTEGRATION

When neuroscientists talk about automaticity in the nervous system, we are referring to the activities of sympathetic and parasympathetic nerves in specific neural networks dubbed the autonomic nervous system, a familiar term from previous chapters. It is also important to note that the activities of these nerves are centred in our human experience of safety and danger, and they are organised in the same way in all of us, although behaving uniquely in every one of us in honour of our unique lived and inherited experiences. In

59

this role, the autonomic nervous system is a faithful keeper of our life stories. However, its vulnerability to dysregulation means that stories it keeps are vulnerable to fragmentation and even corruption.

Consider, for instance, that trauma in our nervous system prevents information from consolidating into accurate declarative memories and distorts our life story. This is ordinarily true under conditions that overwhelm the sympathetic nerves' capacity to process traumatic stress intelligently and safely. Think of chronic poverty, social isolation and environmental disasters that threaten ordinary life and the adaptive defences necessarily intervening to promote survival, like a circuit breaker, instantiating distractions and provisionally anaesthetising the pains of injury and loss—whether emotional, physical or psychological. In the immediate scene, this intervention may involve fragmenting and dampening painful sensations in order to preserve life. But these sensations are liable to resurface in the self as a record of ALEs. I am interested in neuropsychosocial manifestations, so this begins with a trauma in the neural fibres of the brain, spine or prosocial viscera—such as the heart, kidneys and gut. More on this in part III.

To return to memory management, this tells us the nervous system has at its disposal the capacity to fragment and isolate troublesome memories it cannot process or that are unsafe in our consciousness. Hence, the autonomic nerves relegate these troublesome memories to our subconsciousness first for safekeeping, but also to prevent easy access and free flow into consciousness, irrespective of the disturbance these memories may cause in this abeyance. A neural structure called the ventromedial prefrontal cortex (VMPFC) enlists in this task to ensure the nervous system does not register for easy recall sensory cues from the body that are based on adverse lived experiences. This is the area of the brain behind the upper forehead that helps us to make meaning out of sensations and store associations between experience and neurobiological states. By this neurobiological adaptation, survivors of adversity whose lives are besieged by trauma may fail to acknowledge the attendant wounding and bodily disturbance. In addition to the inability to easily access this kind of memory or put language to maladies in their psyche and soma, these survivors' capacity to recall traumatic events may also be compromised by adaptive psychosocial defences that procure a sense of safety, even if only superficially.

Much like the neurobiological, adaptive defences that are psychosocial organise and express themselves physiologically, psychologically and emotionally. In enduring beyond their originating events, these defences are liable to jack the psyche in a state of rigidity and regression, a state wherein the psyche is disposed to avert occasions to move beyond suffering, towards new developmental and in service of resilient growth (Jung, 1992), and inclines towards ALEs in the survivor's past life that feature in maladies that are precise expressions of neuropsychosocial disintegration: a disturbance in the nervous system that cleaves or corrupts body-mind-social synchroneity and undermines the psychosocial impulse to flourish because it distorts social reality and impels the psyche to adapt to the distorted reality. This promotes psychic and somatic maladies by which the survivors' life will be disturbed and from which relief will be sought.

DISINTEGRATION IN THE PSYCHE AND SOMA

Neuropsychosocial disintegration, as defined, leads to psychosomatic maladies. A disturbance in the psyche is liable to cause disturbance and potentially severe disease in the body. The somato-psychologic is equally viable in suggesting that a disturbance or severe disease in the body is liable to cause psychic disturbance and severe psychiatric disease. It is the task of neuropsychology and psychiatry to explore any such event with rigorous research, a task we are equipped to approach with insight into the socioemotional features of neuropsychosocial disintegration, specifically the submission that the nervous system—in its expression of the social and emotional—is not functioning optimally, as nature intends, to keep its host organism safe and well. Therein lies the question of nature's intention and the inference that it is not neuropsychosocial disintegration.

To address this question is to interrogate the neural structures, networks and chemistry involved in promoting nature's intention. At this stage, I think of this as a state of inner peace that characterises neuropsychosocial integration, wherein the organism is anchored in somatic safety, psychological integrity, emotional attunement, relational satisfaction and self-authenticity. You might recognise this as our resilience SPEARS. From a neurobiology point of view, this involves neurosynchroneity and, specifically, the bidirectional flow of information across the cerebral continents in the upper brain, the socioemotional midbrain, the survival instincts and circuits in the brainstem, the spinal chain and peripheral nerves that extend throughout the body.

The nervous system is also bilateral, and the brain, in particular, divides into a left and right hemisphere. In integration, the left hemisphere—associated with logics, reason and thoughts—is in synch with the right hemisphere, which is associated with imagination, creativity and the ability to understand life events without having the facts to understand them—what we call intuition. Think of this as a horizontal axis intersecting a vertical axis along which neural structures are vulnerable to traumas that give rise to autonomic dysregulation that undermines resilience SPEARS.

Naturally, traumatic wounds vary in manifestations in the psyche and soma, including across generations, and as the chapters progress, this will become more evident. In the psyche, for instance, it is not uncommon to find a disturbed sense that one should not exist as one is naturally, or that reality is distorted and experienced like fantasy. In somatoform, disturbance in the body could be experienced as dreadful sensations that trigger native and adaptive defences in response to the slightest pain. This ordinarily begins in the socioemotional midbrain with activation of the stress response hypothalamic-pituitary-adrenal axis (HPAA) and corresponding cascade of survival neurochemicals, that is, corticosteroids, that act to numb disabling pains and protect bodily tissues. However, when this task cannot be managed, it drops down the multilevel neural system, to the brainstem, to the instinctive brain, and into the body. In part IV, we shall learn that cranial nerves are enlisted in this stress management system too.

At this stage, before we can appreciate what might be going on in the body and mind, we will have met with the behavioural features of a chronic autonomic disturbance in the form of the often injurious behaviours and relationships survivors engage in—subconsciously in a drift towards a trauma echo, seemingly seeking a familiar pain and compensating for ungrieved loss. One could argue that the survivor's ability to perceive injurious behaviours and relationships correctly is inhibited by neuropsychosocial disintegration. Similarly, a drift towards a familiar traumatic pain is an expression of a psyche that is stuck in a loop—reacting to traumatic memories that are relegated to the subconscious and, whilst outside of the survivor's awareness, still causing inner disturbance. Hence, in the absence of this awareness, the survivor is not inclined to self-preserve by making behavioural and psychological adjustments to eventuate a more mindful and fulfilling life.

We've learned it could also be that the disturbance in the survivor's mind, body or both is not being perceived. Informally known as psychosocial anosognosia, this malady involves the survivor being unaware of their psychosocial deficit or neuropsychosocial disintegration. In the previous chapters, we learned this could be true for inner disturbances that are subclinical and do not radically impair survivors' capacity to self-preserve. Also, such disturbances range in intensity and expression and are subjected to nuance within the bounds of neuropsychosocial disintegration, so much so that they may not feature as maladies, especially where entangled with a personality trait or proxy self that works to protect a vulnerable authentic self.

In reflecting on vulnerability, there is a strong sense that the role of a proxy self is indispensable to survival under conditions of adversity. This sense that finds resonance in the Caribbean psychoanalyst Lennox Thomas's (2008) reasoning that we are disposed to offer up a defensive proxy when we subconsciously find it hard to relate to our authentic self and in order to feel accepted in our relationships. In this adaptation, the 'proxy' is a false self we develop—from birth—to help us communicate with others and cope in relationships that threaten our sense of safety—in other words, to protect our true self from insults, which is important for our survival.

This false self, however, stokes inner chaos when our body and mind meet society, suppressing the natural drive to express strengths, weaknesses and yearnings, and conflicting with the legitimate sense that we are not invited to express our true self or belong to a collective of vulnerable selves that is bigger than us, such as a faith, family, tribe or the wider world in which we can stand on our own when we need to but also be celebrated and experience being loved and cherished. It may appear when we feel alone—excluded, rejected and ensnared in a triangle of shame, grief and guilt. I find these extremes to be a helpful way to think about a socioemotional compass that ticks away from the positive and towards the negative as it guides disintegration in a dynamic that I shall explore next.

SOCIOEMOTIONALITY IN NEUROPSYCHOSOCIAL DISINTEGRATION

In acknowledging the salience of the socioemotional in neuropsychosocial disintegration, I am compelled to reflect on the triangle of 'shame, grief and guilt' that, incidentally, shows up as a hallmark feature in the narratives of suffering I share in this book, beginning with shame, conveniently, which is ordinarily experienced as a powerful sensation that impels us to change or hide the parts of us that are uninvited and unsupported in our social orbit (Plutchik, 1991). When this is our whole self, as for members of groups that are harmfully stereotyped, the lived experience according to the American social psychologist Claude Steele's insight on *Stereotype Threat* is one of social marginalisation that gives rise to terrible suffering.

Take the exposure to harmful stereotypes, such as 'blacks are capricious' (von Linné, 2018), 'women are inferior' (Fee, 1979) or 'Jews are neurotic' (Stein, 2021), that could inform and reinforce the sense that a survivor's natural self in the social world is defective and undesirable (Steele, 2011). As a result, survivors are liable to endure social scorn for assertiveness, exclusion for cautiousness and contempt for conscientiousness, all instruments of shame coupled with 'normal' and desirable virtues survivors may attempt to hide by, for instance, overextending themselves, bleaching their skin or self-sacrificing. The bigger implication of this hiding, however, is that it features a bid for social acceptance and inclusion, and expresses that shame is not an emotion survivors want those close and dear to know they are gripped by. Much like that of grief and guilt with which it co-occurs, shame shares a high incidence of erosion in and between the psyche and soma that characterises neuropsychosocial disintegration.

This was particularly poignant in the life of the black Caribbean respondents to my ALEs survey, who had a 60 percent chance of living with unresolved grief from having experienced a lasting loss of a parent to adoption, abandonment, death, disease, divorce or other reason before the age of sixteen. We experience this grief as a sensation of intense and chronic suffering, which is amplified by other losses, such as the loss of parts of our self, our vulnerability or authenticity, as well as our unmet relational needs that incline us to think and act in ways that reflect socioemotional deprivation.

In adulthood, we will have adopted defences to protect ourselves from this suffering, but it can be readily observed in young children responding with negative self-talk, anxiety, sadness and even shock when their attachment needs are unfulfilled or they are in other ways hurt by a loved one. This suggests that grief is innate and an important expression of the socioemotional self. For in the grips of grief, it is our socioemotional self that moves to abuse and even destroy the source of our pain, and this could be our own mind and body. In our mind resides oppressive thoughts, such as that of not being worthy of love, protection and respect, and this moves us to resolve this conflict through disordered eating, cutting and other forms of self-sabotage. At the social group level, say in the family or community, this can manifest in destructive envy and random acts of violence against other bodies, which are liable to promote shame and guilt that prevail and even take over consciousness.

Guilt, perhaps the most conflictual of emotions, stokes the sense that we are not deserving of life's gifts and virtues that mark us out as different and which might offend others' sense of inadequacy (Piers & Singer, 2015). This runs the gamut from the physical beauty that decays with time to the authenticity, intelligence and wisdom we acquire in time. Hence, to fall in line with others' expectations and norms, however pernicious, we work to avoid being too anything—too pretty, too intelligent, too confident. We may even overcompensate for our mistakes, deny our misgivings, react excessively to criticism and teasing or accept fault for wrongs and miseries that have nothing to do with us. The chronicity of these irrational whims, fuelled by incipient guilt, typically betray mindfulness.

For guilt deriving from the subconscious is susceptible to denial in the face of exposure. By this susceptibility, guilt, much like shame and grief, works to hide itself, and this was evident among participants in my research, who tended to experience this triune as an antithesis of pride, pride being a deep sense of satisfaction that high self-esteem confers. This can be esteem derived from our own achievement, the achievement of others with whom we are related or esteem derived from possessions that are aspirational, including indomitable ones like self-respect and self-preservation.

This kind of pride is fuelled by a nourishing energy that is protective against the chaotic energies of shame, grief and guilt and attendant maladaptive defences, such as self-abandonment and appropriation of a false self, which we are acquainted with from narratives in previous chapters. These are anthropologically evolved reactions to dangers that are informed by native intelligences but are, nonetheless, vulnerable to pathologies associated with emotions going awry. A helpful example is the inability to provide materially in family life, which is both shamed and criminalised in our society. As one of my research participants put it, 'a man who must be forced by the court', for instance, 'to provide for his children is telling the world he is worthless, and that is not a good thing to be telling the world'. For at the level of the emotional, this life event begets inner disturbance, possibly depression and anxiety that are associated with chronic inflammatory response. This is a shaming inner voice that tells a socialised man that his good citizenship and perhaps worthiness of membership in his family is contingent on his ability to provide something of material or socioeconomic value, such as money, a house or an animal that honours the spirits of enterprise, generosity and provision. Hence, the man who actively works or quietly yearns to provide for his family but finds that his ability to do so is compromised will adjust what he expresses in the world.

I must acknowledge here that the reasons for which a man might find himself in such a dilemma may be endless. However, I am interested in neuropsychosocial events, and a helpful example is a psychosocial legacy that creates this dilemma. More specifically, a history of inadequate provision from adult men in family life that corresponds with the psychic resignation that 'society provides for its children' and that families must not only submit to the mercies of society but also rely on its charity. In reflecting on my work surrounding the psychosocial, I recognise that my sense of this resignation as a shame-deflecting mechanism was first validated by a family friend from Curaçao, whom I shall call Siegfried.

Siegfried was to my father a 'super-cooperator', a descriptor Martin Nowak (2012) used for personalities that 'snuggle' the 'top brass' of a social group in order to survive. Siegfried was a man of little formal education and socioeconomic means. However, in snuggling up to my father, much like a dependant child, his urgent biological need for food, warmth and getting his genes into the next generation was being adequately fulfilled. He was nonetheless troubled in himself.

This I had grasped from his animated defence—with flailing hands, restless legs and admonishing tone—of a certain shamefulness in 'a man's inability to provide for his family', whilst denying in himself any disturbance from his failure to provide for his own four children. Having children, it was clear, was very important to him, more so, it appeared, than the ability to provide children with necessities. Thus, he perceived the reality of childlessness as a greater suffering than the inability to provide adequately for one's family. His defensive posturing, against his expressed denial of shame, seemed to agree. Noticing in vivo his body and mind in this active conflict culminated in an aha moment for me. In recognising the contradiction, I also perceived a proxy self acting to placate an apparent falsity in his psychic resignation that 'society provides for its children'.

This resignation seemed to anaesthetise the suffering that is associated with shame, grief and guilt, especially with its echo of the holy lore that 'God provides' for his children (Philippians 4:19, KJV), which functions to dull the pangs of poverty and, for Siegfried, the pang of not showing up fully for his children in a way being a competent and generous provider assumes. As that pang quietened, it can be said to have descended into his subconsciousness, where, bereft of emotional charge, it kept him safe from the inner chaos that leads to self-abandonment, self-loathing and self-destruction.

In this state of peritraumatic dissociation, in which one could experience disconnection from psychic and somatic pain, Siegfried was ostensibly detached from his own suffering as well as his children's suffering from being inadequately provided for. In this dysautonomic state, one might assume, his proxy self and instinctive unconscious acted to protect his psyche.

Given the psyche's vulnerability to pathologies against which proxy selves guard, this adaptive defence may be necessarily informed by a native intelligence. To appreciate its utility, I must circle back to the self that is driven by survival needs with little regard for consequence, where the infant child is without a perception of self, self-image or an ideal self. Taken together, these acquisitions constitute a self-concept, one to be nurtured in relationship, beginning with the earliest of relationships in family life. In psychoanalysis, as in the second stage of psychosocial development, this developmental stage is safe to regress to in the face of shame and any other oppressive emotion that can evoke in us the sense that we are incompetent or deeply flawed as we are naturally. For it is at this stage we begin to value having at our disposal a competent caregiver to help us fulfil our survival needs. Since this is also the developmental stage at which the nervous system cannot yet safely process oppressive emotions—shame, grief, guilt, despair and so on—the regressor benefits from not being encouraged to draw upon resilience and intelligence SPEARS and psychosocial reserve to navigate adverse life events.

This concept of regression speaks to temporal flexibility in the psyche, to its ability to travel in time and to anchor in earlier stages of development, which is organic and at times appropriate for survival in childhood, when the child is small, mentally immature and has yet to develop capacities to process complex and intense sensations. However, in adulthood, when the concept of self is active, regression betrays norms of autonomy and competence to procure a stable sense of dominion over a world that may not be safe as it is and agency over a self that is not safe as it presents naturally or unnaturally.

Again, much like with showing up in unsafe relationships with inauthenticity and proxy selves, the survivor may be driven to repress unpleasant sensations in order to feel safe or to experience some inner peace, even if only momentarily. This is first a psychic adaptation. But this repression does manifest in adaptive defensive selves too. We were acquainted with dissociation in the self earlier in this chapter, self-abandonment in chapter 2 and self-sacrifice in chapter 3. There is also the abdication of self-worth that can play out in morbid ideation, such as a rogue sense that one is unworthy of love, kindness and peace, which corresponds with perceptions of the self as defective, cursed and unworthy of preservation.

This kind of morbid ideation and its unpleasant sensations are debris of disintegration in the nervous system. We could think of this debris as wounds and lingering pains in the body and mind, sustained by the same chaotic energy that, according to Holmes (2020), fuels adaptive defences to reduce tension between stress and reaction to stress. I have cited chronic activation of the native stress-response axis and dysregulated vigilance as reliable expressions of this energy. But it features behaviourally too. For instance, in the survivor who drinks to a stupor or works into a deadening fatigue to dampen sensations of helplessness. The implication here is that this could be interpreted as a way of self-medicating and preserving oneself. However, crucially, it reflects destructiveness and a battle between an ideal and an inauthentic self.

In this battle, the inauthentic self is satisfied in control and not demanding change, whilst the ideal self wants things to be different and is demanding change. This can be understood, otherwise, as a psychosomatogenic conflict that does not promote well-being, gives rise to inner disturbance that stokes survivors' native and adaptive defences, and requires a free-flowing chaotic energy to express itself, much like would a random emotional, psychological or physical conflict that signals distress and feeds on unbounded energy in the body and mind. The lived experiences of Alex, Amjeet and Siegfried I have drawn upon so far suggest that deployment of adaptive defences under such conditions will not necessarily bring peace or the height which the survivor can get to if awareness and resolve are brought to the inner conflict. And, more insidiously, in the absence of therapeutic intervention, adaptive defences can easily morph into maladaptive, become normalised and masquerade as traditions ancestors pass on to posterity, including traditions that help future generations to survive adversity but are nonetheless traumatic.

PSYCHOSOCIAL TRAUMA IN HIGH DEFINITION

Consider survival in a world in which free family life as we know it is prohibited. Women are callously impregnated by farmers and human traders, and the children they bear are not to be cherished and nurtured into socially secure, psycho-emotionally attuned and relationally fulfilled personalities, but are instead destined to be sold as objects to be exploited in perpetual servitude.

This is an imagery I often invite in my teachings on ancestral trauma, for it is my ancestral legacy and one to which I am particularly sensitised and inclined to protect. My emphasis always is that the vulnerable child cannot depend on its mother for safety, wives cannot depend on husbands for protection from violence—sexual and otherwise—and men cannot depend on a tribe for rescue. In this damned world, one imagines, families that are successful in normalising social insecurity, psycho-emotional privation and relational alienation will also be successful in keeping their children alive and contributing to the next generation. And from this success will emerge a common sense of how to survive in the world, even though couching within this common sense are limited and limiting considerations for long-term well-being. The father of analytical psychology, Carl Jung (1875–1961), used the term *collective consciousness* to emphasise the universal reach of this common sense, particularly in its power to inform norms.

The specific norms that pertain to the psychosocial speak to socially acceptable and unacceptable behaviours. As such, these norms govern expression of the psychosocial—implicitly and explicitly—and inform us of what is appropriate and inappropriate based on sanctions within social contracts, what society will or will not offer in exchange for specific behaviours and adherence to its norms, including the crude norms that are written into crude contracts. Society in this scene is an autonomous subject, but, importantly, it is also a collection of people groups upholding what they are encouraged to perceive as socially safe and perhaps useful tradition.

Tradition is the composite of cultures that transcends generations. A good example in my Caribbean cultural context, of which I can speak confidently, is the use of harsh discipline so as not to 'spoil children', to keep children unheard, subservient, bereft of agency and, crucially, alive. In a practical sense, this may involve depriving babies of comfort by ignoring their cries, whipping children into submissiveness in order to control expression of agency, and shaming child-rearing that deviates from these norms. These norms necessarily evolved in response to a history of dehumanisation in which a child's cry was devoid of value as a signal of distress—say of hunger, anger or aloneness—and a bid for psycho-emotional attunement and regulation. And although the condition under which these norms developed is now firmly in our social history, even if not so distant, the adaptive response, masquerading as tradition, is still held to be useful and perhaps a pragmatic adaptation to difficult family life.

The consequence, in the absence of fulfilling the child's need for comfort that a cry signals, or the cultivation of responsibility the surfacing of agency implies, is that the developing nervous system encodes and expresses in thoughts, emotions and behaviours the message that pain—whether physical or psychic—begets pain and distress is to be ignored or reacted to with distress. Although not readily apparent, this encoding represents a neural template through which the child's social-emotional cells (LeDoux, 1999) and developing social-emotional self will be deprived of nourishment, especially the anointing in endorphins, dopamine, oxytocin and serotonin that facilitates connections across neural networks that mitigate inner crises and promote prosocial behaviour and emotions, such as empathy, compassion and altruism (Schore, 2019).Thus, a deprivation or dysregulation of these neurochemicals in the social-emotional brain—and the nourishment they afford—is associated with social-emotional disorders and antisociality.

The neuroscience of early life is such that the child who comes to the task of life with this deprivation will be forced by biology to adapt and model its doctrines in relationships. Doctrines of deprivation derive from neural assemblies (LeDoux, 1999) and represent physiological records—memories, in other words—of experiences lived, reactions and learning that followed and triggers that have been established. Once installed in the developing nervous system, these memories will influence concepts of self as well as ways of life—socioculture, in one word.

I am talking about adaptations, so this may look like perversions in self-concepts, say a chronic sense that one's self is woeful and undeserving of kindness, protection and general well-being, which extends to a distorted sense of safety. It is distorted in that it functions both as a survival strategy and a neural record of a social-emotional injury. Behaviourally, it might express itself, for instance, as indiscriminate friendliness towards absolute strangers, indifference towards social dis-ease, hostility towards invitation for reflection upon experiences that arise or move in the mind, dis-interest in being comforted and even aversion to having one's anxieties soothed.

In all these manifestations, as well as ones not mentioned, the nervous system will not only act to dampen the inner chaos and attendant neuropsychosocial disintegration but will also function to betray the human need for healthy development from childhood. This includes the need to be equipped with metaphorical SPEARS through which we can develop and refine our senses of danger and safety and explore our world—without excessive fear and overwhelming anxiety. By this, we can be convinced that the acquisition of these SPEARS is an important psychosocial developmental milestone, in the absence of which legacies of social-emotional injury, cognitive retardation and somatic disturbance can get passed across generations in what amounts to psychosocial trauma in high definition: a wound in the self that occurs as a result of protracted exposure to adversity that persists in the environment. At surface level, it presents as unfulfilled psychosocial developmental needs. However, it expresses itself as a chronic disturbance in the nervous system—inconspicuous or otherwise—that produces vulnerability to psychic dis-ease, aversion to mindfulness, volatility in sense of self, distortion in sense of safety and social apathy, all of which undermine the human will to actualise self-authenticity and cultivate psychosocial resourcefulness to live fulfillingly.

I want to reflect briefly on actualised self-authenticity, an important concept in the humanistic psychologies of Maslow and Rogers, both of whom employed it in theories of human potential achievable when the self is undisturbed, say by trauma. Thus, they imply that there is one self to actualise, much like psychoanalysis posits one ego to develop and monotheism believes in one true God to serve. My intention, however, is not to denounce or critique oneness. Rather, it is to acknowledge the remarkable utility of oneness in human orientation, in spite of its dis-sympathy for the multiple selves or configurations of our whole self we juggle and express in service of survival and well-being.

Some such expressions exhibited by participants in my ALEs survey were identified as having originated in protracted exposure to social and economic adversities. For the individual, this is a continuous traumatic stress that could manifest as love for people who hurt them, resentment of people who are kind, pleasure seeking in experiences that harm the body and mind, and resistance to experiences that are nourishing.

These expressions of ALEs tell me that psychosocial trauma, more than events of adversity, is what happens in the nervous system as a result of exposure to such events, how the nervous system processes or does not process adverse experiences that give rise to traumatic wounds and memories, which hijack autonomic regulation and trap it in adaptive patterns of defence and survival. By these events, a prevailing dissociation, roguish in its nature, arises among components of the self, as well as the different neural structures and levels of consciousness I have discussed.

Recall that these include the cerebral-cognitive, social-emotional, instinctive, authentic, inauthentic and ideal selves that are composites of the one body and mind and inform its neurobiological processes. It is at this level that conflict between nature and nurture stymies the potential for growth in the body and mind, where conditions of adversity lingering in the social environment signal that survivors, on their own with natural endowment alone, cannot overcome the adversities that shape their lives. And, by extension, they must be compelled to compromise essential—somatic, psychological, emotional and relational—needs as a necessary response or adaption.

This cue takes me back to the question of how we move through life and learn through experience and feedback that promotes neural connections and psychosomatic adaptations. Take the experience of food shortage, a universal insecurity many of us can relate to, even if only to a limited extent. Imagined alongside the feedback from our family and community that enough food will not be forthcoming however urgently needed, this insecurity is unhelpful in the cerebral conscious. The nervous system, in service of survival, is liable to dampen the distress it stokes.

There is also the repression of painful sensations in the instinctive-unconscious and spawning of psychological narratives to normalise suffering that I cited in previous chapters. In a neurobiological sense, this can be explained as an upregulation in pain threshold and distress tolerance that occurs in response to assured deprivation. The dilemma, however, is that deprivation, especially as it relates to resilience and intelligence SPEARS, chips away at the human capacity for growth, which aligns with both individual and collective pursuits of order and sophistication. By this, deprivation shapes perceptions in favour of the suffering it confers and recruits proxies to protect survivors from the pangs of its symptoms—to mask a fulfilling life that deep down is vacant, incongruent and 'false', to use Winnicott's term.

The idea that such a self leads survivors to entertain perversions in service of survival whilst experiencing inner dread seems an appropriate reflection with which to conclude this part II. The nadir of this reflection is the ALEs that keep people from acting upon natural curiosities and creative impulses, and which leave them feeling inauthentic, unfulfilled and bereft of the resourcefulness they might draw upon to help themselves, and to which they are liable to react and adapt, some by hiding parts of themselves, others by suppressing painful pangs and memories. And then there is neuropsychosocial disintegration that impacts their lives, often unconsciously.

However, the survivor will move through life—thinking, behaving and depleting—in ways that point to psychosocial trauma and its attendant disintegration, presenting themselves to the task of ordinary life, for instance, with cognitive, emotional and social apathy, at times with dreams that are detached from meaningful life changes and talks bereft of meaningful substance. Much like chronic absentmindedness, they present themselves physically but not psychically. Where the trauma is dissociated from its source in their subconsciousness, it is disposed to leak into thoughts, behaviours and dreams across generations. In transgenerational trauma, this is carried forward in implicit memory that holds experiences of the past in the form of emotions and sensations. Some ways this may show up across generations include facial expressions, tones of voice, manners of touch and patterns of attachment relationships between parents and children, thought patterns, behavioural tendencies, approaches to life and vulnerabilities to psychosomatic maladies that defy insight and through which traumatic memories readily express themselves.

By the end of this book, we shall learn that integration and well-being are tasks for nourishing relationships—including with the self. Naturally, this extends to the authentic self that fails to develop during the formative years of early life and where a vacancy sets in, perhaps manifesting itself as a fearful emptiness or even homelessness (Miller, 2008).

Integration brings not only the discovery of this emptiness, which can be filled with authenticity, but also the courage to confront maladies in the body and mind. Survivors can be encouraged to do this by collecting, connecting and correcting their life stories, starting with the story of their genes. We could think of this undertaking as an approach to well-being that promotes intergenerational dialogue as a life-affirming experience that purifies the nervous system. This purification comes with the surfacing of historical trauma, even if only to acknowledge it, and the opening up of the whole self to nourishing connections as integration sets in.

For the survivors who develop the capacity to think clearly, attune emotionally and retain resilience in their response to adversity, this integration is truly transformational. There is also the auxiliary mindfulness that motivates survivors to preserve well-being (Salzberg & Kabat-Zinn, 2020). For, in bringing attention to maladaptations that are preceded by adverse lived experiences and attendant trauma, mindfulness competes with the chaotic energy and allows it to be discharged. Unless, of course, traumas that betray consciousness pose a problem for mindfulness. We have learned this can be true for psychosocial traumas that derive from ancestral legacies. My own family's experience, which I explore in part III, offers an example of this. It is also in this regard that I revisit Alex's experience in therapy and attempt to unravel the implications of the therapist's—unqualified in her social-emotional sensibility—inability to offer qualified validation of his suffering and set him on a path to the well-being he sought.

This is also to appreciate that with Alex the therapeutic relationship suffered from inadequate resonance, which potentially exacerbated his woundedness and activated in him the spirit to entertain behaviours that were inconsistent with his well-being, a consequence against which the therapeutic space should guard, with its import of resonance and representation of the sustenance survivors of trauma rely upon as they undertake to cultivate well-being and authenticity in their whole self, with its metaphorical SPEARS, instincts and strengths. This is an important feature of neuropsychosocial integration, in the absence of which psychosocial trauma embedded in the nervous system is disposed to manifest in psychological, physiological and behavioural adaptations, which constitute legacies that can transcend generations. My exploration continues in part III.

Part III

NEUROPSYCHOSOCIAL (DIS)INTEGRATION IN ANCESTRY

Chapter 6

Ances-Story in Neuropsychosocial (Dis)Integration

In the words of the British social historian Felipe Fernández-Armesto, 'Stories help explain themselves; if you know how something happened, you begin to see why it happened.' As such, the hows and whys of life stories are intimately entwined and cannot be isolated in reconstruction.

Stories are vectors of legacy. In chapter 2, we learned that psychosocial legacy constitutes beliefs, values and wisdom we inherit as well as those we acquire in our lifetime and pass on to future generations. But there is a lot more to stories, and this chapter explores some hows and whys of life stories that bear implications for psychosocial trauma.

I defined this kind of trauma previously as a wound in the self that occurs as a result of protracted exposure to adversity in lived environments. This wound, I have argued, gives rise to disintegration in the nervous system that, for individuals, is liable to reveal its existence in time, often manifesting in psychosomatic maladies. We have learned that psychosomatic maladies are nature's way of alerting us to trauma in our body and mind. That is, as far as nature is concerned, a significant life event or its absence occurred, and this experience has left a deep woundedness.

Ordinarily, the response to this kind of woundedness merges into our way of life, often taking on the characteristics of a norm, as we adapt normally to survive it. Think of the relentless poverty, social marginalisation and domestic violence about which our old folks say 'it's the way it is'. Our protective self—equipped with its intelligence SPEARS—allows us to survive. This is one of the important wonders of our nature. By our natural design, we are response-able to our experience, both lived and inherited, and adapt-able to our environments.

Note the terms are hyphenated. Response-able translates to capacity to respond and adapt-able translates to capacity to adapt. The uniquely remarkable purpose of our response-ability and adapt-ability, evolutionary biology suggests, is the preservation of our species, as a whole, through surviving adversity and promoting ancestral resilience, as the Creator of humanity appears to have intended. I believe in an omnipotent Creator of unadulterated life systems, and to me, this is God. For others, this may be biology or the Big Bang proposed by the Belgian physicist Georges Lemaître. The idea, however spawned, remains that the impulse to survive adversity and promote ancestry is informed by the neurobiological and psychosocial, and this is an important focus throughout the chapters of part III. We begin with the neurobiological—to understand how biological ancestors as well as social parents transfer psychosocial trauma and adaptations to children, grandchildren and future generations more generally.

TRANSGENERATIONAL TRAUMA IN CONTEXT

The first implication of psychosocial trauma, as I have defined it, is that it is not about being born with a hostile genetic mutation or without a limb, although these matters are important. Rather, it is that protracted adverse lived experiences procure disturbance and attendant adaptations in survivors' bodies, minds, behaviours and life outcomes. In outlasting the events from which they derive, such disturbances and attendant adaptations, unless challenged and released of chaotic energy, contribute to suffering in successive generations, much like the originating events the ancestral generations survived. Hence, for future generations, suffering can be wholly inherited. It is, in other words, a legacy of survival that 'didn't start with you,' as Mark Wolynn (2013) argues, and which represents trauma-based adaptations that are maladaptive in the contemporary scene.

Trauma-based adaptations serve as information that is useful for historical reference but, beyond this, clutter rather than serves the bodies and minds they dwell in. This, too, is in addition to inhibiting capacities for well-being, growth and resilience across succeeding generations. We know this as both an axiomatic fact to which life stories point and an empirical fact clinical research allows us to demonstrate. Accordingly, this is transgenerational transmission of trauma, and it is possible because trauma-based adaptations contain resilient neurobiological and psychosocial pieces that are inheritable across generations.

THE NEUROBIOLOGICAL OF TRANSGENERATIONAL TRAUMA

The neurobiological piece in transgenerational trauma speaks to the impact of adversity at the level of the neuron. This impact induces a change in survivors' neural tissues and genetic expression. And by *genetic*, I do not mean changes in the survivor's genetic profile but, rather, changes in how genes in impacted neural cells behave, in how and whether they express themselves or do not express themselves. Another way to appreciate this event is by interrogating our genetic potential to ascertain whether it is optimised in service of our well-being or compromised by adaptations to adversity that occurred somewhere along our ancestry. These patterns bear utility for survival and—understandably—are passed on to descendants in ancestral cells that are hereditary and from which entire genetic profiles and nervous systems develop.

Thus, beginning our life story in our ancestral cells is a nod to the seemingly ancient thesis on the origin of our species in which the English naturalist Charles Darwin (2019) suggested that 'heredity' factors are passed on from generation to generation, controlling the traits of offspring. This is, in a word, an ancestral legacy that reflects biological adaptations. To appreciate its hows and whys, however, I must circle back to the pertinence of biochemicals through which cells in the body—including in the nervous system—connect and influence the story of life. That life, as does the story of ancestry, begins with chemical molecules interacting with each other.

More precisely, our ancestral story begins with four biochemicals—identified as adenine (A), thymine (T), cytosine (C) and guanine (G)—twisted into two spirals and folded around a protein called histone. These proteinous twists, known as deoxyribonucleic acid, or DNA, were unravelled in a sophisticated study that the American biologist James Watson and English physicist Francis Crick (1953) undertook. The content of DNA, it has since been discovered, is the biological information we inherit from our ancestors.

A global consortium of research labs mapped this biological heritage in 2001, unveiling a 'data pack' of approximately twenty thousand genes and three billion DNA base pairs identifiable by the first letters of the four originating biochemicals. The sequence of these letters in the map is as important to the proper functioning of the body and mind as the order of letters in a word is to understanding its meaning. We could think of this map as a book of instructions to make a human without nature's input—an incredible feat if it were possible. Nonetheless, this respectable work, or the Human Genome Project as it is formally called, remains an important reference in our understanding of how genes shape us and influence the unfolding of our life story. A part of this understanding is that genes contain ancestral instructions for our development, functioning and reproduction. As such, our ancestry lives in us. All of our estimated thirty-seven trillion cells that rely on energy from intracellular catalysts, known as mitochondria, we inherit from our mother through the egg cell in an unbroken genealogy. Mitochondrial energy is used by cells in our body in all tasks, from preserving our DNA to enabling our physical, mental and biological functions.

In nature, the sperm and the egg cells that join to form the zygote that develops into a child contain the DNA of both parents and contribute equally to a new DNA sequence. This never-existed-before sequence, now defining one—or more for monozygotic siblings—as unique, will begin the life story of a new generation with the ancestral biological information it retains, including that of the parents.

Importantly, this includes codes for information that stay constant throughout the life cycle—such as eye colour, blood type and natural sex—which often match those of the parents. it also includes codes for information that are less sturdy, such as psychological traits, emotional disposition and vulnerability to maladies. Vulnerability to maladies, in particular, retains saliency in clinical research that focuses on genetic therapy and ancestry in making sense of health outcomes. A good example is the extent to which children of chronically sick parents carry in their genes an elevated vulnerability for adverse health.

I am compelled here to reference schizophrenia, a fairly rare but severe neuropsychiatric malady. Schizophrenia is rare in that a random person in the general population bears a 1 percent risk of diagnosis. However, for the children of the afflicted biological mother, that risk increases to 10 percent and to 50 percent where both biological parents are afflicted. This tells us that ancestral legacy plays a role in the risk for adverse neuropsychic health outcomes, and in the case of schizophrenia, that risk is substantial (Hilker et al., 2018).

Reference to a risk as substantial, as it relates to intergenerational vulnerability to adverse health, psychosocial trauma and neuropsychosocial disintegration, invites valid questions about quantifiability. For answers, I turned to the Centre of Excellence in Complex Disease Genetics at the University of Helsinki, where a research team identified numerous genes that conferred 'substantial risk' for the disease in twenty-four thousand cases (Singh et al., 2022). Notably, among these genes were disabling mutants of two glutamate ionotropic receptor subunits—identified as GRIN2A and GRIA3—that promoted dysfunction in the glutamatergic system. These genes, in a word, are involved in regulating the behaviour of glutamate in the brain. We learned in part II that glutamate is an abundant excitatory neurochemical in the nervous system, and it is vital for cognition, relationality and prosociality, the very capacities impaired in schizophrenia and which the disabling genetic mutants disrupt. But this is not the full story.

Beyond its psychiatric features, schizophrenia is largely neuropsychosocial. It is a complex malady that binds the psychosocial and neurobiological. We have, for instance, deviant activities occurring in synaptic pathways and neural circuitries in the prefrontal cortex that lead to the onset of social behaviour deficits—largely in adolescence and early adulthood (Dempster et al., 2011). Interestingly, a paper published in *PLOS Biology* in 2020

(Comer et al., 2020) linked social behaviour deficit at this stage in the life cycle to a mutation of an immune-system-regulating gene. Precisely, an over-expression of Complement component 4 genes (mutant C4A) in the synapses of certain cortical interneurons corresponds with microglial engulfment of synaptic fibre and reduced cortical density.

Recall my remark in chapter 4 that tidily kept synapses promote neuronal communication. This is an important job neural immune-system microglial cells carry out. However, when these cells are overstimulated, such as in the case of C4A overexpression, they engulf the synapses instead of maintaining a debris-free cleft. This action poses a significant risk for schizophrenia, so much so that an individual with two copies of the C4A mutant, inherited from both parents, bears a risk of up to 50 percent. Beyond this, the risk of developing the disease is environmental.

This tells us the risk of developing schizophrenia and similarly complex clinical conditions is as much societal as it is genetic. Equally important, staying with schizophrenia as our example, is that these statistics show a greater or equal chance that children of severely ailing parents will not develop their parents' ailment. Their genetic predisposition to poor health outcomes is not necessarily deterministic. This is attributed to nongenetic factors, the chief of which is the process by which genes encode instructions and express themselves. It is here helpful to emphasise that genes reside in DNA molecules, which are within cells packed inside the twenty-three pairs of chromosomes that make up our entire genome. Twenty-two of these paired chromosomes—called autosomes—are identical in males and females. The twenty-third pair consists of the X and Y chromosomes that differentiate the male and female sexes. The female organism has two copies of the X chromosome, while the male has one X and one Y chromosome. Each autosome is assigned a number based on its size, with unique genes found on each. The C4 genes, for instance, are located in chromosome 21, and GRIN2A and GRIA3 are located in chromosomes 16 and X, respectively. As such, in order for these genes to express themselves, say in physiology and behaviour, they must be accessed and their codes must be transcribed and translated, a process that involves deference to transcription factors, messenger ribonucleic acids (mRNA) and a system of regulation that is epigenetic (i.e., above genetic).

In speaking to the relationship between genetics and the environment, nature versus nurture, the field of epigenetics is as dynamic as it is enormous. For my purpose here, it suffices that epigenetic research confirms that ancestral information in genes is response-able and adapt-able to environmental influence, which is regulated by epigenetics. This was established by geneticists Eva Jablonka and Marion Lamb in an elaborate body of work that combines evolutionary biology with social history. Their book *Epigenetic Inheritance and Evolution* (1995), in particular, argues that every individual experiences the environment in a unique way. However, interaction with our environment is foremost about producing in us behavioural and physiological modifications that promote our survival, a task overseen by our adaptive intelligence, as you will recall from chapter 4. To reflect the unique ways each one of us experiences the environment, this capacity to change ourselves in response to environmental demands reflects epigenetic regulations that are unique to each of us, including monozygotic siblings sharing the same DNA sequence.

Hence, unlike the DNA sequence, which stays constant throughout the life cycle, epigenetic regulations respond to and reflect the ever-changing demands of environmental input, such as nutrition, lifestyle and psychosocial trauma. For instance, in response to persistent hunger brought on by famine, epigenetic regulations can alter the DNA molecules in which reside the genes that encode instructions for expression of hunger (Heijmans et al., 2008), thus modifying the behaviour of those genes to promote survival with little demand for calories. Beyond hunger, however, this is really about the capacity to change the behaviour of genes in ways that impact survival and well-being. An event that occurs when chemical tags attach to or detach from DNA molecules, changing the molecules' structure and access to the genes inside. Tags from methyl chemical groups, for instance, can change the ways regulatory chromosomal proteins bind to DNA molecules so that the sheath of a tightly bounded protein cannot be easily removed to allow access to the genes. This activity, known as methylation, is involved in a range of vital biological processes, such as neuroregeneration, neurochemical synthesis, cells' repair and growth management, as well as genetic expression and epigenetics.

More than functional, methylation is necessary for life. However, methylation of, say, the cytosine base in our DNA to make 5-Methylcytosine, necessary for regulation of gene transcription, attracts free proteins that attach to methyl tags. Roguish tags attached to DNA molecules by toxic proteins, such as those associated with unhealthy diet and dysregulated endocrines, could mean that methylation blocks transcriptor molecules from accessing the genes inside. By this, genes in fully methylated DNA molecules are inaccessible, or silenced. This implication also extends to methyl tags attached to DNA histones, which cause the histones to fold and hide parts of DNA, rendering genes inside inaccessible. Acetyl group tags attached to histones confer the reverse effect by causing the histones to unfold to render genes accessible for transcription and expression.

With this level of insight into the process by which epigenetics causes changes to DNA and genetics, we can consider pre-embryo genesis when the sperm and egg cells are packed with parental epigenetic tags, which will be deleted when they form the embryo that develops into a child. However, it is believed that about 30 percent will pass to the next generation, and this epigenetic inheritance can go back into distant ancestry (Heine, 2017). These are like the voice of ancestors telling stories of their lived experiences and adaptations they pass on, should their descendants need them to survive. We can begin to make sense of this inheritance with the first cell of all the children a woman will bear forming in her ovaries while she is a four-month-old foetus in her mother's womb. This is to say that our cellular life began in the womb of our grandmothers. Half of every one of us, as a full-term baby, will have spent five months in our grandmother's womb, and half of her in the womb of her grandmother. I delight in telling my grandmother I began life in her womb and was nourished by her organic diet I still enjoy today.

This is remarkable when one considers the utility in being forewarned about the world in which we might live our life before our mothers are even born. As the adage has it, being forewarned is being forearmed, and this cannot be a bad thing where our safety and peril are concerned. However, it is not only signals and regulations about what food, safety and peril await us that we receive from our grandmothers. We also vibe to the rhythm of their heart, lungs and blood flow, and this rhythm vibrates all the way back to the very first mother. Hence, it is not odd to experience life as a deep orchestra of vibes that we react to but cannot always explain. For me, it is the vibes of my distant nomadic ancestors who wandered the lands of premodern Africa, Britania, Iberia and Greco-Albania, whose mitochondrial energy I have inherited. We know this energy to be a reliable biological inheritance through which ancestral legacy can be traced, since the mitochondrial DNA in our cells retains the genetic features of its originating oocyte, believed to be that of Mitochondria Eve (Stoneking, 1993), the mother of contemporary humanity, whose epigenetic sensibility all mothers are disposed to inherit and pass on to future generations of mothers.

Much like family cognomens in matrilineal cultures, mitochondrial DNA allows for the tracing of ancestral heritage, including the energy blueprint for responding to adversity. When cells divide, epigenetic tags carrying this information are transmitted to the next generation of cells to help them remain specialised. I noted earlier that each cell will contain two copies of ancestral genes, one from each natural parent. In the sex-defining X and Y chromosomes, however, one copy of the unique Y chromosome is available to be transmitted patrilineally. The genes in the twenty-two autosomes, which come in pairs, generally perform the same functions, but it is not unusual for the copy inherited from only one parent to be active. This is another type of mutation known as imprinting, and epigenetic regulations differentiate the two copies of the genes and determine which is active and which is inactive. It is possible to lead a fulfilled life with imprinted genes that do not cause problems, providing the active copy is sufficiently healthy. However, development disorders, severe disease and even premature death can occur in cases of abnormal imprinting, or any other type of mutation for that matter.

An incident of acute myeloid leukaemia (AML) that ended the life of two of my distant cousins in childhood, and which, incidentally, acquainted me with premature death, brings this implication to reality. Exposure to death invokes negative emotional states, intensely, and premature death is a life event that hardly makes sense from the point of view of the nervous system, which by design promotes life and acts in service of survival, safety and fulfilment. With this in mind, hereditary AML appears to be among the most insidious of diseases, for it is marked by a difficulty in producing life-promoting blood cells beginning in early childhood, as opposed to acquired AML that begins in adolescence and adulthood. The aetiology of both variants, nonetheless, is a genetic mutation, a loss in function on the GATA2 gene on chromosome 3 and the CEBPA gene on chromosome 19. Both of these genes express themselves in embryonic stem cells that perform duties necessary to produce leukocytes—white blood cells—that are germane to our native immune defence system (Hahn et al., 2011).

When the native defence system cannot protect the body and mind from environmental toxicity or protracted adversity, survival is compromised. An undefended body is as good as a dead body, to talk in a not-so-sensitive way about the chronic poverty, inadequate healthcare provision and little prospect to overcome deprivation that characterise life in the village community in which my young cousins lived and died. The neurobiology of these psychosocial traumas, as with the AML that killed them, dysregulates the whole immune system and leaves it vulnerable to depletion that compounds in time. It is in this sense that such a virulent genetic mutation occurring long after birth speaks to the vulnerability of genetics in an adverse environment. More precisely, we become increasingly vulnerable to genetic mutations as epigenetics act to promote our survival in the face of protracted adversity, such as to allow us to get sustenance from the food we eat, however little; to function in relationships, however poor; and to weather traumatic stresses that tax our genetics and give rise to mutations and dysregulations we are disposed to pass on to our descendants.

At this stage, with adverse lived experiences and environmental stress in focus, we can be satisfied that epigenetics plays a role in the risk of developing maladies for which a genetic predisposition exists. This can be gleaned from the epigenetics of schizophrenia and AML. However, the crucial question remains: how can we reverse deviant epigenetic regulations that lead to poor health, or rather, how can epigenetics promote good health outcomes in spite of genetic vulnerability?

The answer comes from a 2003 study involving agouti rodents by Duke University researchers that was featured on the cover of *Molecular and*

Cellular Biology (Waterland & Jirtle, 2003). 'For the first time ever, we have shown precisely how nutritional supplementation to the mother can permanently alter gene expression in her offspring without altering the genes themselves,' shared Randy Jirtle, professor of oncology and senior investigator on the study, in a follow-up article in *ScienceDaily* (Duke University Medical Center, 2003).

I was an undergraduate student in the Netherlands, and it was around this time I became a pescetarian in earnest, not least because the agouti rodent is a delicacy on the island of Dominica, where my maternal family hail from, but because of my awakening to how our environmental source of sustenance and nutrition shapes our life story. The study, fascinating as it was groundbreaking, began with curiosities surrounding how environmental influence can be adapted to control the genetic mutation and epigenetic regulation that cause chronic disease.

Diet, our source of sustenance and energy and the internal body's direct contact with the external environment, was adapted for the experiment that followed. The diet of chronically sick pregnant agouti rodents were supplemented with folic acid, vitamin B12, betaine and choline enriched with methyl group chemicals, based on a hypothesis that the pups would be healthier than peers whose mothers were not fed the enriched diet. A genetic mutation on the agouti gene manifests in a yellow coat and extreme obesity, which predisposes carriers to a range of severe diseases that include cardiopathy, diabetes and cancers. Granted, rodents are not humans, but they share with us a lot in terms of how their nervous system and genetics behave. So there is value to us in such an experiment in terms of understanding how environment influences genetics and, in particular, how methyl group chemicals involved in epigenetic regulations modify or silence roguish genetic activity. In this regard, the agouti pups' experience was enlightening, giving legitimacy to the idea that parents transmit acquired genetic modification and characteristics from their own life to their children, an old consideration associated with the French naturalist Jean-Baptiste Lamarck (1744–1829). The effect on the pups' genetics when their yellow-coated obese mothers were fed the methyl-enriched diet before and during pregnancy was remarkable: they were born lean with a healthy brown coat, even though they had the same agouti gene as their mothers. How? The overexpressed agouti gene, the study revealed, acts in the hypothalamus to interfere with signals of satiation, as well as the behaviour of other genes that code for colour and cell renewal. The extra nutrients, one or several, caused the agouti gene to become methylated, presumably during the early stages of embryonic development, thereby reducing its expression and potentially that of other genes implicated in adverse health risk for agouti rodents. Methylating the agouti gene thus reduced the pups' susceptibility to obesity, diabetes and cancer. Their peers whose mothers were not deficient in the selected-for nutrients but had not been fed the methyl-enriched diet, however, were born yellow-coated, ate excessively and wound up obese, diabetic and cardiopathic.

The first implication for us is that we can influence the expression of our children's genes, to correct for vulnerabilities in genetics and epigenetics we inherit and can pass on to posterity. But this must be intentional. Secondly, this tells us something about the nature of DNA. Call it the sacred domain of nature that allows the randomness of genetic mutation in response to environmental demands that are unpredictable. In this category falls adverse lived experiences that cause genetic mutations. Mutations, though, are not all bad. In fact, it is nature's way of ensuring variations and diversity in populations. When natural selection draws on variations, they can become rather stable, and this involves the replication of viable cells, repairing of damaged cells and deactivating junk DNA by a process that is not at all random. For instance, cells employ methylation mechanisms to deactivate or prevent the replication of viral remnants known as transposons that insert themselves randomly into our genome and cause maladies. However, when transposons attach to a DNA molecule, inserting themselves in or near a functional gene, there is a risk of the gene being methylated or mutating in some other way.

Cellular transfer and replication include autocorrection for rogue mutations and fragments on DNA molecules. This means the more fundamental a gene is to the functioning of our organism, the higher the probability that mutations will be corrected so that its expression returns to a natural state. This is the sacredness of well-being preserved in our DNA that feeds into the hows and whys of epigenetics and assures us that chronic maladies in life stories that include ancestral heritage are the antithesis of nature's mandate.

Hence, whilst epigenetics is involved with the risk of 'genetic' maladies by determining whether the promoter and suppressor genes are active or silenced, the genome that promotes the healthy functioning of the body and mind retains sacred capacity to self-repair, in spite of epigenetic regulations that impact the genes contained within it. There are, of course, the questions of what life events within a generation affect the genome, specific experiences that promote rogue epigenetic regulations, and in addition to epigenetic regulations, what other legacies may be implicated. These are important questions to consider in making sense of transgenerational trauma, adaptations and maladaptations that cause suffering, which is not in any way to suggest they are easy to answer.

However, contemporary life is replete with major events of adversity and stories of survival from which we can draw valuable insight. In my research for this chapter, I was lucky to gain such an insight from the story of a close relative of a dear friend. I shall call him Jake, who, with his family, survived the Great Ice Storm that struck North America in 1998. What sensations whirled inside the survivors' bodies, and what thoughts persisted in their minds during the days and weeks that millions of people were forced to survive with too little heat and without electricity? Jake was twenty years old at the time and, as he remembers:

> The ice storm was an experience I'll never forget. The beauty of the ice on the trees and plants captured a winter image, but for us living through it, it was dreadful. The first day the storm started, we lost power where I lived in Laval. Laval is a neighbouring city of Montreal. Both cities are actual islands. My parents and I stayed home without power and heat the first night. We had a kerosene heater in the hallway to heat the bedrooms, but the fumes from the heater almost killed us, lol. Bad idea to keep warm.
>
> The following day we were forced due to the cold in the house to go to a family friend's house in Montreal. They had electricity. They were fortunate to live near a grid where there was electricity. I also stayed with a friend who had a fireplace. It was eight days before we got power at my house. Some places further up north in Quebec got power a month after. The rural areas were hit the most. Some milk farmers had to throw away millions of gallons of milk due to no power for refrigeration. The key thing I witnessed is . . . people stayed together and helped the people that lost everything. At the time, all schools were closed. So my mind was at ease without worrying to travel to school. At my age and younger, a lot of kids were mostly happy staying at home. But for our parents it was another ordeal. All the food in fridges and freezers were wasted. My mind was in distress, but my body experienced the cold, the wetness, and mixed sensations of content and frustration, not knowing when things will get back to normal, but keeping faith things will get better. (Jake, 2022)

The dread, frustration and distress of which Jake speaks echo the findings of researchers who studied the effects of maternal stress occasioned by the Ice Storm on children's development from birth through adolescence. They were able to show that—in addition to epigenetics—neurobiological and psychosocial factors are equally consequential in foetal development and the first two decades of life. A team of researchers at McGill University tasked with this work was able to effectively isolate objective stressors, subjective reactions and personality factors among 178 pregnant women who survived the Ice Storm. Objective stressors included the days without heat and electricity, and the subjective reactions included traumatic stress and neurobiological expressions.

The neurobiological factors included elevated cortisol levels sustained over twenty-four hours and somatic symptoms of severe stress. For my purpose, which will become apparent later, I am compelled to highlight the difference between stress and severe stress, as they pertain to suffering. We learned in chapter 4 that stress ranges from the virtuous to the mundane of daily life, from which we recover fairly quickly. These stresses, however, can become chronic and accumulate into what the American neuroendocrinologist Bruce McEwen (2000) calls an allostatic burden, which can give rise to neuro-chemical imbalances, perturbation in psychosomatic rhythms and accelerated disease processes. Severe stress, or distress, however, is pathological—dis-ease producing—stress that accompanies excessive adaptive demands. This can occur when survival demands upon the body and mind are overwhelming and leading to bodily and mental dysregulation that persists outside the scope of survivors' intelligence SPEAR—I'd say the precise state in which the pregnant women and gestating babies found themselves during the storm: the cold, entrapment, lack of access to midwife care, the uncertainly surround-ing how long this suffering would last, the mother's worries for their babies. The consequence? Follow-up studies with the children from the ages of six months to nineteen years revealed lingering effects on attention, behaviour, intelligence and physical development that persisted into adulthood. Higher incidences of allergies, asthma and autism disorders than is found in the gen-eral population were also pronounced and concerning.

Allergies, asthma and autism are distinct clinical conditions that are treated in unique ways in contemporary medicine. The similarities and differences in presentations, however, point to autonomic dysregulations that intersect mul-tiple and overlapping survival systems. Namely, the native immune system, the stress response system and the endocrine system. Allergies, for instance, are associated with the immune system's hyperreactivity to constituents in the environment. This could be anything from harmless pollens the immune system misperceives as antibody pathogens that cause infections, to chronic stress that summons an immune system response and arrests the autonomic nerves in that state. As such, allergic diseases are normally treated in clinical medicine with psychotropics that suppress the immune system's autorelease of defensive neurochemicals. The chief of these chemicals is histamine, a stress-regulatory hormone that prepares the body to cope with injury and inflammation when the stress-response system is activated (Branco et al., 2018).

Ordinarily, histamine is released by immune system cells to defend the body against allergens, such as dust, mould and certain foods that cause maladies. By this understanding, allergic disease is a condition of autoim-munity. This is also true for asthma, a psychosomatic condition in which chronic inflammation restricts the respiratory tubes (Muramatsu et al., 2003). Inflammation is a natural immune system response to injury and, in the respi-ratory pathway, is indicative of trauma. I'll have more to say about asthma as a manifestation of psychosocial trauma in chapter 8. Here it suffices to say that, in clinical medicine, asthma responds well to synthetic copies of stress-regulatory hormones. We learned in part II these were corticosteroids, mainly cortisol, which acts to suppress the inflammation, and adrenaline, which dilates the respiratory tubes. Like cortisol, adrenaline is produced by the adrenal glands, in its medulla.

Recall the adrenal glands alight atop the kidneys and that active secretion of corticosteroids is a response to signals of stress from the social-emotional brain. This is essentially the neurobiology of stress, and it tells us asthma is a manifestation of chronic stress as much as it is of autoimmunity, fitting tidily into the conversation about psychosomatic maladies that reflect protracted exposure to adversity, attendant psychosocial trauma in bodies and minds, and a high incidence of such maladies in a population that was exposed to a very particular event of adversity.

There is also the incidence of autism. From *auto*, the Greek word for 'oneself', and *ism*, which translates to 'bias', autism emerged in the clinical literature as early as 1908, when it was introduced by the Swiss psychiatrist Eugen Bleuler in an account of what he perceived was a morbid retreat into the self, characterised by limited social curiosity and obsession with self-stimulating behaviour that made it seem like the autistic personalities were disconnected from the social world.

More contemporary research establishes the pathogenesis of autism before the nervous system debuts in the social world (Greenspan & Wieder, 2008). In that sense, autism seems out of place in a conversation about exposure to adversity in the social environment. Until it is not. In fact, the high incidence of autism among the children who survived the Ice Storm reminds me of the high incidence of schizophrenia in Caribbean-derived populations (Pinto et al., 2008). Schizophrenia, as we learned earlier, is a rare neuropsychiatric disease with a discernible epigenetic profile. There is the question of what environmental adversity has befallen the Caribbean people, what collective trauma underlies this incidence, a valid question I shall explore in the next chapter. Here my task is to examine the possibility that autism is a neuropsychosocial phenomenon: as the American psychiatrist William Singletary put it, 'a neurobiological disorder of experienced environmental deprivation, early life stress, and allostatic overload' (2015). This is the precise experience of babies developing in utero during the Ice Storm, who would be advantaged by an epigenetic profile that equipped them with a deficit in social-emotionality and a proclivity for self-stimulation suited for survival in a world that was cold, dark and dreadful. This is autism, an arguably intelligent trauma-based adaptation that intersects with the neurobiological and psychosocial. The neurobiological dimension points to deficits and mutations in a diversity of neurocircuitries, neurochemicals and genes that do not translate to a distinctive neural structure, but together they contribute to anomalies in social-emotional processes and a range of cognitive, motor and sensory abilities.

Neuroimaging and genetic studies commonly highlight deficits in oxytocin, glutamate and serotonin chemistry in the mirror neuron circuitry, in the emotional empathy system (Dapretto et al., 2006). Mirror neurons allow us to mirror the actions, behaviours and emotions of others and are implicated in a range of neurocognitive functions, such as social cognition, language, empathy and theory of mind. In short-circuiting this social-emotional system, an unfiltered view of the world emerges, expressing itself in a discernible straightforwardness that can be experienced as the indifference I recognise in my autistic students in the classroom. As in other areas of their lives, this straightforwardness is often accompanied by very little tolerance for disorder and disgust and a high degree of conscientiousness.

There are also the mutations of synaptic scaffolding (SHANK) and fragile mental retardation (FMR1) genes on chromosomes 22 and X, respectively, which are associated with mental retardation and glutaminergic transmission anomalies (Nisar et al., 2022). Recall that glutamate transmission in the synaptic cleft is important for cognition, learning and prosociality. Thus, its deficit in autism gives rise to suffering that expresses itself on a spectrum of severity, from debilitating social-emotional deficits, disordered cognition and stuckness in distorted perceptions of reality to the mild, albeit unconscious withdrawal into the self that is an adaptive response to a social world that is chaotic, unpredictable and at times unfriendly.

These features, incidentally, are also characteristic of schizophrenia, which share a high incidence of comorbidity with autism (Zheng et al., 2018). Where co-occurring, however, the uniquely schizophrenic symptoms present themselves relatively early in chilhood, which satisfies the classification of autism as an early childhood condition (American Psychiatric Association, 2013; World Health Organization, 2022), unlike in schizophrenia, where symptoms tend to show up in late adolescence to early adulthood when the executive brain—prefrontal cortex—takes its final leap to maturity. By this feature, schizophrenia is a malady that promises a crash in executive function, which occurs at a stage of a significant demand on executive capacity—the demand for maturity and to assimilate social reality fully.

This insight coils back to my question on epigenetics that promote good health. Recall that epigenetics is about nurture, how we experience our world. In ordinary reality, we have an accurate perception of our self, our world and our place in the world, all of which demand substantial social input by adolescence. This is a natural state for which we are adapted—in which we live, suffer, heal and perish. But it is also one a distorted perception of self and reality betrays. As such, there is a sense that autism disorders, as are schizophrenia, are maladies of the genome's inability to self-repair that reflects in the disintegrated self. This would also transfer to the intelligence SPEARS not promoting the resilience SPEARS of somatic harmony, psychological integrity, emotional attunement and relational satisfaction. This is conceivably a maladaptive response to psychosocial trauma, which leads to neuropsychosocial disintegration. An advanced state is one of neuropsycho-social collapse into which what is left of the severely traumatised—abused, taunted, neglected, terrified and ailing—self descends when it is unable to competently invoke the neuropsychosocial system in service of its survival. And the body—poorly cared for—serves as a container of a dis-abled and unsalvageable psyche.

Another observation is that the severely ailing self presents with a history of ALEs and traumatic wounds that elicit neuroinflammation. Neuropsy-chosocial collapse, hence, is an extreme manifestation of chronic traumatic stress and autoimmunity, both of which are reliable features of trauma-based adaptations that transmit across generations. In this light, we can begin to appreciate more fully the extent to which exposure to adversity that gives rise to psychosocial trauma corresponds with psychosomatic maladies across generations. But this is a nuanced relationship and one best explored in a separate quantitative study on ALEs and transgenerational pain. For there are also, at a surface level, maladies through which psychosocial trauma expresses itself appearing to share little common, but which are indeed linked by origin. It is in teasing out this origin that we could access a more comprehensive under-standing of how a specific psychosocial trauma or a stack of such traumas might manifest in life and health outcomes. There is the inevitable intergen-erational transmission of inner strengths—psychosocial resources—that are important too, and which I am yet to explore. Before that, I want to turn my attention to maladaptations of a psychosocial nature that are inherited across generations, the psychosocial stress that sustain them and some implications for neuropsychosocial disintegration.

Chapter 7

Psychosocial Trauma as Legacy

Beginning in Early Life

The previous chapter explored psychosocial trauma within the context of biological legacies that offer us a sense of belonging and relatedness. Whether that is to a family, tribe, nation or any other affiliation, it remains true that we are relational creatures as much as we are creatures of legacy; we experience life in relationships, and legacy alerts us to our strengths as well as our vulnerabilities in our relatedness. This includes vulnerabilities to ALEs and trauma that feature in developmental disorders and psychosomatic maladies.

Granted, there is so much that goes on in the psyche—in terms of how we engage with and respond to society—that begs to be understood and to which research brings clarity, especially about vulnerabilities and pathologies that originate with ALEs and show up across generations, at times far removed from the originating events. This chapter undertakes to explore the psychosocial dimension of this legacy and establishes personality as an essential component.

THE NEUROPSYCHOSOCIAL OF
TRANSGENERATIONAL TRAUMA

A good place to begin this conversation about transgenerational trauma is with the experience of parents who lived through tragedy upon tragedy in the social world and imagine this shaped their worldview and affected how they parented their children.

For example, imagine first-generation great-grandparents who lived in dire poverty and of whom the great-grandfather, the breadwinner, died prematurely from an acute disease. The second generation's upbringing was dispersed among extended families, friends and strangers in households where they were alienated, neglected, sexually abused and invalidated. This generation learned that children are deprived of agency over their labour and bodies, are beaten for the slightest of transgression, and adults' physical strength, parental privilege and conditional regards are misused on children in their care.

The third and fourth generations experienced much the same. They were brought up, largely, by in lone-parent households with educational and socioeconomic limitations alongside emotional and psychological dis-ease that persisted throughout their lives. In a clinical sense, these generations are encumbered with a host of autoimmune diseases—including asthma, juvenile diabetes and hypertension—that dysregulate the heart, lungs and vasculature, in addition to the mind. Thus, there is a sense that the bodies and minds 'inherited' across the generations are defective and undeserving of considered protection. A palpable vacancy of authenticity in the self also gives rise to chronic grief, and for those who appear to cope better, there is the sense of guilt.

Summarily, in this family, life begins with unrelenting poverty and the penalty of the loss of a significant security figure. Ordinary life is defined by emotional and material insecurities that give rise to a chronic lack affecting four generations. These experiences are traumatising, and we could argue that there are necessary epigenetic and neurobiological adaptations. However, equally important is that the children are socialised to become the parents they have. And this involves acquiring patterns of behaviour and expectation that reflect the persistent state of adversity in which life is lived. Across the generations, this is expressed in

1. little to no achievement in education and socioeconomic domains, as measured by credentials and material possession that can be traded for advantages and opportunities;
2. an impulse to attack kernels of agency in the self, as implied by physical, psychological and emotional responsibility and resourcefulness; and
3. a proclivity to invalidate, dismiss and mock authenticity in the self.

These patterns of behaviour and expectations serve the members of this family as they remain bonded by a collective trauma in a relationship with themselves and each other in which there is little demand and encouragement for self-reflection and differentiation. We may even say that the collective trauma is functional, in that it fulfils a need for commonness and togetherness. However, such trauma-based adaptations are fuelled by the same chaotic energy that sustains all maladaptive defences and, as we learned in chapter 4, stymies native intelligences—the intelligence SPEARS—upon which core needs and resiliencies depend. We may then say that the capacity to retire trauma-based adaptations and recover from psychosocial trauma across the generations in this family is truncated. These adaptations, now maladaptive, are sustaining the conditions in which they arose and are recycled and transmitted psycho-socially. But why?

This is in fact an anecdote from my family history, to which I shall return later. It is important here insofar as it speaks to the focus in this chapter. The psychosocial dimension in transgenerational trauma as it is preserved in family life and social history. Beginning with the social cues and patterns of behaviour that are passed from one generation to the next, from parents to children, in social, psychological and behavioural systems that prepare them to survive in a world in which the trauma originated—a world of suffering, that is.

Structurally, these systems function to take care of the generational need to survive the sequelae of old traumas. Recall that this includes vulnerabilities to psychosomatic maladies and neuropsychosocial disintegration that call upon the native adaptability of the body and mind. Hence, the capacity to recycle trauma-based adaptations in bodies and minds across generations is an ancestral legacy that, in addition to woes, bears wisdom. In part II, we learned this wisdom inheres in the entire scope of life experiences, which includes lived and inherited experiences as well as native and divine intel-ligences that can be shared with others or applied in practice to overcome ordinary life challenges.

The virtues of these intelligences—inscribe in social history—point to the utility of ancestral legacy in protecting surviving generations from the sequelae of psychosocial trauma. Think of the disabling stings of a 'whoop-ing' in childhood. This might feel archaic to some people, but nearly half (47 percent) of the respondents in my ALEs survey before the age of sixteen were often beaten or made to feel afraid that an adult in their household might physically hurt them. How might the child survive this assault? First, there is the inherent disadvantage of childhood in that the child is unable to prevent the whooping or protect their body from violence in general. You might find respite in the belief that a 'whooping' by a loved one in early life prepares the child to survive more severe and inevitable assaults by those they love as well as those who do not love them in adult life.

Equally important, too, are the delayed consequences. I've talked about schizophrenia and cancers, but there are other ways neuropsychosocial disin-tegration expresses itself in time. In my family, and in the Caribbean experi-ence upon which I draw in this book, this includes psychosocial deficits and maladaptations derived from surviving ancestral legacies of dehumanisation and disaffection that are handed down across generations in ancestral epi-genetics and sustained across the life cycle by psychosocial stress.

SOCIAL HISTORY OF PSYCHOSOCIAL STRESS:
BEGINNING IN UTERO

Having established ancestral legacy as a vector of psychosocial trauma, it behoves me to untangle what I believe is the psychosocial knot that makes this trauma wickedly transgenerational. I'll begin with the admission that this is no small task, especially as it appeals to our evolutionary response to adversity, that is, the activation of our instinctive response to stress. Put differently, the task of parsing intergenerational trauma demands interrogation of our native defence system, which is self-initiating in moving us to protect our body and mind from assault. The 'defensive dragon' I talked about in chapter 3, that which we all in some way behold within us, is an agent of this system. Interrogating its volatile spirit, however, is messy and complex. My start is the prenatal nervous system, which debuts around the fifteenth day of gestation, when a sliver of the few dozen cell that is the developing embryo, called the neuroderm, invaginates into a tube that develops into the big brain and spinal cord. From then on, it also begins to be vulnerable to influence from the psychosocial world. That is, to stress.

At this stage, the neuroderm is only a few unspecialised neurons. But even by then, its reaction to psychosocial stress can shed light on the intergenerational transmission of psychosocial impulse, the mechanism by which parents confer psychosocial stress and adaptive responses onto their prenatal children. Distinct from the trauma to which it could give rise, psychosocial stress is best understood as tension in the body and mind that derives from interaction with the social world. A crude manifestation is the increased pressure upon the heart, lungs and musculature that arises from exposure to cold wind. Corticosteroids will move the mother to wrap up in a warm blanket and tuck her hands between her thighs. Oxytocin, endorphins and glutamate will move her to cuddle up to the nearest limbic creature that is receptive of her bid for warmth. Thus, in the absence of overwhelm, the mother's native defence system takes care of this tension with the help of a precise neurochemistry, and the baby gets the signal that mother is protected, safe and sufficiently resourced in the world.

The opposite message, however, is received when survival demands upon the mother are excessive, such that her protective defences or resources are inaccessible or inadequate. For example, if she is homeless, afflicted by a disease or isolated in the conditions of a storm and feels depleted in energy, hopelessly pessimistic, unsupported in her family and unsparingly unsafe. Copious studies—including the McGill University study cited earlier—have charted how toxic levels of stress regulatory hormones secreted under such conditions in pregnant mothers travel to their womb and infuse the amnic fluid in which their growing babies are cushioned and experience life (Bergman et al., 2010; Coussons-Read, 2013).

Naturally, this experience includes the exchange of life signals and biochemical products between mother and baby, much of which would be ingested by the growing baby in the ounces of fluid gulped daily. In addition to nutrients and flavours, any toxins it contains are ingested too, processed by the baby's developing organs and excreted into the womb's ecosystem.

This is important to emphasise, for it tells us that amnic fluid, which comes from babies' kidneys, will give a reliable indication of well-being in utero, including a lack thereof in cases of exposure to toxins and deviant levels of neurochemicals that increase babies' risk of being born dis-eased, prematurely and underweight (Coussons-Read, 2013). A helpful measure of this risk is the 20 percent variation in newborn babies' weight that ties to levels of cortisol in pregnant women exceeding the two times above average that is normal (Shriyan et al., 2023). This makes sense when one considers that chronically excess levels of cortisol reflects chronic distress, which shifts the mother-and-baby state from growth to protection. The growth-inhibiting effect of excess cortisol in the womb causes the baby to be born smaller than the norm. This tells us—foremost—that excess cortisol from chronic distress in pregnant women can cause low birth weight in their babies. This is a trauma-based adaptation, perhaps to inadequate nutrition and other psychosocial stresses that cortisol reacts to. But this is not the full story.

Recall from part II that cortisol is the chief stress-regulatory hormone and gets its signal for release from the hypothalamus, in the social-emotional brain. This signal will initiate a series of neurochemical releases and reactivity. Upon receiving a stress signal, from say the amygdala or cerebrum, the hypothalamus secretes corticotrophin-releasing hormone (CRH) to its inferior pituitary gland. This is to induce the pituitary gland to secrete adrenocorticotrophin-releasing hormone (ARH) to the bloodstream, that then travels to the adrenal glands and, in the adrenal cortices, the outer layer of the adrenal glands, prompts the release of cortisol and the mobilisation of an appropriate stress response. Such a response may be to flee from a stressor, fight an aggressor or whatever other defence is opportune. Although, according to the American neuroscientist Joseph LeDoux (2022), our evolutionary adaptation tends to favour an adrenalised fight or flight, which is another way to say a sympathetic spinal-chain activation.

In principle, the sympathetic chain is a complex network of neural fibres that run alongside the spinal cord and exit the thoracic and Lumbar spines to activate muscles throughout the body in service of our defence and protection. Figure 7.1 shows these nerves, a total of twelve from the thorax and the first two from the Lumbar, which innervate specific muscles in the body and organs in the viscera upon receiving a signal from the 'protective dragon' of our native defence system.

HUMAN NERVOUS SYSTEM

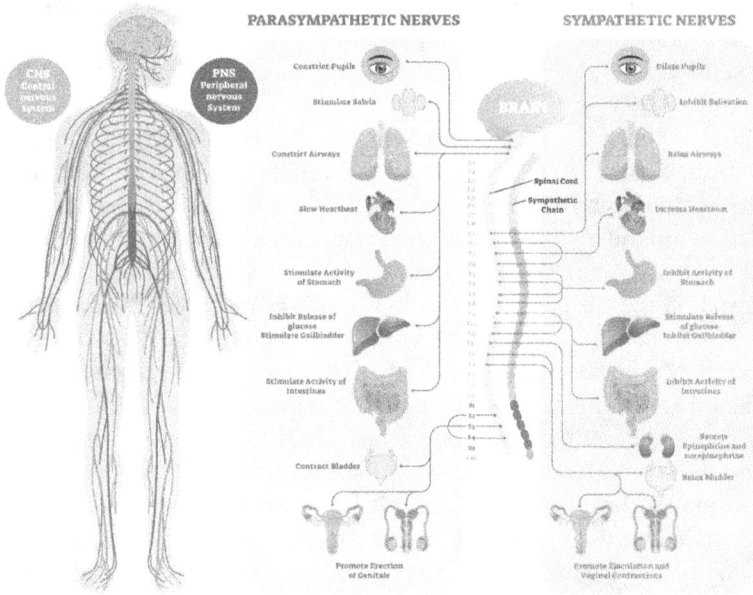

Figure 7.1. Autonomic Nervous System. *Image © VectorMine / iStock / Getty.*

With the help of figure 7.1, my interpretation of the relationship between the sympathetic chain and our adaptive defences is that, in a state of activation, the first of the twelve nerves from the thorax, the T1 to be exact, innervates the eyes to dilate the pupils, the mouth to inhibit salivation, and the lungs to relax the airways. Dilation of the pupils allows the eyes to take in more information about a threat and survival opportunities in the environment, inhibition of the salivary glands suppresses digestion to preserve energy, and relaxation of the airways allows for more oxygen to be taken in to facilitate the increased demands of sympathetic activation. The next three nerves, T2, T3 and T4, innervate the heart to increase the rate of its beats. This is to push oxygenated blood more quickly throughout the body. T5, T6, T7 and T8 inhibit activities in the stomach to preserve energy. T9, T10 and T11 go to the kidneys' cortices to invoke cortisol release, the gall bladder to inhibit digestive enzymes and the intestines to inhibit excretion. T12 innervates the medulla in the kidneys to stimulate release of adrenaline and noradrenaline that are needed for alertness, endurance and vigour. L1 and L2 from the Lumbar spine go to the bladder and genital organs, but also to the head, to suppress a range of parasympathetic activities. Excretion, copulation and empathy are examples of such activities.

This is the body's natural setup to respond to psychosocial stress in the environment, however perceived. We could also think of this dynamic as an expression of somatic intelligence, wherein the nerves of the sympathetic chain, against which the innards fall, deploy autonomously when we feel unsafe, to be accompanied to their target by energy-carrying vessels that fuel the body in service of survival. So the lungs open up to increase intake of oxygen that sustains the body in a fight or flight; heart rate increases to gets oxygenated and adrenalised blood to vessels and muscles more quickly; and muscles stiffen to help the body move quickly. These are all appropriate responses to psychosocial stress that have been refined by evolution to promote survival for a sufficiently resourced and flexible adult, but not so much for a young child or an incubating baby, whose exposure to toxic levels of stress is not inconsequential.

Beginning with the release of cortisol into the bloodstream, which we have learned is a faithful servant to our native defence system. In the developing baby exposed to toxic levels of stress in the pregnant mother, this translates to toxic levels of cortisol that prioritise survival over growth, and by this response, the baby experiences deprivation of growth-promoting nourishment. By toxic, I mean a sustained level of excess or inadequate cortisol that warns of distress in the social world and encodes or stays in reserve in the body system until it can be encoded into the baby's native self-rescue and stress-response circuitries. In a simple sense, to encode an experience is to process it. Thus, one can think of these codes as formulas to survive distress in the social world—to which the baby will begin to react from the fourth month of gestation, when limbs and facial muscles can be coordinated to express sensations.

The American radiologist Jason Birnholz observed babies in utero at this stage of their development making animated faces, kicking about and sucking their limbs. The limb-sucking in utero, in particular, is a self-soothing impulse that also happens to explain prenatal ulcers (Verny & Kelly, 1982). Immediately apparent is that these are all adrenalised expressions of how the baby is experiencing and reacting to life events, and when it comes to suffering, this is traumatic stress. One could think here of the pangs of hunger, grief and chemical toxicity that reflect maternal adverse lived experiences and reaction to an unsafe social world more generally. The Kuwaiti America spiritual healer A. H. Almaas spoke to this incidence when he wrote that 'The child is very open, and can feel the pain and suffering going on in its immediate environment. The child is aware of its own body and can also feel the tension, rigidity, and pain in the mother's body or anyone else it is with. If the parents are suffering, the child feels it. If the mother is suffering, the baby suffers too. The pain never gets discharged' (2000, p. 85).

To discharge the pain is to bind and contextualise the chaotic energy that sustains it, an undertaking that requires a reworking of the survivor's life story with quivers of SPEARS that I shall explore in part V. Here I want to emphasise that, under conditions of adversity, the pain inside of the mother is really an announcement of lingering psychosocial stress. This is the kind of stress that accompanies being displaced, contemplating an abortion, being abused, starvation, chronic disease, a relationship with the father that leaves her worried about her ability to provide enough for herself and her baby, and just about any other prolonging adverse life event from which relief is not immediately conceivable.

Whatever the source of this stress, lingering elevated levels of stress-regulatory chemicals will concentrate in the same target bodily tissues in both mother and baby. In muscle groups in the arms and legs, to serve bodily defence, and in neural substructures in the hindbrain, from where defensive reflexes originate. I have mentioned relational worries, disease affliction and isolation, including in the conditions of a storm or war, that could bring about this stress response. But incidents of psychosocial stress could be endless and less articulable too.

Consider her little-perceived psychological pain and emotional insecurity surrounding her child's health or addicted, homeless, unknown or unwaged father that are equally expressed through neurochemistry that disturbs nerves and encode in her developing baby's nervous system. In old Greek, 'nerve' translates to *neuro* and 'disturbance' to *sis*, tying together as 'neurosis'. This is not the cluster of unconscious anxieties and phobias of psychoanalysis. Rather, it is that chronic sense of the world not being safe as it is, and that one must be equipped with adaptive defences—codes—to protect the self and feel safe enough.

For the child in utero, life does not begin with a sense of safety or the conditions for a healthy sense of self. However, informed and prepared by the mother, the child arrives in the relational world equipped with predispositions and inclined to compensate for these vulnerabilities. My work with preschool children in Basseterre, St. Kitts, in the Caribbean between 1997 and 1999 and primary school children across the Midlands in England between 2015 and 2016 alerted me to these dispositions falling into five discernible and consistent patterns as they informed personality and response to stress by the age of three.

We are acquainted with some of these dispositions and how they may predict survivors' reaction to psychosocial stressors from the life stories in previous chapters. For instance, the warrior disposition engages sources of stress in conflict and reflects a fight response pattern. There is the nomadic disposition to dart away from signals of adversity and sources of stress that inheres a flight response. The third, also a nomadic disposition, is to wonder aimlessly and even mindlessly around signals of adversity and sources of stress, which defines a float response. I have also cited the fold and furrow response patterns, both of which are features of a settler personality that kindles a disposition to shape-shift in the face of stress and the disposition to collapse under the weight of stress, respectively. Since observing these dispositions in small children, I found them exhibited consistently too among my high school, college and university students and mental healthcare practitioners who attend my workshops. Let's explore them in some depth.

PSYCHOSOCIAL STRESS IN ADAPTIVE DEFENCES AND PERSONALITY

The Disposition to Engage Signals and Sources of Stress in Conflict: A Warrior Fight Response Pattern to Psychosocial Stress

Watts's important work on 'discovering who we are and what we can be' offers a reliable profile of the warrior-fighter (2000, p. 19). It is that forceful personality who 'can always make their presence felt and comes to the task of life with high tenacity and ability to execute plans' but, alas, also an 'impulse—an ancestral memory—to always be in control', leaving little room to cultivate compassion and emotionality in the self. Thus, the fight pattern of response to psychosocial stress is akin to a fire fighter constantly engaged with fire. In addition to accidental fires, this includes malevolent fires, imagined fires and fires started simply to satisfy the impulse to fight, all pointing to a hyperreactive amygdala and neurons in the thoracic spine on alert to innervate the visceral organs and muscles for a fight.

In the three-year-old child, this is the readiness to strike a playmate for reasons ranging from 'I'm bored' to 'I want a toy'. This is the ten-year-old who surveys the playground with clenched jaws and hands curled into a fist. And the police officer who reaches for a lethal firearm with her nondominant hand when it would serve her to reach for a taser gun with her dominant one. In this state of hyperarousal, the sympathetic chain is chronically activated, and the body is mobilised to confront stressors and perceived threats. By extension, core bodily functions—such as breathing, digestion and immune defence—stay inhibited or disorganised as inner resources are redirected to physical defence. Thus, levels of adrenaline and noradrenaline stay high to sustain strength and alertness, as will cortisol to control inflammation. Glucose levels, too, will be high in order to sustain high energy, and endorphin secretion constant to numb the pain from injury—whether physical, emotional or psychological.

Evolutionarily speaking, this is an autonomic regulated response to acute stress, and it is meant to last whilst a stressor persists and there is a sense of real danger (Sapolsky, 2004). However, as with the conditions of adversity that derive psychosocial trauma, when this adaptation is protracted, suggesting chronic psychosocial stress, the autonomic regulations will default to this state. In a clinical sense, this is the state of dysautonomia in which survival impulses and adaptive defences are playing out in personality.

The Disposition to Dart Away from Signals and Sources of Stress: A Nomadic Flight Response Pattern to Psychosocial Stress

The flight response pattern to psychosocial stress, much like the fight pattern, is a highly adrenalised disposition. However, rather than confront a stressor, it is one to escape in a nomadic way. Watts (2000) profiled the nomad as the restless personality who 'must always have something going on', the archetype that approaches life with curiosity and naked authenticity—what you see is what you get—but, alas, bears the untiring impulse—the ancestral memory—for exploration and perceived stimulation in the unknown. In the three-year-old child, this is the constant need for 'the restroom', to know 'what you doing' or to 'go outside to look for' something. It is the need for life infused with uncertainly, and, in the face of a stressor or aggressor—whether real or imagined—it is a variation of the impulse to run, jump or dart away unencumbered.

There is this interesting analogy with birds, their long life being ascribed to a natural tendency to fly away from predators, although in the wild juvenile birds can have high mortality rates and their approach to life—their aimless wandering, more precisely—is reminiscent of the float response. The flight response, nonetheless, is unique in that it is purposeful and directive, as the nomadic survivor takes flight away from a source of stress to a place that is not perceived as unsafe. The purpose of this flight being to avoid or mitigate stress, but there is also the soul-nourishing pleasure of finding new things and experiences.

Think of the teenager who runs away from a violent home, not into the streets, but to the safety of a friend's family and PlayStation; the battered spouse who seeks refuge in a safe haven and gets to make cookies for appreciative children there; and the migrant who seeks opportunity in a new country to provide for a family, build a community or experiment with different ideas of civilisation. Whilst these are virtuous adaptive responses to acute psychosocial stress, they can become maladaptive when hijacked by chronic psychosocial distress. The child who comes into the world bearing this disposition could find herself stuck in a chronic state of flight, wandering aimlessly through life, much like the juvenile birds in the wild that are vulnerable to predation and premature death.

The Disposition to Wander Aimlessly around Signals and Sources of Stress: A Nomadic Float Response Pattern to Psychosocial Stress

The third disposition with which the child might emerge from life in utero is to float through life untethered, but not in a directed or purposeful way. I had this idea when I was about ten years old on a field trip in the Commonwealth of Dominica with my peers. We were playing with my latex volleyball, one of my favourite childhood things I had purchased in St Maarten with money I had earned myself. It wouldn't be an understatement to say it meant a lot to me, perhaps because it was my only toy, or the only toy I was allowed to own and play with. On that day, we were playing in the sea, wildly volleying the ball to each other with all our muscle power, having good ten-year-old-kids kind of fun under the watchful eyes of our teacher, when at one point it was hit with so much force that it spawned out of our reach and floated away into the ocean, evading all efforts—including that of the adults—to fetch it back. Decades later and alive in memory, I still wonder about that ball. Whatever happened to it? Did it encountered peril in a storm, overwhelming heat or get a puncture against a sharp object? Was it found on an island beach by a child who gave it a home, appreciation and gentle play? And, above all, what other fate could have befallen it had it not escaped our aggression?

Although losing the ball was a difficult experience for us children, especially me, the reality is that it floated away aimlessly from our aggression and symbolic unkindness, indifferent to what good or evil lay ahead. This is how I am often led to think of chronic and cumulative psychosocial stress in survivors who float through life untethered emotionally, relationally and somatically. Or, more intimately, as I discovered among the young people who call the streets of Seattle, Washington, their home, of that baby deserted by her father at the news of her conception, who survived attempted abortions, institutionalisation and abuse at the hands of caregivers in childhood, trafficking and prostitution in adolescence, and survives unhoused in adulthood. This is a rather crude example of how adrenalised untetheredness and a float response to psychosocial stress play out for many survivors, but important is that it speaks to the reality of some people we interact with in our ordinary life, people in our families, communities and workplaces who are morbidly individualistic and depend on their enterprise and wits to survive adversity. According to Watts's theory, encouraged by the memory of ancestors who wandered from place to place alone or in small bands, averse to combat and unhindered by uncertainty, this nomad comes to the task of life with very little patience and tolerance for psychosocial stress.

In the three-year-old child, this is the offering of a tale of an imagined adventure as a distraction from a challenging task. In the ten-year-old, it is the involuntary escape into mind-wonderland in response to the drama of school, family life and prepubescence. Among the traits with which she will survive adolescence and adulthood, some are liable to be magical thinking, spiritedness, calculated super-cooperation and superficial charm that will inevitably cause tension in the relationships she is impulsed to end and leave behind. For, although fraught with uncertainty and unimaginable stress, this untetheredness—seasoned in utero—is familiar, and familiarity augurs respite, a sense of peace that is reinforced by poor self-esteem and a general apathy towards deprivation. In the absence of connection to a purpose, relationship or self-worth, survivors show aversion to mindful activities that bring awareness to conditions about which one may feel helpless and are so replaced by magical ideas that feel safer and reassuring.

The Disposition to Shape-Shift in the Face of Signals and Sources of Stress: A Settler Fold Response Pattern to Psychosocial Stress

The disposition to fold, or shape-shift, in response to psychosocial stress with which the child emerges from uterine life serves the need to survive in a group. This would be an especially crucial need in a society in which group-based identities are bases for disadvantage, or even persecution, as they are for survival. According to Watts (2000), this settler personality 'gets on well with almost everybody', and achieves this with an impulse to make the best of any given situation but, alas, also with an almost desperate need to belong and be 'liked'. As such, relational security is important to this settler personality, who comes to the task of life with remarkable tolerance for adversity and diversity among those with whom they share, as well as the ancestral memory to tolerate psychosocial stress in the hope of better times ahead. The fold, thus, is about adapting behaviour patterns to conform with what others seem to want. This could involve being a particular kind of person, equipped to survive a particular kind of experience and bear a particular kind of pain.

The three-year-old folder child, who perceives coldness and indifference in a caregiver, might react by offering a joke or trick in a bid to change the caregiver's mood. At the heart of this behaviour is an understanding of emotions and the impulse to problem-solve. Ordinarily, these are the very 'nice' people who are attuned to their surroundings, responsive and stick with a problem until it is resolved, even at their own peril. However, the disposition to shape-shift or fold in response to stress appeals to inauthenticity in the self that is primed for adversity and suffering, and the self may actively seek out these states. In adult life, this self could manifest as indispensable, overbearing, dangerous—or the absolute obverse: trifling, trivial and harmless.

In chapter 3, I talked about Amjeet, the brilliant ayurvedic doctor who was stuck between the need to provide for his family and the need to protect himself from the insults his disproving employer meted out towards him, folding himself into an apparent people pleaser—shape-shifting and fawning his way through toxic relationships in which he suffered but felt bound to persevere. In staying quiet, seemingly unimportant and unthreatening, he succeeded in deflecting negative attention from himself but at the cost of his integrity and professional regard. For, in the grips of a fold, the survivor is acting in the role of a servant, one whose safety is contingent on folding into a personality that accommodates the needs of a master and survives the attendant ALE. This could be battery, neglect, abandonment or any other form of violence that exacts obedience and servility through infliction of suffering.

In her work on 'posttraumatic slave syndrome', the American psychologist Joy DeGruy (2017) explored the extent to which this is largely true for melanated peoples of the Americas, among whose ancestors the fold was a protective adaptation for five centuries in response to protracted racialisation, dehumanisation and 'legalised' subjugation. For such people, whose blackness in its myriad shades was designated a target for condemnation, the wages of expressing sovereignty and body autonomy was death. Today, whilst these consequences are no longer sanctioned legally, the ancestral disposition to fold in response to psychosocial stress is inherited across generations. At the group level, we continue to be socialised in ways to survive our ancestor's suffering, to accept that we do not belong among high achievers, among those who are respectable and respected and whose successes—however small—are celebrated. Love, kindness and security in relationships are not given by birth right, and as such we cannot afford to imagine a life free from limitations, even if only to express our self and our needs authentically. We learn in our families, communities and feedback from other social groups that to exhibit intelligence, competence and sovereignty is to be socialised white, or act white, and that by virtue of our blackness, we must work twice as hard to achieve half the reward (Eddo-Lodge, 2018), our reference being white identified groups and increasingly non-black-identified groups. These ALEs speak to a psychosocial stress that undermines psychological fortitude, but importantly for survivors, it is a reflective life story.

Among the autonomic nerves that regulate this state, one is liable to find a hybrid that intersects with sympathetic activation and parasympathetic calmness, which is held in place by that volatile neurobiology I discussed in chapter 3, wherein cortisol, adrenalines, enkephalin and dynorphins released to the spinal chain clash with the dopamine, serotonin, oxytocin and endorphins of social-emotional connection. This is a state in which the ancient reptilian instinct to freeze in the face of imminent danger faces off with the evolved mammalian instinct to stay relationally competent, because to fight, flee or float away is not a safe choice.

This is reminiscence of the double consciousness W. E. B. Du Bois (2016) explored in *The Souls of Black Folk*. Unable to change their skin colour that is a target for assault, 'black folk' have learned they can fold their body, offering only parts or distorted version of themselves, their feelings, thoughts and culture, in ways that distract the racist and release endorphins to numb the pain. Endorphins are implicated in this relational competency in a way that helps us to cope with despair and the intense pain that is associated with psychosocial distress.

The Disposition to Submit to Despair in the Face of Signals and Sources of Stress: A Settler Furrow Response Pattern to Psychosocial Stress

Featured earlier as a disposition to collapse under the weight of psychosocial stress, the furrow response speaks to descension into the depth of aloneness and despair. This is the three-year-old child who faints at the sight of a caregiver's angry face, or the fifteen-year-old who drinks bleach in response to a chaotic home life that is beyond her capacity to cope with. Furrowing, thus, is about relief from a painful reality. At a group level, this is a social reality suffused with violence and chaos, but at the individual level it is typically an interpersonal relationship in which feedback invokes a sense that one does not belong, is not good enough, gets half as far for working twice as hard and cannot be seen as weak or in need of help. According to Watts's (2000) profiling, this is liable to lead the settler to self-betray in exchange for acceptance and belonging, perhaps driven by an 'all or nothing' impulse that leads to the 'cutting off of their nose to spite their face', or to the masking of their despair with token identities that are revered, even if inauthentic.

Acceptance, belonging, masking despair, token identities, reverence and inauthenticity all point to an inherent flexibility in our perceptions and use of language that serves us when our needs are in conflict with our reality and we must reconcile what is nourishing and what is harmful to us in a way that is acceptable. Examples of what I mean can be found in cultures in which children are encouraged to perceive themselves as worthy and loved, but only insofar as they serve the needs of adults who provide for them. Women are encouraged to perceive themselves as 'independent' and 'strong queens', unlike the revered sovereign of an empire who has at her disposal necessary wealth and an army of resourced personnel to carry out her bidding and ensure she is safe, but as in 'a personality who lives through unthinkable suffering with little if any resource, and somehow manages to stay alive, even if bruised and broken'. Men can perceive themselves as fearsome kings and warriors, but not in the sense that they are equipped with strategies and tools to build kingdoms, families, communities and enterprises they are proud to protect. Rather, it is that they are hustlers. As one of research participants put it, 'Our culture where we come from, life has always been a hustle. We are hustlers. When you are a hustler, there are only certain things that you know about and that's hustling' (Lloyd/Hyde, Greater Manchester, 2009).

Hustling is a term loosely used to mean a competitive struggle to survive by means of a special scheme to earn money. In village cultures of the Americas, for instance, hustling schemes are typically unregulated and often—though not always—of an underworld nature. One might find unregulated food provision, housing and self-care services offered by personalities identifying as mamas, cooks and stylists. But hustling schemes could also include gambling, drug dealing and prostitution, to which younger generations and especially boys and men are introduced by relatives and contacts in their community who identify as entrepreneurs, bosses and dons. What all these schemes point to, however, is the human need for safety and the esteem and reverence that enterprise and status identities confer.

In the face of despair, these identities bear utility in that they are protective, even if only in imagination or in an alternate reality where, as one of my students put it, 'we are all valued and protected by God'. Protected means as little as being kept alive, even if in a state wherein the 'knowns' that stoke confusion, dejectedness, fear, anxiety, depression and myalgia in settler populations are suppressed and curiosity in the 'unknowns that won't kill' survivors quickly is vacated. In this reality, the SPEAR-less survivor is liable to self-loaf, self-destruct or self-medicate inner dis-ease as a way to make the relational world appear less adverse and unsafe.

Recall the experience of Alex, the father of three, who fell into isolation and alcoholism in an attempt to gain relief from his distress during the pandemic. Incidentally, this is not an uncommon response to psychosocial distress among survivors, who move through life with a disposition to furrow into the depth of despair, seeking relief in psychoactive depressants and stimulants that summon a sense of pleasure, at the exclusion of social conditions that promote well-being (Inaba & Cohen, 2007). For instance, alcohol, benzodiazepines and opioids are used to caress the socioemotional brain and inhibit the consciousness of pain and amphetamines and narcotics are used to inhibit neural activities and promote calm in the prefrontal cortex. These depressants and stimulants, however, work as they do by hijacking organic processes in the nervous system and, in so doing, leave the survivor vulnerable to unpleasant psychosis, somatic mutilations and self-abandonment. So at the cognitive level, the appeal in this kind of self-medication is counterindicative, until one considers that the objective is to dampen the sensation of suffering, to survive psychosocial distress and—by implication—to preserve the survivor's capacity to contribute to the progression of our species. This can be readily achieved in the depth of a furrow when the survivor is moved—neurochemically speaking—towards what is pleasurable and feels good, however bad in actuality. For the impulse to furrow is fuelled by a powerful neurochemistry—the precise chemistry of psychodepressants and stimulants—that masks suffering.

SPECTRUM OF AUTONOMIC ACTIVATION IN ADAPTIVE DEFENCES

The adaptive defences to psychosocial stress with which we navigate the social world point to dynamism and democracy in the personalities with which they align. Thus, my reference to the warrior-fighter does not preclude the warrior-nomadic floater, the warrior-settler folder or any other configurations of the warrior, settler, and nomad personalities, which are differentiated by subconscious processes that allow them to respond and react to life events in predictable ways that derive from ancestral memories and cultures. Memories and cultures inherited from ancient ancestors who lived incestuously in highly endogamous groups that preserved their personalities and survival dispositions—whether aggressive, peaceful or wandering. Whilst civilisation has brought these groups together, forcing coexistence, these personalities and dispositions converge and persist in 'the three main tribes of man', as Watts (2000) put it. Their resilient neurobiology and psychosocial endowments having been inherited by successive generations to help them adapt to their environments. This is the essence of genetic memory—the actual or failed reaction to a life event that is remembered by neural cells and retained in a memory that is passed to posterity via the reproductive cells.

Assimilation, which is a condition of our relatively modern civilisation, means we cannot claim to be a pure specimen of any one tribe, but our ancestral instincts are preserved in our rather stable although randomly selected genetics, and those of one group will usually be dominant, giving rise to predictable behaviour patterns that govern the ways we live, or would live if our way of being were not modified by our lived experience. This begins, naturally, with our genetic selection, which is a fairly random process that could mean settler parents produce warrior children and warrior parents produce nomadic children. This means we can be born to and socialised by parents from whom we have very different survival instincts and personality traits, and this is important insofar as it has a clouding effect on our authentic self and what strengths and weaknesses come to us naturally.

Consider the settler parents who—consciously or unconsciously—socialise their warrior child to 'go with the flow and roll with the punches', whereas the child's disposition is to go against the flow and intercept the punches. Or the warrior parents who condition their settler child to 'hit back against the bully', whereas reporting the bully to an adult—say a parent, coach or teacher—with responsibilities for child safety feels more natural to the child. Or the settler grandparent who encourages the nomadic grandchild to apologise for misgivings and to make peace in relationships, when what comes naturally to the grandchild is to terminate stressful relationships and move on to others, presumably less stressful ones.

The idea is that, beginning with life in utero, we are primed for the social world in which our genetics anticipate we will live, and the personality disposition with which a child exposed to psychosocial stress in utero debuts in the world will inform that child's adaptive defences to adversity throughout the life cycle. Moreover, when psychosocial stress lingers and qualifies as trauma, adaptive defences can undermine well-being and promote suffering. It is in this sense that predispositions to compensate for vulnerabilities and survive adversity with which children come into the social world are maladaptive. In a world of unrelenting stress, these maladaptive defences run the gamut from the highly adrenalised hyperreactive fight-or-flight responses to the moderately adrenalised hyporeactive float, fold, and furrow that inform and predict the life outcome of the surviving generation but are no less communicable across generations. It is this communicability that winds up the conversation on how the legacy of psychosocial trauma happens and introduces the conversation on where and why it happens.

Chapter 8

Psychosocial Trauma across Generations

In Practice

We have explored how adaptive defences to psychosocial stress are primed before we are born, beginning with the energy-catalysing mitochondrion that power every cell in our body and continuing with the sensibility we derive from our parents' reaction to psychosocial stress, which, incidentally, seasons our own native stress response circuitry. We affirmed that our need for somato-psycho-emotional attunement and relational safety—our native SPEARS—is also established before birth and fulfilling this need is essential for resilient well-being as well as recovery from psychosocial trauma, a mandate that connects us to our ancestry. This addressed the 'how' question of intergenerational transmission of wisdom, psychosocial trauma and vulnerability to disintegration, but not quite why psychosocial legacies that set up vulnerabilities to adverse life outcomes are sustained and at times revered among survivors. In exploring this question, I turn to my own ancestry for insight.

I am fortunate to have, as my bequest, precise events of adversity across five generations of my family that I can interrogate to make sense of psychosocial trauma and dispositions that predict and promote specific life outcomes. I'll begin this interrogation here, with a goal in this chapter to explore psychosocial trauma as it persists across generations, entwined with the spirits of family, religiosity, community and schooling that establish in us a necessary sense of connection and belonging, and, as such, are important forces of socialisation. This sense of connection and belonging addresses the two important questions of why trauma happens and why psychosocial legacies that set up vulnerabilities to adverse life outcomes are sustained and at times revered among survivors.

PSYCHOSOCIAL TRAUMA IN INTERGENERATIONAL
FAMILY LIFE

The Spirit of Family: Vector of Psychosocial Trauma

My aunt Shona scored 14 out of 21 on the ALEs scale. As you will recall from the preface, a score of 12 out of 21 or higher corresponds with a particularly difficult childhood, and where it includes the loss of a father through abandonment or premature death, it corelates with unrelenting poverty and suicidality, in addition to a nearly 500 percent increased chance of suffering with a debilitating disease—such as asthma, diabetes, hypertension and mental disorder. This score also suggests that as Shona moved through life, she or a close relative would be hospitalised or medicated for a severe psychiatric condition, such as alcoholism, anxiety, depression, eating disorder or schizophrenia, and would require adjustments for a special need because of severe disease or disability.

Shona's first son, Shem, who like me was brought up until early teenage years mainly by our grandmother, had an ALEs score of 7, half of which came from childhood psychosocial traumas that included premature separation and abandonment by natural parents and, until the age of six, suffering with asthma. His total score, however, points to a degree of adversity throughout his life from which he could recover with support and nourishing SPEARS. Two of Shem's four daughters, being raised by their mother in a single-parent household, suffer with asthma and, incidentally, premature separation and abandonment by a natural parent.

Shona was one month gestating in 1962 when her mother, my grandmother—whom I call Nan—twenty-six years old and already a mother of six, married Shona's father, my grandfather, Nixon, then thirty-two. Nan tells me this marriage was a haphazard event against her mother's wishes and her own instincts. Her godmother and Nixon's father were the guests. My mother, Lily, was ten months old, and Shona would arrive eight months later. Nan tells me this was a time of grief and uncertainty. The sudden death in 1957 of her fifteen-month-old baby son, Marcel, had left her awfully worried about her children's safety.

Nan and grandfather were step-siblings, connected in an extended family when Nan's mother, Christina, married Nixon's father, Laurence. Both Christina and Laurence were casual labourers on British colonial estates but they also owned fertile lands, which they had inherited informally from their slave-holding Scottish ancestors. They were able to farm subsistently, and for themselves and their children there was enough to eat. Children were plentiful and helpful on the farm, and Laurance practiced spiritual medicine, from which he earned a little as a healer.

Nixon lost his own mother when he was four years old and was for the most part cared for by his teenage sister. Through this experience, he was acquainted with the trauma of losing a significant attachment figure in early childhood. By the age of thirty-two and after seven children with Nan (including Shona in utero), he was eager to marry and build a home and threatened to desert the family in this bid, a threat that echoed the vulnerability to sexual predation, childhood pregnancy and education and socioeconomic underachievement he knew to be associated with fatherlessness in families and against which he was confident Nan would want to protect her children. Nan was encouraged to marry him as a way to ensure he stayed present and available to their children, as a father who would keep them safe and whose ways they would follow, even though his ways—in line with his time—were hash, often injurious and adapted to securing obedience and submission. This shaped submissive, suggestible and otherwise manageable children through a regime of discipline that did little to acknowledge or promote the children's agency and authenticity and did more to value the lack of inconvenience in his parenting. My uncle Antoine recalled, 'He was a nice man, very nice. He would take me places. To garden, to fish with him. But he was always ready to beat us. If I'd do something wrong, he'd make me kneel down on a [aluminium] grater until my knees bleed' (interview, 2022).

At this level of the psychosocial, the children in relationship with their parent are learning that self-expression portends pain. There is also the equally potent emotional messaging that people who love them also hurt them, people who provide for them materially inflict pain upon their body, and to avoid being hurt further, they should not fight back. We might argue that this messaging is harmful to a child's sense of self and explore it at the level where, for the warrior child in particular, it undermines his authentic self, which may never develop fully.

Equally importantly, however, is that this socialisation serves a model of life wherein people are violent in relationships, and more so when the offender is resourced, whether materially, physically or relationally. Small children, whatever their disposition, are limited in capacity to protect their mind and body from assault. Escaping from the stressor is also not ordinarily a safe choice. Their native defence system under these conditions, nonetheless, is compelled to promote their survival, and one way it might do this is by flooding their bloodstream with endogenic opioids to numb the pain. Through this measure, the child survives this protracted state of adversity as a settler.

This occurs at the intersection of the psychosocial and neurobiological, where the need for somato-psycho-emotional attunement and relational safety (native SPEARS) is forfeited at the expense of survival. Every cell in the child's body is enlisted and energised to fulfil this native need. Now disrupted, somato-psycho-emotionality becomes informed by violence and woundedness, and a perverse blend of love and loathing sets up the developing child's relational expectations. Among those expectations is that relationships in which love and provisions are exchanged are ones in which pain and loathing are experienced.

Incidentally, this is the condition in which confusion, disintegration and inauthenticity in the self sets in and normalises. As the American psychologist Janina Fisher (2017) puts it, children experiencing harm at the hands of loved ones are disposed to split their minds—and self by extension—in order to survive. Part of them is forced to carry on masking their woundedness while the part hosting the wound remains guarded, hidden, ashamed and even hopeless.

This trauma-based adaptation allows the child to survive protracted adversity and remain connected to loved ones, and by extension sources of provision. But this is occurring at the expense of the child's wounded self that retains the sense of deficit and shamefulness and, as such, is alienated and uninvited to belong. The wounded self's alienation from the rest of the self reflects neuropsychosocial disintegration, which is how the child will move through life, strung out, in a sense, on a toxic neurochemical cocktail of love and loathing. Love as in emotional connection and sustenance, and loathing is about emotional disconnection and starvation, a state of safety and danger that, when activated, forces love and loathing to follow each other, much like left and right. For the social-emotional nerves that regulate sensations of safety and danger, this is a dysregulated state in which confusion occurs. In a neural sense, love is invoking the neurochemistry of hate, and hate is invoking the neurochemistry of love. Think of the paradox 'I hurt you because I love you'. The nervous system remembers, stores and automates this association as it is repeated over time, frequently triggered and enthused with an unbounded flow of chaotic energy. When triggered, the survivor is reacting to the pain as it is inscribed in memory in the wounded, alienated self, first at the emotional level but also in the soma.

Incidentally, the familiar neurochemistry of shame, grief and guilt that fuels this reaction also acts to suppress virtuous and resilient personality traits. The child, thus, is not only cheated in the development of emotional, psychological and relational competencies but is also disposed to respond to life events with maladaptive traits. This provides another aha moment that helps me make sense of Shona's ALEs score, which reflects her generational experience and that of her eleven siblings. Given their childhood experience of severe relational distress and neuroses surrounding death, desertion and poverty, their vulnerability to severe disease and disability seems predestined, emerging behaviourally in their early life. We've met my mother earlier. Born a healthy baby, she didn't learn to walk until she was two years old. As childhood egoism has it, this might have been her way of expressing she wasn't ready for this life and the autonomy to survive on her own feet it demanded of her. But, more importantly, it confirms that prenatal baby Shona's and postnatal baby Lily's neural systems developed under conditions of prolonged distress.

They were nursed throughout the entire year following Nan's marriage, a time when newlyweds, in a contemporary sense, would be in a phase of bliss and sweetness. Nonetheless, life was fairly optimistic, certainly with unconditional love in the home, essential anointing in herbal baths and homemade castor oil, and enough health-promoting food to eat. Nan nurtured her children, and my grandfather provided within his means, until he died suddenly in 1970, at the age of forty, from viral dysentery, leaving Nan with nine young children. The eldest, daughter Monnet, was fifteen years old, and the youngest, baby Dian, was six months old. The neurosis surrounding death and paternal desertion noted earlier may have indeed been a prescience of what was to come.

The Spirit of Religiosity: Vector of Psychosocial Trauma

My grandfather was buried within twenty-four hours of his passing. And, without delay, Nan managed to pay the Catholic Church in the nearest town of Portsmouth the ten Eastern Caribbean dollars for a Mass she was led to believe was necessary before his soul could make its way to heaven. The French priest, Fr. Rene Parry (1920–2012), accepted to oversee this sacred task. However, on learning of the circumstance surrounding my grandfather's passing and the misery that was about to unfold in the family, he offered to help Nan with provisions in exchange for sex. In shame and confusion from her perception of the 'Holy Father' as undefiled by intimacy with women, she politely declined but 'held it for him'. In her words:

> I was so ashamed, I know they not supposed to have sex with women, and they not supposed to get married, so I said no, I said no. He had it [his erect penis] in front of him, so he asked me to hold it in my hand for him. So, I hold it in my hand for him until it went back normal, and he gave me a Bible, the best gift I've ever had. But I never went back, I don't even know if he did the Mass. But I gave him the money. (Interview, 2022)

Recall that shame is a depletive emotion that responds to the sense that we are defective as we are naturally. Along with confusion, wherein expectation and reality are in conflict, shame gives rise to disintegration in the self, which splits to hide it and survive in its grip. As in much of the Americas, religiosity and its conduits—churches, Bobo Shanti houses, mosques—offer recourse for this misery, playing a significant role in Caribbean life and welfare through inspiring hope and offering of provisions that cannot be overlooked (Gilbert & Coyte, 2007).

Believers' psychological health, for instance, benefits from the offering of 'confession' therapy in church. Religious authorities, such as the 'fathers' of the Catholic Church, although unlikely to be trained mental health professionals, are psychologically savvy and competent in counselling, even if only in a pious sense. This is especially true for those inclined to promote faith and reliance on a compassionate God in times of hardship. God—the generous, merciful and loving—represents a distraction from feelings that are upsetting and dysregulating, which is what we understand as emotional distress. In this spirit of religiosity, there is a sense that God's grace is enough to overcome hardship. There is also the moral token in the self-sacrifice of Jesus that inspires believers in times of distress to appeal to the Almighty for guidance and mercies. As such, it would not be insensible for a grief-stricken widow to seek out mercy and 'confess' her woes to her 'father' in a bid for compassion, hope and perhaps catharsis. My grandmother, however, was sexually abused and had her trust in this sacred relationship shattered, a traumatic spell that, she'd say, not only hijacked the spirit of her religiosity but also compounded the layers of unmetabolised psychosocial trauma already besieging the family. This event occurred because the other conditions were present.

The Spirit of Community: Vector of Psychosocial Trauma

The cruel and overwhelming experience of lack that quickly took root in the family was distinct in that, unlike the women of her descent, Nan had never worked as an income generator.[1] In itself, this was not unfavourable. However, alongside her lack of education in the then not-so-distantly emancipated British slave colony, her prospect for respite was pitiful. With little access to resources and in service of her children's welfare, she could only channel her ancestral adaptive impulse to relinquish parental response-ability and 'shifted' the care of some of her children to extended family members whom she considered decent and 'better off'. Customarily, this is a practice that functions to nourish the spirit of community, which she felt would serve her children well, for it is the community that embraces and raises the child, who will not burn it down to feel its warmth. In reality, however, the children's experience was one of maltreatment, including neglect and sexual abuse.

Incidentally, the maltreatment of children is inscribed in our ancestral memory, and children of the Americas, 'stamped from the beginning' (Kendi, 2017), are ordinarily exposed to cruelty in family and community life. We

---

[1] I use this term to account for the enslaved women of my ancestry who laboured to generate income and wealth not for themselves and their families but for their enslavers.

could think of this memory as a collection of secrets, strategies and practices bequeathed to us by our ancestors that we can use in order to survive. But it appears that we often cannot distinguish between what is good or necessary and what is not.

My aunt Monnet's first experience of sexual abuse came at the hands of her grandfather, my great-grandfather, and is a poignant example I have the misfortune of eliciting from my ancestry to speak to this reality. She was eight years old when it happened and was warned by him that he would cause her father, his son, to whip her should she disobey or reveal the 'secret'. This kind of 'secret event' is traumatic for a child, but what it highlights is that the child's socialisation surrounding self-worth, body autonomy and safety—or lack thereof—in caregiving relationships in her family and community is consistent with a need to survive conditions of dehumanisation. This occurs in conditions wherein she is not perceived as vulnerable and in need of protection, in which her value is in her body and her body is a source of pain and suffering, which she bears in service of her caregiver's gratification. This message contradicts the nascent need for healthy, caring and attentive relationship in which a child develops intelligence SPEARS that promote self-regulation and neuropsychosocial integration. Moreover, as she cannot prevent nor be protected from this suffering, she learns to negotiate its intensity by adapting her behaviour and folding herself in ways that aligned with the expectations of others, especially the expectation that she would be subjected to abuse and violence in her relationships as she moves through life. This would play out with remarkable precision, for instance, in her relationship with the man by whom she would become pregnant at the age of seventeen and go on to have five children. It was an injurious attachment relationship that mirrored the ones she had with her father and grandfather, in which she and her young children were exposed to sexual abuse and battery before being deserted. In this case, they were deserted not because of premature death but by calculated abandonment.

ALEs scores ranging from 10 to 16 out of 21 across the two generations correspond with incidences of aloneness, difficulty building close and trusting relationships, self-harm, suicidality and clinical intervention for severe psychiatric conditions such as alcoholism, schizophrenia and eating and mood disorders. Loss of a father, submission to a predatory community spirit, and protracted exposure to violence—physical and sexual—in childhood predict a lifetime of misery. In addition to the recycling of abuse and violence upon bodies and minds across the generations, trauma-based adaptations play out in caregiving relationships in which it is not safe to express authentic emotions. However, the attendant sadness, fear and anger from being betrayed and violated are real and—charged with unbounded chaotic energy—these implant in the nervous system as psychosocial trauma. Until this energy is bounded and discharged, the trauma will be a source of disease the inauthentic self will be inclined to hide, and it will disturb and hurt the body. It may express itself perceptively, such as in body aches, diabetes and hypertension, or psychologically, as dissociative cognition, wherein the survivor's own thoughts are alien to them. Behaviourally, it may be expressed in self-loathing, self-harm and misadventures that point to self-abandonment for the sake of attending to the needs of others. In disposition, one could also think of this as an expression of the settler's fold-fawn response. What is also evident is how its power is sustained and encouraged in social relationships, which leads me to the relationship with the Judaeo-Christian ministries that provided basic schooling in the community in exchange for observance of religious doctrines they promote.

The Spirit of Education: Vector of Psychosocial Trauma

This was the educational opportunity to which my mother and some of her siblings had access. In its design, the prescribed tradition of servitude and subjugation it enforced left a legacy designed to exact obedience and subjugation whilst suppressing the free thought, imagination, curiosity and agency to problem-solve that are conducive to progressive citizenship and actualisation of authenticity in the self. The implications of this tradition continue to echo in my family life in socioeconomic marginalisation and psychosomatic maladies. For instance, Shona explains the chronic anxiety she has suffered with since her father's passing as a 'disabling sensation' in her chest cavity. Uncle Antoine describes his lifelong nocturnal enuresis as 'something' he will 'never talk about'. And morbid ideations across the generations reflect a hopeless sense of lack and helplessness that are characteristic of the settler's furrow and nomad's float. These maladies are clearly sequelae of inadequate and perhaps inappropriate education surrounding well-being across the generations, but they are also telling of an ancestral legacy that holds reverence.

The Spirit of Ancestral Legacy: Vector of Psychosocial Trauma and Recovery

Whilst a diversity of experiences has contributed to poor life outcomes across the five generations in my family, I want to circle back to two events with which I believe these outcomes originate: Nan's marriage in 1962 and her husband's death in 1970. This is to acknowledge, first, that premature marriage and death are ALEs that are overwhelming and deeply traumatising, and, second, they evoke psychosocial adaptations that sustain misery across generations. The first of these traumas, Nan's premature marriage, set her up with a sense of security as a vulnerable mother of young children. And the

second, when that security was shattered, brought loss that continued to surface in the life of her children, grandchildren and great-grandchildren, manifesting, for instance, as chronic anxiety in Shona and Dian, who were infants
at the time, as asthma in 50 percent of their children and grandchildren, and
in a palpable apathy towards the brute limitations of being poor lone parents
across the generations.

All of this points to the specific life events that overwhelmed Nan's native
and adaptive defences and betrayed her ancestral wisdom, which, incidentally, were primed to effectively contextualise and respond to psychosocial
stress and to promote self-agency, as evident in her recounting of Shona's son
Shem's last asthma attack in 1986:

> He woke up and was calling, 'Granny? Granny?' He couldn't breathe, and his
> medicine had finish. So, I picked him up and put him on my chest. He was four
> years old, but he had it from since he was three months. He was breathing heavy,
> so I put him on my lap and started rubbing him, rubbing him. Then his breathing
> started to get better, so I started to pray, and he fell asleep on my lap. When he
> fell asleep, I put him down and went to bed, but still waiting to hear if he gets
> up. All of you were there sleeping on the floor. I was tired, but I was waiting.
> Then a few hours later, I heard him call again, 'Granny? Granny?' I get up, he
> was coughing this time. I pick him up again, put him on my chest. I had some
> soft candle [container wax]. I melted some in a teaspoon and give him to drink,
> and continue rubbing him, rubbing him, until he coughed up the thing [sputum].
> Then I put him on my chest again until he fall sleep. That was the last time, he
> never had it again and he never needed the medicine. (Interview, 2022)

Over three decades later, now at age forty-one, Shem remains asthma free
and hardly ever unwell. Even as an active husband, a father of five and crafts-
man, he has Nan present in his life as his safe person. Happenstance, magic
or advanced science? The answer is all three. For in addition to good old
luck, 'any advance in science is indistinguishable from magic', as science
fiction writer Arthur Clarke wrote (2000). To make sense of this life event,
we must look to ancestry for insight into childcare rituals that bring recovery
from childhood disorders and disease and the science of how mammals care
for their babies in ways that promote resilient well-being. Beginning with the
understanding that children who experience premature separation, isolation
or neglect or who are caused to suffer unnecessarily in any other way by their
natural parents and other caregivers are prone to develop chronic diseases and
disorders from the inevitable distress and protracted internal dysregulation
brought on by their suffering. Recovery and resilience come with internal
regulation and reversing these ALEs.

It turns out that a caregiver's regulated nervous system can be engaged
to co-regulate a care recipient's dysregulated nervous system. The calming

rhythms of a caregiver's body promote energy transfer to the care recipient and proffer somato-psycho-emotional regulation, an antidote to the nervous system hyperactivation that gives rise to psychosomatic diseases, such as asthma. This is the mammalian way to soothe anxious babies, bring calm and reassurance to those with whom they are securely attached, and build resilience in their body and mind. By instinct, Nan enlisted her nervous system to effectively acquaint Shem with his three essential SPEARS: first, his native need for somato-psycho-emotional attunement and relational safety; second, his somatic, psychological, emotional, adaptive, reflective and social intelligences; and third, his somatic harmony, psychological integrity, emotional attunement, relational satisfaction and self-authenticity. This is the nervous system anchored in safety as chemistry is exchanged in neural networks to evoke and fortify sensations of resilient well-being. But also to fuel inner motivations and sensations of fulfilment that affect bodily functions, movement and memory.

The motivation and fulfilment system, known otherwise as the mesocortical limbic pathway, connects the ventral tegmental area (VTA) with the nucleus accumbens and ventral striatum in a dopamine circuitry that moves us to do more of what fulfils us and helps us to stay vigilant when our safety or the safety of our loved ones might be in peril. It rewards us, too, when we find comfort in prayer. This was Nan's experience after her sacred appeals in

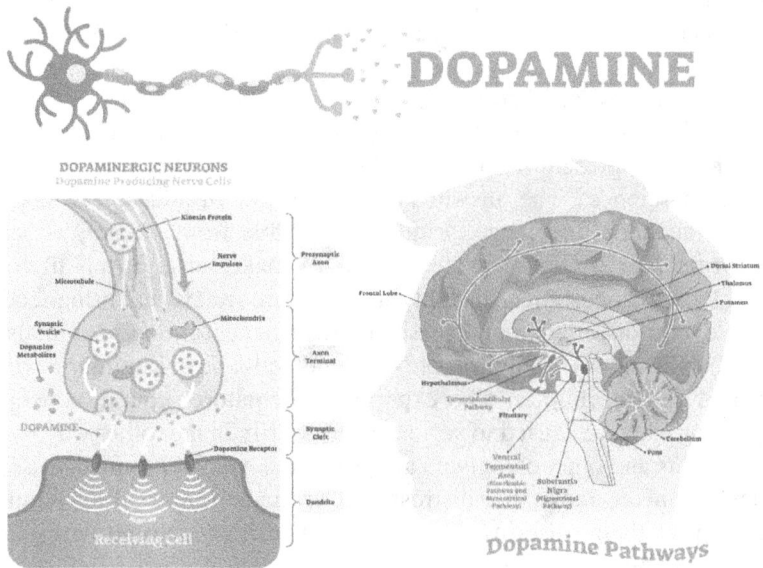

Figure 8.1. Motivation and Fulfilment Neural Circuitry. Functions include reward motivation, motor function, compulsion and perseveration. *Image © VectorMine / iStock / Getty.*

times of need, not only to keep her grandson alive in the midst of a vicious asthma attack but also for answers about my selective mutism and childhood autism, my younger sister's unspecified developmental delays and just about any malady with which we turned up in childhood. By providing us with a consistent and reliable emotionally nourishing relationship within which we learned to relate with joy and warmth and develop the important skills of meaningful communication and problem-solving, Nan effectively eliminated our neuroses—psychosocial trauma, neurobiological dysregulation and deviant epigenetic regulations—and in so doing reversed not only our psychosomatic maladies but also our insecurities and neurodevelopmental disorders that coloured our experience in the social world.

When at age eleven I was struck by a careless cyclist and sustained a hindbrain injury that was thought to have impaired my declarative memory system permanently, with prayer and resilience SPEARS Nan found a fix for that too. What she tells me about prayer is that it is a reach inside, into the depth of vulnerability, to connect with the divine Spirit in a space where the unknown becomes known and what cannot be known is accepted as such. Thus, praying to a compassionate, forgiving and loving divine God is in itself cathartic, as it is evocative of a comforting psycho-emotional state wherein solutions to difficult and seemingly unsolvable problems are found.

This is self-possession, and to acknowledge it is to invoke one's own divinity and courage to reach deep inside and discover sacred wisdom that might even be ancestral. Like the very kind that led Nan to the wax candle and its miracle healing powers. Incidentally, wax candle is a staple medicine in Caribbean healing that originated with our ancestors, who believed it helped to release tension in soft body tissues, increase blood flow and minimize muscle spasms. This wisdom—passed on to their descendants—prevailed in keeping baby Shem alive and, as Nan says, 'curing his asthma'. But there is also the ordinary 'I don't know how, I know I prayed and then I had the mind to try certain things, and you all were cured . . . that's it'.

LEGACY OF TRANSGENERATIONAL TRAUMA IN DESTINY

I mentioned earlier that Nan, at eighty-eight, is in remarkably good health, which is reflected in her vitality, mobility, freedom and deep sense of purpose. She is also sufficiently literate from having used the Bible given to her by Fr. Parry to teach herself to read, and she has since read her Bible daily. This fondness for reading and engaging with literary information daily is a habit I picked up from her early in our relationship, and to this day it is often the subject of our conversations, much like everything health related. When I asked her how she is in better health than her children, she tells me first 'it's God's work'. But, more importantly, she believes stress 'defiles' the body, and she is not inclined to retain stress beyond what is necessary. To appreciate this adaptation, in itself a trauma response, is to appreciate the social history that prepared her for the life she leads, a history in which her ancestors were enslaved in the Caribbean under conditions of structured dehumanisation that wounded their bodies, minds and spirits for hundreds of years. By all measure, this is the most protracted adverse lived experience in contemporary history.

So deeply destructive was the experience of chattel slavery in the Caribbean that survival rates among the enslaved were frighteningly low, with over 50 percent in some territories being dead within a year of arrival from Africa (Kendi, 2017). A mere ten miles from the village of Woodford Hill where I spent my childhood with Nan, the old Castle Bruce Sugar Estate in the northeast of Dominica continues to preserve this memory. 'Something terrible must have happened' there before emancipation in 1834, Joseph Sturge and Thomas Harvey (2007) wrote in *The West Indies in 1837*. Along with 224 deaths and 51 births, the record of enslaved persons had fallen from 281 to 162, for whom the absentee owner, Sir Lawrence Dundas, Earl of Zetland, was compensated £3,317 at the loss of their servitude. This reward reflected the prevalent but nonetheless cruel idea that the value of life, as of relationships, is in the currency and capital it generates.

The more disturbing reality, however, remains that the fewness of births as well as the fearful number of deaths on that estate reflect the unforgiving condition of slavery in the Caribbean. I am bound to imagine that our enslaved ancestors who survived long enough—since we are here—did so with exceptional adaptations in their psyche, epigenetics and neurobiology. I could begin with the uterine environment in which the slave child was introduced to this world, but more appropriate is the sense the child's nervous system made of this world with the help of mothers' stress-regulatory corticosteroids (Buss et al., 2012), which of course reflected the reality that the child could die prematurely, would eventually be enslaved and the mother's worry about relinquishment and the attendant lost opportunity to nurture in her child the positive self-image necessary for relational competency. The emotional, psychological and relational adaptations to these traumas point to disintegration that preserves survival and allows for the conceptualisation of psychosocial trauma as a life event that fulfils the need to preserve life in the face of adversity. This happens, and with this there is also the necessary radical acceptance rooted in ancient traditions of letting go of expectations and not overinvesting in experiences that stoke pain and over which we do not have control. This speaks to a need to accept harsh conditions of life for what they are, even when accountability is unassigned, conditions such as children and parents sold apart at the whim of enslavers, and so creating traumas that betray intimacy and promote emotional apathy as an appropriate adaptation.

Today, the practice of shifting childcare responsibility from natural parents to relatives, neighbours or even friends is an established pattern of family life in the Caribbean that is believed to promote a spirit of community (Russell-Brown et al., 1996). But it is a practice that clinical psychologists persuasively argue is traumatic for a child and no longer serves the purpose for which it was entertained by our ancestors. It is a risk factor for suffering in young children—when they are separated from their natural family for extended and uncertain periods of time—associated with poor health, economic and social outcomes. The consensus in developmental psychology is that this setup occurs within the first three years of life. Hence, not getting those early years right is not only linked to noncommunicable psychosomatic maladies but also to violent behaviours, poverty and, at a national level, lower rates of economic growth and social development.

Even so, the value in 'child shifting'—though established under the conditions of slavery—cannot be overlooked, especially since it retains ancestral wisdom, in much the same way as ancestral medicine does. Consider how the wax candle the enslaved used to fuel fire lamps was leveraged as medicine to save life. This wisdom was invaluable in healthcare at the time of emancipation and thereafter, for the impoverished formerly enslaved would not have access to the limited conventional medicine and certainly not a penny of the twenty million pounds Britain awarded to slave owners for 'loss of property' (Slavery Abolition Act, 1833, sec. 24). Today, this wisdom and tradition continue to serve descendants, and it would be unkind and arbitrary to give them up, much like the raising of grandchildren, which brings bliss and fulfilment to grandparents in our cultures.

Beyond the will to survive—bearing ancestral wisdom—this is also about freedom and purpose, for example, to assemble, dance, drink rum, join religion and gain literacy, and ultimately to love and raise their children and grandchildren with self-determination, even if tainted with the sense that material security involves surmounting multigenerational layers of grief and overcoming a multigenerational legacy of impoverishment. Where this security is achieved, it will be marginal, fragile and easily lost, for absolute material security is false. To the initiated, this sense can be frustrating but not at all alien, for it is grounded in our ancestral story, which cautions contemporary generations and empowers them for the future.

This is perhaps the best way to appreciate the value in ancestral history that is reinforced by psychosocialisation, the process by which we refine our SPEARS and strengthen across generations, overcoming our frightening experiences that are liable to influence our sense of self and the parents we become. Again, in my family, the violent whoopings, exclusions from schooling and emotional neglect that are extant in the lives of the third, fourth and fifth generations can be taken as inherited expressions of dehumanisation and subjugation that are out of place in our time, having originated in our legacy of slavery and serving only to preserve ancestral trauma and trauma-based adaptations.

However, in revisiting my ancestry, I am relieved to perceive a profound—even if quiet—yearning for change, beginning with my grandfather's effort to ensure he was a valiant protector and provider whom his children would know and be proud of. It continued in Nan's marriage as an undertaking to protect her children, her commitment to raising her children, her acquisition of literacy from which I would benefit and her commitment to raising her grandchildren and ensuring we were somatically safe, psychologically integrous, emotionally attuned and relationally fulfilled. These efforts reflect in a diversity of lived experiences in the population of her seventy descendants across four generations. However, the chaotic energy of specific events of adversity in her life signalled to her children that the social world is nerve-wrecking and that being a nervous wreck is one way to survive. Incidentally, the social world in which they would live their childhood and adult lives is one that is besieged by nerve-wrecking experiences of poverty, racism and socioeconomic marginalisation, in the face of which their adaptive defences were inadequate.

I have talked about chronic anxiety afflicting this generation and asthma among their children and grandchildren to suggest that a vulnerability was inherited, rather than the diseases per se. This vulnerability was embedded in their nervous system, the master host of our entire human story that allows us to navigate the terrains of life, meandering around adversities to arrive in relationships with ourselves, our environment and others. But every so often, the nervous system falls short in its adaptability, and we come to these relationships frightened, bruised and at times broken. Whatever our condition, it will be transmitted in one form or another to our posterity. Perhaps in the body as a disease, in the mind as dis-ease or in the spirit as the quiet yet desperate yearning for relief from sufferings, whether inherited from our ancestors or the ones we acquire in our own lifetime. That is the source of deficits in our stress response, which manifests as psychosomatic maladies, which are expressions of neuropsychosocial disintegration.

TRANSGENERATIONAL NEUROPSYCHOSOCIAL DISINTEGRATION

Summarily, neuropsychosocial disintegration begins with a disturbance in the nervous system and moves on to how we show up in the social world, how we function and respond to life events. This disturbance contains biological and psychosocial components, and it is the psychosocial that I have conceptualised as a trauma embedded in the nervous system that is sustained by unbounded chaotic energy. My insight into my ancestral story tells me that unless this kind of trauma is surfaced and discharged of its energy, it will not only make its way across generations but will also block access to authentic self-expressions. Social history that honours ancestry is important in parsing this trauma, and the consequence of disregarding it can be severe. It may mean that survivors get the message they cannot be understood and—for Alex—the sense that the relationship with his therapist is in deficit. In other words, he is not encouraged to evoke his inner wisdom and capacities on his journey of authentic self-discovery; hence, the therapeutic relationship cannot sufficiently meet the goal of wellness he seeks.

This experience can be further psychologically wounding and inhibiting in the pursuit of recovery. It is truly a cycle of trauma-traumatised-trauma that plays out within the context of relationship. This includes the relationship one has with one's own self as well as with other entities and the world. Relationships, it is clear, are central to the functioning of life, and the way that survivors of trauma and disintegration experience relationships is central to their success in accessing recovery, integration and resilient well-being, a process that is not without tension. Undertaking to recover authenticity in the self and integrate the body and mind is one event; to achieve these outcomes is quite another. The chapters in part IV discuss structures, principles and processes that are implicated in this task.

Part IV

NEUROPSYCHOSOCIAL INTEGRATION IN PROCESS

Chapter 9

Neuropsychosocial Integration

Structures, Resources and Processes

Part III explored psychosocial trauma as it gives occasion to psychosomatic maladies and neuropsychosocial disintegration that persist across generations. Psychosocial trauma is also understood to manifest in the self by inhibiting authentic expression and congruity with the first purpose of life—the preservation of life itself. In this chapter, we shall learn how this comes together in the expression of life, beginning with an exploration of discernible structures that are enlisted to bring about a transformation in the mind and body, followed by the resources and principles that are implicated in this course and along the journey from neuropsychosocial disintegration to integration.

NEUROPSYCHOSOCIAL INTEGRATION
ESSENTIAL STRUCTURES

The essential structures for neuropsychosocial integration encompass social history, social psyche, social environment and the social engagement nerve that intersects the neurobiological and psychosocial.

Social History in Neuropsychosocial Integration

Social history encompasses social and historical narratives and templates that promote our survival. Naturally, this includes surviving protracted ALEs— whether psychosocial trauma in childhood, environmental disasters, social exclusion or even chattel slavery. The important question for the sufferer is, 'How did those before me survive comparable situations?' The intelligence SPEARS help to answer this important question. But much of the response will be recycled in allegories and received wisdom and inscribed in the social psyche to be recalled and deployed when needs arise. According to Maduro (2018), the psyche functions like a central storage facility for resources that can be drawn upon to survive the inevitable challenges life brings. These are resources—aptly conceptualised as psychosocial—that bear implications for how we show up in the world, make sense of our experiences and respond to life events. More precisely, psychosocial resources encompass skills, beliefs, talents, personality factors, sense of mastery, agency, esteem and social support with which we appraise psychosocial stressors and manage psychosocial stress, in a way that promotes well-being and resilience in the body and mind.

Thus, psychosocial resources, whether native or adaptive, are fuelled by the same mitochondrial energy that sustains the body and mind, an energy so important to life that it is elevated to the status of a deity in some cultures. In Hindu theology, for instance (Singer, 2007), this is the goddess Shakti, who fuels survival instincts and links descendants across generations in an unbroken chain. We inherit the catalyst for this energy from our mother, and she will, for up to the first ten months of our life, co-regulate the rhythm of this energy as she holds us inside of her body and prepares us for the social world in which we will live.

This is a good place from which we can begin to appreciate the import of social history as it structures our life and promotes our survival. We have at this stage a mother sharing with her developing child—as they are deeply connected and exist as one—the emotions and sensations whirling inside her body and mind. These may be love, gratitude and hopefulness, but this is a book about psychosocial trauma, so it could also be anger, sadness, shame, grief and guilt. Sensations of psychosocial stress she will share with her child, and the impact of these will show up in psychosocial capacities and behavioural impulses with which the child moves through the social world, absorbing its history but also creating a story that will be passed to future generations in neurobiology and socialisation. Directorship in how this story develops and transmits is a feat of agency that I strive to encourage in my students. In my own story, it began with the emotions and sensations that were whirling inside my own mother, which she directly shared with me as a developing foetus. These included her sadness at finding out she was pregnant with a child for whom she could not sufficiently provide emotionally or materially; anger from finding out she was deceived by my much older father, who had his own nuclear family in a different country; anxiety at being a vulnerable teenager in a country very different from her own; and other sensations of stresses both inside her body and in her social environment.

These are experiences for which she prepared me when I was developing inside her body and the impact of which would show up in my childhood autism, but also in my psychosocial resourcefulness and behavioural patterns in adult life, as I arrived in the world primed for adversity with a desperate need for solutions, intolerance for my own vulnerability and the neural conditions for the fiercely self-directed and cautious nomad that I am. It is a personality I happen to share with the wise barn owl that thinks deeply and hunts quietly far and away for solutions to difficult problems. So dominant is this personality since my childhood that when I was struck by a cyclist at age eleven, my upset upon regaining consciousness was not that I had been hurt but that the experience had left me incapacitated in my task to solve my own life problems, and to this day I cannot recall the event that led up to that state. In service of my survival, my nervous system, it appears, safely tucked away the memory in my unconsciousness or failed to lay it down in support of my personality. My grandmother's available wisdom in overcoming aversity and commitment to my recovery and well-being beyond this event certainly helped. She would ensure that she stayed attuned to my bodily as well as my psychological and social needs, to fulfil them in a way that prevented dysregulation and disintegration from taking root in my still developing nervous system. This brings me back to the neuropsychosocial, which we learned in the opening chapter binds the neurobiological and psychosocial in a structured relationship, and their synchroneity preserves a degree of functional integration. But before social history can play its part in this process, it must be accurately integrated into the psyche, from where it must be expressed to promote this integration.

Social Psyche in Neuropsychosocial Integration

In social neuroscience, the psyche is perceived as a self-organising system that differentiates and contextualises energy—whether creative and life sustaining or destructive—that flows inward to bodily structures and outward from the body. By this fluid energy flow is not restricted to substructures within the skull or skin. The psyche acts within the body, transducing information into energy; it is intrasomatic. But it is also social in that it exchanges information between bodies; it is intersomatic, and carries out this task without descending into chaos. When it comes to neuropsychosocial integration, this is a state in which the psyche correctly discerns information—such as social-historical events—and appropriately contextualises such information. The opposite is true for disintegration, wherein the psyche fails to appropriately contextualise information or altogether inappropriately differentiates and contextualises information. These are adverse intrapsychic events that ordinarily correspond to psychosocial stress, the kind that precedes psychosomatic maladies, relational conflicts and social disturbance, such as social riots and civil warfare.

An optimally functioning psyche, however, appropriately differentiates and contextualises information in a way that maintains integrity in information flow within and between nervous systems and does not provoke dis-ease or promote disintegration. For these events are occurring within the bounds of our cumulative capacity to tolerate psychosocial stress, what the interpersonal neurobiologist Dan Siegel (2020) calls our 'window of tolerance' for adversity that we develop in our relationships as an extension of our social environment.

Social Environment in Neuropsychosocial Integration

This encompasses the relational experiences—both good and bad—that are reacted upon in the body and mind to shape the psyche and by extension the entire nervous system. I explored some such reactions in the previous chapter as they relate to psychosocial expression. But there is still a lot to say about how life events feature in the body and its neural networks.

We are familiar with the functions of neurons in the brain and spine, but there are also the cranial nerves that exit the brainstem to innervate muscular and sensory processes in service of our survival as we move through life. These nerves are constructed by individual neural cells that bundle together as they travel away from the brain, giving rise to an extensive network of connectivity throughout the body. The literature that explores the diversity of functions carried out by these special nerves is vast, but much of it agrees that they all contribute in some way to our ability to find food, digest, excrete and crucially stay alive and safe. However, in considering the contribution of the social environment to these tasks, we must become acquainted with the activities of the tenth cranial nerve, which I refer to interchangeably as the vagus nerve and the social engagement nerve.

Social Engagement Nerve in Neuropsychosocial Integration

The story of the vagus nerve in contemporary neuropsychology began in 1921 in the dream of the German physiologist Otto Loewi, who discovered its role in the transmission of impulses through the excitatory neurotransmitter we know as acetylcholine. Acetylcholine, in other words, is important for communication in the nervous system, and this includes both motor and sensory signals. It serves the vagus nerve as it carries out its important task of transporting information between the body, brain and the spinal chain. Eighty percent of that information is sensory, moving toward the brain and spine, whilst 20 percent is efferent, moving away from the brain and spine to muscle activities in the peripheral nervous system, that is, in our diaphragm, lungs, gut and similar organs.

Structurally, the vagus nerve is a twin bundle of fibres that divides into a ventral and dorsal branch of the parasympathetic nervous system. *Ventral* means front side; hence, the ventral fibres originate in the front of the brainstem in a neural structure called the nucleus ambiguous. This structure, as is the ventral vagal fibres, is associated with cues of safety and activities that are innervated from the sacral spine in the lower back (see figure 7.1). Through this association, the nerves from the sacral spine inform emotions, behaviours and bodily functions that occur naturally in a state of well-being. This includes the desire to connect and grow in relationship as well as to rest and regenerate, feed, heal, self-care and procreate.

Dorsal, from medieval Latin *dorsalis*, means the back side and lends its name to the vagal circuit that couches behind the fluid-filled third ventricle in the socioemotional midbrain, between the thalamus and hypothalamus and above the pituitary gland. This is a hypothalamic region from where immobilisation originates and in neuropsychosocial disintegration is associated with anergia, hypotension and the attendant chronic fatigue, lethargy and withdrawal of consciousness.

Incidentally, these physiological states are also associated with psychosocial trauma that features social apathy, helplessness, absentmindedness and lack of curiosity that inhibit the survivor via the parasympathetic pathway, creating a state of chronic stuckness in which neuroinflammation inhibits the synthesis of prosocial serotonin, dopamine and noradrenaline. This disease state is a reliable indicator of vagal dysregulation that originates in the cholinergic pathway, as in addition to its responsibility for voluntary movement, acetylcholine is also the chief neurochemical that regulates inflammation in the nervous system by suppressing reactivity in the immune system.

When this unbounded energy is distributed throughout the body, the survivor is liable to lose contact with authenticity and move through life as if absent to him- or herself, a state inversely related to the hypervigilance an activated spinal chain invokes (Rosenberg, 2017). I might refer to this survival state otherwise as sympathetic activation, stress response or simply fight-or-flight. Its neural circuit, in addition to the two vagal circuits, actively regulates somatic and emotional states that reflect in behaviour and reaction to life events, although via different pathways. Consider, for instance, visceral organs in the body cavity that are innervated by the ventral vagal fibres (see figure 9.1).

True to its name, this vagrant wanders down the brainstem, along the side of the neck reaching into the inner ear, behind the carotid artery, down the throat, and around to the front of the body, hugging the lungs, diaphragm, spleen, thymus and intestines on its way to the colon. Meandering in the chest and stomach cavities, it decreases the heart rate and vascular tone to reduce blood pressure; regulates glucose in the liver, insulin secretion from the pancreas and acidity and motility in the gut; suppresses inflammation via the cholinergic pathway; and opposes sympathetic response to stress. In engaging visceral organs on its way from the neck to the colon, the ventral

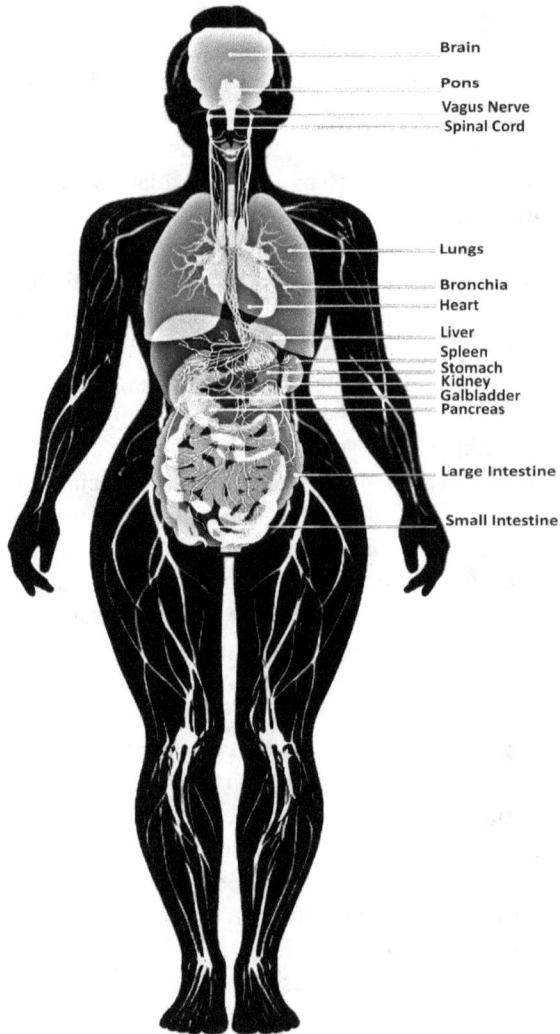

Figure 9.1. The Social Engagement Nerve. Figure courtesy of Dagmar Roelfsema.

nerve also introduces appropriate breaks to do either of two things, to excite or relax visceral tissue to promote life and prosocial behaviour, a necessary condition for neuropsychosocial integration, until otherwise.

The ventral nerve's extensive fibres and critical reach attract and transport pro-inflammatory molecules that circulate in the body. Collectively known as cytokines, these molecules are released by the immune system in response to actual or perceived injury in the body and mind that needs to be limited and signposted for internal therapy. However, in a chronic state of immune defence activation, the state of autoimmunity I talked about earlier and in previous chapters, these molecules are known to cross the blood-brain barrier (BBB) and impact prosocial behaviour by inhibiting serotonin, dopamine and noradrenaline release from neuronal synapses.

There is a big question surrounding the conditions under which the blood-brain barrier can be breached, especially as breaching it goes against the course of nature. In other words, how our brain power comes under siege, when it is meant to be protected by layers of specialized cells that supply the brain tissues with nutrients, shield the brain from toxins in the blood, and filter harmful compounds from the brain back to the bloodstream, to be detoxified by the liver or filtered out of the blood into urine by the kidneys. The answer to this question points to cytokine storms hijacking the ventral vagus nerve under conditions of chronic inflammation to which the barrier is vulnerable. But there are also the neural structures with permeable membranes that allow them to transmit information to and from the brain. The circumventricular organs, for instance, play a role in physiological health by monitoring the content of the bloodstream and relaying this information to the brain so that it can do its job of promoting order and integration in the body and mind. However, by this permeability, free radicals and toxins in the bloodstream can access the brain and evoke pro-inflammatory immune responses from microglial cells—the most prominent resident immune cells of the central nervous system—that protect the synapses.

Also crucial is the vagus nerve's task of informing the psoas nerve in the lumbar area. This is the chief nerve that enables the pelvis to move and is therefore invaluable in allowing us to move voluntarily across environments. There can be any number of reasons for which people move and change environments. There is the obvious reasons of finding provisions, escaping from danger and protecting ourselves and our loved ones from adversity, which can look like hurricanes in the Caribbean, civil war in Yemen, famine in Somalia or a rape culture. In this sense, the psoas is arguably the most emotional muscle in the body since it hosts deep secrets and traumatic memories of failed escapes from danger (Francis, 2018). There's more to say about this role in my exploration of neurosomatic well-being in part V. My point here is that, whatever the reason to undertake a major change in our life, coming to such decision typically involves uncertainty that we depend on our brainpower to resolve, much like all else life throws our way. And major changes, whether behavioural, environmental or in personality, reflect in our body and mind at the cellular level, which will be reinforced by the environment. When it comes to adversity, this may be behaviour change in the direction of being less social. Think of Alex in chapter 2. The first implication is that of adverse health outcomes to which social isolation leads, which can be exacerbated by insensitivities and negative feedback—say psychosocial stress—in the environment. Thankfully, these outcomes are often the kind that can be improved by turning to the integrated self, cultivating its resources and engaging it as a source of its own healing and sustained integration. The essential resources in this process are explored next.

NEUROPSYCHOSOCIAL INTEGRATION
ESSENTIAL RESOURCES

Scores of variables are involved in how psychosocial trauma is processed in the body and mind. For instance, social history and biological vulnerabilities that are beyond our control will mean some people are more resilient and cope better. However, the human capacity to withstand and overcome psychosocial stress, even when we are disintegrated, is one that we can act to strengthen throughout our life cycle, drawing on the idea in neuropsychology that we can turn into our self to harness psychosocial resources that promote integration and resilience. Such resources, Erikson (1995) argued, are the output of a psyche that is inclusive and inclined to self-heal. This is to say the psyche is by design integrative in its task to promote life and well-being, both at the structural level where it integrates input from biology and the environment and at the functional level where it integrates the self, social history and adaptive defence.

The nervous system is at the intersection of all this integration, acting as an axle that joins the psyche, soma and society, holding them together in that dance of life I talked about in part II. Nonetheless, the nervous system remains incredibly vulnerable to dysregulation under conditions of adversity, particularly the kind that gives rise to psychosocial trauma that depletes or overwhelms the survivor's capacity to cope or move adaptively through the adversity and discharge the energy that builds up in the nervous system. Bring to mind, for instance, the event of being hunted in the wilds of West Africa for the sake of being enslaved in a strange land. The nervous system is liable to mobilise its sympathetic chain to fight or flee from this menace, increasing the secretion of adrenaline, cortisol and glucose to facilitate this reaction. But if this fails and you are seized, your nervous system may react as if its demise is imminent, by invoking an adaptive parasympathetic state of immobilisation or unconsciousness. This is what we call a freeze or faint response, both of which bring a release of endo-opioids that are implicated in pain-free deaths. Hence, this is an adaptive state that is quite distinct from the dispositions I discussed in chapter 7 and one in which, insight in neuroscience warns, the nervous system can stay stuck in the absence of death. For it is an adaptive response to chronic trauma, which, incidentally, allows me to make sense of the survival of my ancestors beyond their seizure in Africa, enduring of the dreadful Middle Passage and enslavement in the Caribbean and wider Americas.

This adaptive response to trauma is one in which integration is suspended and the consequent vacancy produces distinct symptoms, such as inflammation and fog in the psyche and agitation and fatigue in the soma. As such, the psyche and soma can behave differently and independently on trauma time. Both are self-regulating, and like the psyche, the soma has a trove of capacities—including those that are incongruous—that jostle in service of its survival.

However, when the psyche and soma are out of synch, as in a state of disintegration, one can dominate the other. In fact, psychic energy can dampen somatic energy—such as that which fuels gut instinct—and thereby suppress its contribution in the evaluation of ALEs that gives rise to trauma. This is how, for instance, the rationalisation that 'sparing the rod spoils the child' encourages a caregiver to physically abuse a child. We might say a deep cleave between the soma and psyche is inhibiting the caregiver's ability to attune to the child in such a way as to sense in their own body the child's pain and deter their impulse to inflict that pain. We met this impulse earlier in the warrior-fighter archetype who needs to 'always be in control' and comes to the task of life emotionally inhibited and empathically vacant. I'd go further to say this vacancy results in a dysregulation in the emotional-empathy circuitry, which gives rise to a dysempathy that blocks neuropsychosocial integration. Thus, the course from disintegration to integration must necessarily be informed by the principle of integrous empathy.

Integrous Empathy

Deriving from interpersonal neurobiology, where Siegel's concept of 'mwe' resides (2022), integrous empathy speaks to the sense that 'I can see me and you, and you can see me; I can feel me and you, and you can feel me; I can relate to me and you, and you can relate to me; I am not alone, and you are not alone.' We are with others and others are with us in a shared humanity. And this is possible because our minds' eyes, heart and soul as well as our gut instincts are synched, relational and promoting of life and well-being both inside and outside ourselves.

By these features, integrous empathy involves attuning both emotionally and cognitively to sensations whirling inside our own body as well as those others are experiencing from within their frame of reference. This is natural to us when information reaching our cognition for interpretation is uncorrupted by psychic dis-ease or somatic disease and is filtered deep in the neocortex and limbic system, where the insula is active, playing a role in autonomic control and somatic sensations. Under conditions of psychosocial stress and trauma, to which these processes are vulnerable and by which they can be inhibited, it is easy to think of empathy as something we either have or do not have. The fact, however, is that empathy—originating in the insula cortex (Gu et al., 2012)—is a neurobiological state that executes naturally when the soma and psyche are ordered and synched.

In chapter 13, we shall learn it is the third feature of our neuro-emotional SPEAR that promotes well-being and integration in the self. This is a state in which we can relate to ourselves and others with authenticity, are readily able to access curiosities surrounding our self as well as other selves, and attune to the deeper layers of experience that impact life, both our own and that of others. This includes the influences of liberties, culture, ancestral legacy and social history that shape the intricate patchworks that we are and inform the ways we show up to the task of life and wend through its marvels and miseries. It is like that humble stream in a rugged mountain that leads to a river that leads to the ocean and all the wonders and dangers the ocean contains.

Integrous empathy gets us to appreciate these wonders and dangers, but also the vulnerability, suffering and quiet yearnings inside of us and among us. We experience it in our mind and body because it involves cognitive, emotional, somatic and divine processes that underlie the human capacity to attune emotionally and respond to suffering. This is compassion, the term coming to English by way of its Latin root *passio*, which means 'to suffer', and the prefix *com-*, translating as 'together'. As the American psychologist Rick Hanson put it, this is 'suffering together' (2018), the gift of having others invested in our well-being with kindness and sincerity and not having to suffer alone when depletion and pain present in our body, mind or soul. This also encompasses being aware of our internal needs—including the need for integration and authenticity—and undertaking to satisfy those needs, which takes me to mind-heart-soulfulness.

Embodied Mind-Heart-Soulfulness

I would be the first to agree that embodied mind-heart-soulfulness has a somewhat counterintuitive ring, thanks to the neuroscience that establishes the heart as an autonomous host of our loves, emotional bonds and fears; the mind as what the brain does, what psychoanalysts call the psyche; and the soul as esoteric. However, by my definition, being mindful and soulful is about being in tune with what is ongoing in the heart, mind and gut as well as the divine—moment by moment.

Mind-heart-soulfulness is a state unfettered by chaotic energy. I am here referring to the kind of energy that sustains adaptive defences to reduce tension between stress and reaction to stress and which, incidentally, is associated with idle sensations, subconscious ideations, unregulated pangs and visceral butterflies that can hijack the mind and the gut and freeze the nervous system in a state of dis-ease.

From the perspective of integration, this state of dis-ease is momentary, an appropriate reaction to a difficult experience but still one in which energy is redirected from the newer and most sophisticated continent of the nervous system. We know this as the frontal lobe, mainly its prefrontal cortex, where we think clearly and solve complex problems. Thus, cognitive disengagement and ineffectiveness is what we experience when it is impaired by insufficient life-affirming energy. When this occurs, we can seek guidance in our *heart-gut-soul axis* (see figure 9.2), which in its own way behaves like a brain system (Blake, 2019).

In fact, the ancestral religion of which my great-grandfather Laurence (1888–1976) was a master promotes the belief that the soul has a mind that is mindful, a will that is free and emotions that motivate its actions. Much like the gut and heart, the soul is distinct but not isolated from the psyche and is a part of us—a source—we can turn to when cognition does not

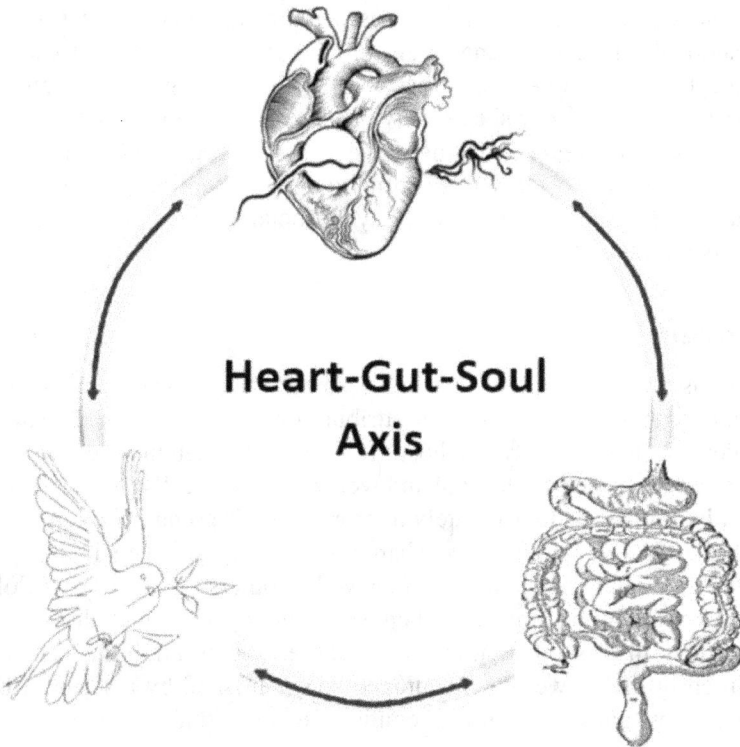

Figure 9.2. Heart-Gut-Soul Axis

provide the resolve we seek. It is, for instance, the source through which Nan appealed to the divine in prayer for guidance as she undertook to cure asthma, autism and unspecified developmental delays in her grandchildren. It is not about religion but the sanctuary of unconscious wisdom from which healing energy derives and that we can tap into for guidance to solve difficult problems.

The way I tend to put this to my students is to have them appeal to their unconscious resourcefulness and recall a problem, question or a curiosity that they grapple with, to play it out to their soul's mind, to direct energy to it and bring clarity, before going into a place of wonder. This may not necessarily be a place; it could be a state of ignorance in which some elucidation, guidance, perhaps even a fix might emerge. This may come as an image, a potion, a taste, a sound, a smell or a feeling or in some other way. The idea is to wait with patience and allow it to come into consciousness.

This may sound like a mindfulness exercise or even soulfulness, and it could be, for it works to bring clarity to problems and solutions to consciousness, in much the same way as the craft of prayer through which my elders reached into their soul—where they held the divine—to engage with its purity and fullness and to find relief in times of hardship. This relief sometimes came suddenly, forcefully and often quietly. But importantly, it came and was accepted in the conscious mind. The way Nan engages with it emits the sense that the soul is nourished by divinity. When it is full, it is free, and the free soul is calming and nourishing to the heart and gut, which in turn sustain the soul in its fullness. All of this is offered up for discernment in a mind that is dynamic, open and unimpaired by psychosocial trauma, which leads me to psychosocial integrity.

Psychosocial Integrity

Integrity is fundamentally about wholesomeness and truthfulness. Recall from part II that truthfulness is an attribute of the authentic self that accurately detects cues of safety and hostility in the social environment and motivates action in service of survival and well-being. Naturally, for us, this calls for trust in our psyche to accurately interpret what is going on around us, and also trust in those with whom we share our social world. This is to say that, with trust, we can depend on ourself as well as others to act in service of life and well-being, our natural state when we are not dysregulated, disordered or disintegrated. In Eriksonian developmental theory, it is a trait that establishes itself in early life as we are encouraged and nourished by a sense of being cared about, which sets us up with confidence in our self, in others and in the world of relationships.

This is the kind of socialisation that promotes psychosocial integrity. However, by virtue of our responsiveness to feedback from our relationships, and our social environment more generally, we are vulnerable to insecurity and confusion in our self-perception when the feedback we get is guilting, shaming or in any other way incongruent with how we are naturally. This poses a problem for psychosocial integrity, which I'd say is a precursor to neurosis: the ever-present sensation that the world as it is unsafe, and we are better off if we fold into a personality that fits in.

In our social as well as professional lives, wherein we are vulnerable to excessive disapproval, rejection and too little encouragement, this could feel like a corrosive tension between our psyche and socialisation, and it might well be. In his exploration of the 'biology of belief', the American cellular biologist Bruce Lipton (2015, p. 169) demonstrated a weakening in bodily muscles that accompanies a conflict between conscious belief and formerly learned 'truths' stored in the subconscious. The American psychologist Leon Festinger felt this experience was necessarily cognitively injurious and coined the phrase 'cognitive dissonance' to speak to its incidence. Another word for dissonance is *incongruity*, a state in which the psyche is in conflict with the social and adapts by avoiding difficult reflection in order to align with the messages the nervous system receives. The implication is that the self depletes in confidence and loses trust in the utility of its native SPEARS.

This tells me that self-confidence, as also is courage to defend one's true self, is important for preserving psychosocial integrity, even when we are actively wounded in our body, mind and soul. This wounding could come from, say, a disease in the body, social marginalisation or even a sense of aloneness that stokes inflammation in the psyche (Van Susteren & Colino, 2020). Psychosocial integrity, however, is what will allow us to recognise this woundedness or threat of being wounded and act so that we do not stay stuck in a disintegrated neural state, the kind that gives rise to emotional vacancy, irritation and hopelessness, for instance. It bears out that these sensations are normal in the face of adversity, and experiencing them from time to time can help us build resilience with which we can weather the impact of psychosocial stress. So this is not all bad. When presaged by sensations of satisfaction, such as pride, reverence and hopefulness, they can in fact keep us interested and motivated. With sustained ventral vagal input, this is the passion and eagerness we recognise and value in people who are aspirational and relational and whose psychosocial integrity is underpinned by resilience SPEARS.

This applies even to those whose quality of life is depleted by factors such as ancestry, genetics or place of birth that influence their life paths but over which they do not have control. In fact, such factors will account for about 20 to 30 percent of how our life turns out. Promising, I'd say, as it tells me that up to 80 percent of how our life turns out—how our life story unfolds—is within our influence. This is our gift as intelligent sentients, and in addition to our heart-gut-soul axis, it makes us uniquely human. The impulse to seek safety and well-being within integrous and nourishing relationships, including with our own self, is sacred.

We all need nurturing and resonant relationships in which we feel congruent and can heal fully when we are wounded or recover when we are depleted in resilience. We can be vulnerable and authentic because we are integrated in how we function as individuals as well as how we are received relationally. Essentially, this is about how we move through life and draw upon our resilience SPEARS, but such relationships can be with a mentor, a teacher or a therapist, anyone who promotes our well-being and helps us to actualise our liberties, such as the liberty to love and relate in healthful and meaningful ways, as our ancestors ensured we have. Ordinarily, this is a bequest that can be cultivated or recovered with well-being SPEARS along the course of integration and actualisation of authenticity in the self. I shall explore this course in part V. Before then, it helps to reflect on the incidence of psychosocial trauma to which it is vulnerable and liable to submit.

Recall from part II that this trauma derives from protracted exposure to adversity. This could be anything from dispossession of one's body as with chattel slavery, economic poverty, social-emotional deprivation or any one of endless other examples of which our history is replete. Each of these circumstances will be subjectively experienced and reacted to along a spectrum from acute to chronic. The ALEs study and family history from which I draw this assumption sheds light on the extent to which this trauma wreaks havoc across generations, and not only in my family. Its analogue of a wild forest fire that will burn every tree in its path until one turns around and courageously blows out the flame is relatable.

One could think of the burnt shards as the scars that will remain as a testament to suffering but also of inner capacities to overcome adversity, integrate the attendant trauma and stabilise the body and mind. It is in this sense alone that scars left by psychosocial trauma—after a successful therapeutic intervention—are meaningful ancestral legacies and invaluable representations of wounds, now healed. Wounds in bodies and minds—perhaps inherited—are reminders of what once happened that was not conducive to wellness and needed to be accepted fully and forgiven. This kind of radical acceptance along with resilient well-being and authenticity in the self are expressions of neuropsychosocial integration and its distinct neural processes and state, to which I shall now turn.

NEUROPSYCHOSOCIAL INTEGRATION
FUNDAMENTAL PROCESSES

Neuropsychosocial integration involves the circulation of information in the entire nervous system in service of well-being. The American neuroscientist Stephen Porges (2020) coined the term *neuroception* to speak to the nature of this information, when it is generated in the body, separate from the brain and the psyche. By this definition, neuroception occurs below the brainstem. Naturally, there is the question of how the cognitive and emotional continents and structures get the information they need or use to play their part in a bid for integration. This happens to be one of my favourite neuro-questions, and the answer begins with three key sources from which this information derives:

1. The first is the visceral organs—such as the gut, kidneys and heart—which express discernible inner body activities. These expressions, also known as interoceptions, includes, for example, the gut's rumble that warns of hunger, the kidneys' secretion of adrenaline in response to stress and the heart's slowed rate that affirms a sense of being loved.
2. The second source of information that informs cognition and emotion is the sacred soul. This is the esoteric self that connects our nervous system to other souls, divine entities and the nervous systems of other sentient organisms. We acknowledge this when we say, for instance, that we 'can feel our ancestors', 'God talks to us' or 'we are spiritual'.
3. The auditory, gustatory, olfactory, tactile and visual systems that take information to the nervous system from outside the body via sensory receptors in the ears, tongue, nose, skin and eyes constitute the third source that informs cognition and emotion. Another term for this information is *exteroceptions*, which derive from social interaction.

I cannot here do justice to the complexity of these systems in their important task of keeping us informed and responsive to all that goes on in our world. However, as I mentioned earlier, the cranial nerves are integral to this process, and this will be more clearly true as we come to understand how we receive and process information from inside and outside of us in service to our survival and well-being.

The first job of these nerves, naturally, is to stimulate native instincts that promote survival. This includes basal instincts such as attachment and foraging, but also subconscious functions, such as heart rate, breathing and orientation in space at any given time. These instincts and functions are regulated in the brainstem—in the ancient reptilian complex—from where the vagus nerve projects its neuroceptions to the cerebral cortex via the thalamus.

The thalamus—from the Greek *thalamos* or 'inner chamber'—sits atop the brainstem and is the only neural structure that relays information directly to the cerebral cortex (Halassa, 2022). This includes up to 98 percent of sensory information, so the thalamus has the important task of filtering what gets through for interpretation and what doesn't. This bears pertinence on the course towards integration as the transfer of accurate information is important for authentic expressions. All this mean is that, upon receiving a true neuroception, say of safety, the neocortex will return an affirmation to the autonomic nerves via the ventral pathway that leads to the heart. Incidentally, this pathway interconnects with cranial nerves V, VII, IX and XI in the brainstem to bring social engagement to life and activate the impulse to broadcast and respond to invitation for contact and relationship.

Cranial nerve V, known as the trigeminal nerve, innervates movement of our eyes, mouth and jaws in service of friendly communication—something seen, spoken or heard and reacted to favourably. Cranial nerve VII is the facial nerve that innervates our facial expressions and taste. It is what enables

Cranial nerves

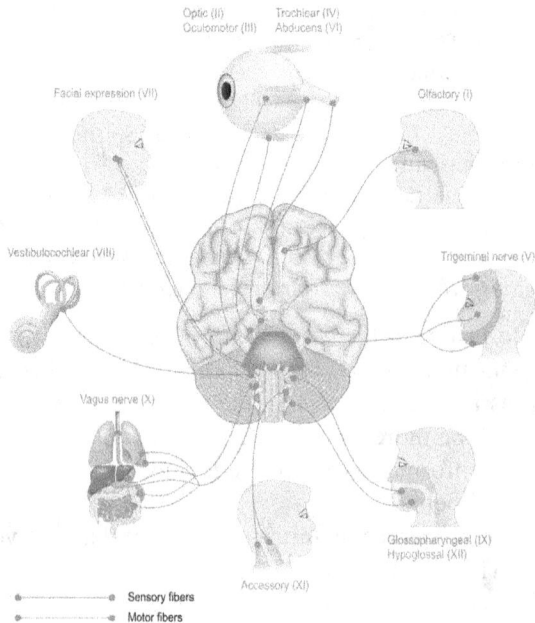

Figure 9.3. The Cranial Nerves. A collection of twelve paired nerves that emerge from the brain. The first two, the olfactory and optic nerves, originate from the cerebrum, while the other ten come from the brainstem. The function of the cranial nerves determines their names, which are assigned using Roman numerals (I–XII). *Image © ttsz / iStock / Getty Images.*

us to express warm and positive emotions on our face. Cranial nerve IX, the glossopharyngeal nerve, innervates the warm tone and sweet variations in rhythms in our voice. Another word for this feature is prosody, from Greek pros, 'towards', and ōidē, 'song'. And lastly, cranial nerve XI, the accessory nerve, innervates movement of the head, neck and shoulders to allow us to show that we are interested and interesting. These true exteroceptions reaching the vagus nerve create or reinforce neural connection between experience and response.

The proper functioning of these nerves is therefore crucial for our experience in relationships, for they broadcast on our face and in our behaviour how we are experiencing our social environment. Needless to say, disturbance and disease in the body and mind that impair the ventral pathway could mean the broadcast they emit is inauthentic or even perilous, which reminds me of a conversation I had with a friend in Moscow who had struggled with relational security since childhood. Her dominant experience was of relationships that left her feeling vacant, inadequate and unwanted. An ALEs score of 10 out of 21 reflected a family history of drug-misuse addiction and a personal history of domestic violence, loneliness, abandonment and incompetency in building close and trusting relationships, quite discernible psychosocial traumas that seemed to block her ventral vagal pathway and inhibit neuroceptions from reaching accurate interpretation in her brain. Stuck in her body, below her brainstem, these neuroceptions were susceptible to faulty interpretations that gave rise to disabling neurosis. Her restless legs, shallow breath, chest tightness and chronic hypertension are examples of how these faulty neuroceptions were expressed.

This is where perception does not reconcile with reality, and it is a symptom of disintegration in and between the body and mind. Her mind may know she is not in imminent danger, but this perception of reality does not cascade down into her body. This is all psychogenic and tells us that it is possible to perceive without neuroception, a condition well explored in the psychiatric literature.

Consider, for example, the perception and corresponding painful sensation of being 'eaten by bugs' that do not match reality. This is known as delusional parasitosis (DP), and it is a psychosomatic disorder where the perception is without a true neuroception and the mind cannot discern this. It may also be that bodily sensations do not reach perception. In this case, these sensations are somatogenic and may do things like evoke reflexes and disturbance in the body. Nonetheless, this is a challenge for perception and raises questions about interpretation and expression of bodily and mental states. For example, what happens to neural signals the brain gets, or does not get from the body for interpretation, and what does this mean?

Damasio's (2002, 2021) exploration of the relationship between cognitive and subcortical processes has been an immense influence in my appreciation of the neural processes that underlie perception and neuroception, in showing that the neural structure involved in cognition also regulates emotions, instincts and visceral experience. Accordingly, higher mental processes of which perception is an example are informed by emotions and neuroceptions whirling inside the body. In positioning the body first within the chain of processes that generate thoughts, imagination and social behaviour, we are feeling organisms that think, as opposed to thinking organisms that feel, resolving the controversy of whether emotion comes from the body or the body state comes from the emotion. It is like the chicken and egg debate, where we try to determine which came first.

My work with incredibly savvy young people who live on the streets and sleep under bridges in the city of Seattle, Washington, helps me to put this into perspective. The question there is whether these young people, generally teenagers, run away from home into the perils of homelessness because they are terrified of the abuse they have experienced in their family, or is it that they are terrified the perceived possibility of being abused by their family and, therefore, they run away from home and are homeless? Which of the two is true? The answer is probably both, and probably neither. The events are informed by a bidirectional flow of information between the body and the mind. So body and mental expressions reflect each other, and under normal condition the body and mind produce one state. The terror, anxiety and muscle tension in children who are habitually abused by caregivers tell us about a body-mind state in which fear is expressed somatically as anxiety and muscle tension. However, I have talked about the body and mind not always working with each other, which is what might be happening with delusional parasitosis or even the more familiar anxiety attacks and 'running away from home' because of a perceived threat of abuse, which may not even exist.

The body and mind are in a state of disintegration, and neuroceptions traveling towards the brain to be interpreted are corrupted or even disrupted, and you get a blown-up somatic arousal. Ordinarily, this looks like a legitimate reaction to a threat, as if it is instinctive. And sometimes it is instinctive, where the information from inside the body making its way up for interpretation is stuck in the instinctive brain and defines not only how we react to what is happening internally on an emotional and physiological level but also how we engage with the world. To appreciate this, consider how often you regret ignoring your gut about something that caused you trouble. Or the obverse, when you felt pleased you honoured your gut feeling and then found out it was the right thing for you.

The instinctive brain complements activities in the cognitive brain, but it is also there to compensate for cognitive impairment, and it is absolutely valid. When we ignore our instincts, whether that is a gut feeling or a physical impulse to move our body to a different place or keep it in a familiar place, we do that at our own peril. This is often a symptom of trauma that cleaves the mind-body connection. However, ALEs that fail to reach cognition and perception will stay in the body and in time impair the capacity to engage with the body in an intelligent way. The cognitive and emotional brain systems will also adapt to the reduced input from the body, and a number of neural processes—including the insula activities deep in between the frontal, parietal and temporal lobes—will be affected. Think poor insulation.

I have discussed the role of the insula in empathy, but its helpful to emphasise that throughout the teenage years, as the brain develops and matures, it shrinks to reflect this maturation (Wierenga et al., 2014). It ends up being a tiny ribbon with a big responsibility in the execution of perception of what's going on inside the body. This is largely neuroceptions but also sensations and emotions, such as hunger, heartache and love, about which it exchanges information with, say, the amygdala and hypothalamus in the socioemotional brain's limbic system, the cerebral cortex via the thalamus and the organs in the viscera. This network facilitates awareness of what is going on both inside the body and around us. For instance, it enables us to associate palpitations with anxiety, anxiety with fear of being abused by our family and being abused by our family with the decision to run away from our family home, towards the uncertainly of homelessness. So it is sensitive to ALEs that gives rise to trauma. However, according to a multidisciplinary study by research teams from Iowa State and Stanford Universities (Klabunde et al., 2017), this vulnerability shows up differently in female and male brains. More precisely, the team found that the anterior section of muscle that encircles the insula—called the anterior circular sulcus—was larger in boys who had survived at least three adverse life events that gave rise to trauma than in their nontraumatised peers. The opposite effect on the insula was true for girls. The same cortical section was smaller in volume and surface in the traumatised girl than in their nontraumatised peers.

This abnormal difference in size and volume in the insula among child survivors of trauma affirms that trauma manifests itself differently in the capacity to perceive and interpret neuroceptions. More precisely, trauma accelerates insula aging in the female brain but delays it in the male brain, giving rise to a number of consequences. For instance, an abnormally large insula in boys is consistent with cognitive immaturity and a disposition to underestimate danger; hence, motorcycle scooting is fun, not unsafe, and car or train surfing is about having a laugh. We could argue that this delay in maturation is functional in that is allows traumatised boys to retain innocence and perhaps develop psychosocial resources to face off the perils of poverty, disability and premature death to which they are disproportionately vulnerable in adult life.

An abnormally small insula in girls, on the other hand, translates to accelerated maturation and premature puberty. We might think of this as a neurodevelopmental adaptation that is protective against threats to which the fragility of childhood is vulnerable. The idea is that, in childhood, girls are especially vulnerable to sexual predation and parentification, against which nature may act to protect them by advancing their maturation. But with this adaptation also comes a worrying disposition to exaggerate danger. For instance, a headache is reacted to as if it is a fatal brain tumour, a sniffle equates to imminent death from COVID-19 and constipation is interpreted as bowel cancer.

An abnormal insula that is linked to psychosocial trauma can also mean that survivors' capacity to cope with adversity is compromised and their nervous systems is more easily hijacked and held in a state of paralysis by ordinary stress. This is a state in which the stress response system ordinarily fails to stimulate the survivor to act to self-protect and a chronic deviation from homeostasis and the consequent allostatic overload ensue. This consequence expresses itself in cumulative wear and tear the body and mind are not designed for and the impact of which can be catastrophic for the insula (Waterland & Jirtle, 2003).

For instance, the effect of an allostatic overload in an underactive insula may mean difficulty with perceiving neuroceptions. The survivor may not remember to eat because neuroceptions of hunger are not reaching the insula and may not bathe because neuroceptions of disgust or the need to clean the body are not being perceived in a neurotypical way. The survivor may even self-harm because pain signals are not being interpreted in the insula, or it could be that they are seeking to activate their insula. A thing about self-harm—and this is especially true for the cutting I see in teenagers with whom I work—is that the self-infliction of physical pain is an insula-activation strategy, a stimulus to reconnect their body and mind to allow them to perceive more of what's going on in their body. Not always, but this is often the case. Acute physical injury, it turns out, forces the nervous system to oscillate between sympathetic activation and a parasympathetic nonpain state in which GABA and endorphins help them to cope with the pain. In this state, both the pain and the capacity to cope with it are perceived and this is the objective, but it is a state that also inhibits their capacity to engage in the present and solve real problem, because the ventral and cognitive circuit are dulled out.

This event can profoundly distort the survivor's senses of safety and danger as the disintegrated nervous system is flooded by the chaotic energy of this maladaptive state and the insula stays stuck on the perception of the world as a dangerous place. Excess secretion of GABA that suppresses neuronal activity in the insula and leads to its underactivity may look like absentmindedness that can lead to hypersomnia, or daytime sleepiness. On the flip side, a lack of GABA can mean uninhibited neuronal signalling and an overactive insula that can feel like the chronic anxiety that is associated with mood disorders and paranoia. Wherein, for instance, an innocuous rash is interpreted as leprotic, a friendly touch from a peer is interpreted as a sexual violation, misfortunes are manifestations of witchcraft, and the survivor is unable to shift their attention away from these interpretations because the insula is stuck exaggerating or falsifying neuroceptions that activate the sympathetic chain, and the brain cannot send a true interpretation back. It is all somatic, and the survivor feels as if something unsafe is happening in their body.

Faulty neuroceptions are problematic for the brain, which cannot send signals via the ventral track's myelinated fibres, designed to transmit signals to the body and mind more quickly than, say, the signals from the unmyelinated dorsal fibres. When these signals are blocked, the nervous system is liable to return a false neuroception or an inconclusive interpretation that triggers a maladaptive response. This may range from a warrior's foolish fight to a settler's fuzzy furrow that reflects vagal dysregulation. In a word, this is a stuckness in a chronically activated sympathetic chain that gives rise to the chronic inflammation I talked about in part III.

As I revisit this idea with vagal dysregulation in mind, I am inclined to consider that these adaptations originate in a sympathetic state that predisposes the survivor to autoimmune maladies, such as asthma, as well as severe and complex psychiatric and somatic injuries that do not respond to vagal flexibility, by which I mean where the ventral vagal inhibits dorsal and spinal sympathetic activities to bring about an active ventral state that corrects this dysregulation and mitigates symptom severity. Fortunately, this is something survivors can be encouraged to do to help themselves out of dysautonomia and into presence and social engagement.

This is the foundational processes that curves back to perception, and it is what the psyche does as it draws information from the brain, and the brain from the rest of the body. From perception we derive the more sophisticated psychic activity of discernment, both of which can be cultivated in a nourishing relationship in which the survivor is encouraged to tune into their own body and mind, where they are sure to find psychosocial traumas, including those inherited from ancestors, that give rise to disintegration and to which they are subconsciously reacting. The object, nonetheless, is that, however ancient, deep and problematic traumas are, we have the capacity within us to facilitate their contextualisation, to achieve neuropsychosocial integration and, as we grow in integration, also to repurpose the old scars and memories as legacy. This will help us to cope with adversity and move through life purposefully and with resilience.

Chapter 10

Neuropsychosocial Integration

Aims and Steps

Like the forest fire that burns every tree in its path—reducing the forest to ashes—until it is put out, psychosocial trauma stokes neuropsychosocial disintegration and its psychic, somatic, emotional and relational sequelae, which get passed from generation to generation and wreck lives until interrupted and contextualised. Until one survivor in an active generation wields their native, intelligence and resilience SPEARS to bring integration to his- or herself. That one survivor may bring peace to their ancestors, share healing with the current generation and spare future generations.

This reconciling of experiences from social history with those of current times and projecting for the future is central to cultivating inner capacities to restore naturalness in the body and mind and authenticity in the whole self—an event that involves synchronising the body-mind-social axis by confronting and discharging the chaotic energy of psychosocial trauma and freeing the survivor from a life riddled with disintegration and in-authenticity. At the end of this chapter, we shall come to appreciate the centredness of authenticity, as well as the aims and steps of neuropsychological integration.

CENTERING AUTHENTICITY IN NEUROPSYCHOSOCIAL INTEGRATION

The notion of centering bears a therapeutic tone that I want to acknowledge from the outset. This is my influence, derived from the principles of personality psychology and psychotherapy a la Rogers. I have undertaken to enhance this influence with the neurobiology of the psychosocial and polyvagal theory, which emphasise interdependency among the social-emotional, behavioural, psychological and therapeutic. At the heart of this approach lies the body-mind-social axis and a nonhierarchical alliance with survivors based on trust in the human will to live through what is important, both in body and mind.

For survivors, this begins with native needs and capacities, the native and intelligence SPEARS that inform goals and reactions to life events. Importantly, this involves the somatic or physiological reaction in their body, as well as the psychological that derives from their thoughts and the emotional that constitutes their feelings. And then there might also be a spiritual, which would encompass the esoteric and unknowns that exist independently of their body and mind. With the psychological dimension, we are looking at ideas, opinions and thought process, whilst the other dimensions involve a less judgemental exploration of lived experience that comes from a place of openness, congruence and empathy.

At this stage, from a place of disintegration, the authentic self is beginning to emerge with curiosity towards a future uninhibited by trauma and an orientation focussed on nourishing relationships in which it experiences kindness, attentiveness and unconditional acceptance. This authenticity encompasses knowing thyself deeply, so it comes from deep within the self, where it can stay protected from uncomfortable exposure. This is a place free of delusions, exaggerations or false narratives. Thus, the authentic self is congruent with reality and does not entertain shape-shifting in the social world, even if that means disapproval of the world. Hence, discovering this self is also about discovering these core needs, along with emotional, psychological, somatic and relational strengths. Such a discovery, one imagines, begins in the depths of the nervous system, in between states of autonomic activation in the deep unconscious. And, ultimately, it surfaces in the ventral vagal complex. This is where the sympathetic and parasympathetic fibres of the nervous system are affirming each other and promoting authentic self-expression and well-being.

To actualise this experience is to employ neuropsychotherapy in the freeing of its content, surfacing the 'repressed'—to borrow a Freudian expression—and encouraging the survivor to fully bring into acceptance their shamed, hidden or rejected experiences and sensations, so they can be transformed into sources of strength and healing energy. Healing comes naturally as all that does not serve the body and mind is released, in much the same way as psychoanalysis elucidates the triumph of mental health when chaos and rigidity in the unconscious are confronted and repurposed. It is by bringing these inner tensions to consciousness that pathologies to which they give rise are released and health is transformed. This is important for therapy that takes place at the level of the cerebral-cognitive and social-emotional selves and works to improve synchronicity between the two. For neuropsychosocial integration, however, we are working deeper. We are working at the level of cellular tissues, in the depth of the nervous system, where cells across vast cortical surfaces are encouraged to signal together, to create waves and synchronies that stabilise into neural networks.

Networks of cells that activate at the same time in a pattern can be reinforced with repetition and installed in character. The precept is that as neurons in differing parts of the nervous system are encouraged to signal together repeatedly in authentic and healing states, authenticity and positive character traits will emerge. This is neuropsychosocial therapy, and its process begins with some understanding of neuroanatomy and works to establish the presence and capacity of the authentic self. For it is authenticity in the self that will be engaged to carry out the contextualisation of trauma and bring integration to the nervous system. Naturally, the inauthentic self, doing its job of protecting the survivor's deep secrets, will tender resistance, and the authentic self may well retreat. This may look like regression or even descension into a furrow, challenges the authentic self could face in its important task of overseeing synchronicity between the survivor's inner world and outer world and surfacing itself from suppressions and pathologies that characterise a bad life. With this in mind, there are key aims to consider.

ESSENTIAL AIMS AND STEPS IN NEUROPSYCHOSOCIAL INTEGRATION

1. To surface and process unmetabolised traumatic stress, traumatic wounds and trauma-based adaptations that are embedded in the nervous system.
2. To retire neural encodings of psychosocial traumas and de-autonomise the behavioural expressions that disguise as traditions and psychosocial resources.
3. To encourage and integrate a neuropsychosocial system to emerge with resilience that is reinforced by life-affirming psychosocial resources.

The survivor who achieves these aims is an effective operator of the nervous system at both the intrapersonal and interpersonal level, one who is competent in and committed to actualising change in their life when actionable opportunities arise. As Rogers (1995) observed, 'there are some very special moments in a person's life when they feel able to change'. Change that favours integration calls for such moments and depends on the therapeutic experience to nurture inner capacities and create them. However, until polyvagal theory, there was little clarity on how this works at a neural level—the level of neuroanatomy. This extends to how we can reorient the default settings in our nervous system that are in place before we are even born.

The idea in neuropsychosocial integration and specifically neuropsycho-therapy is that we can learn to retire connections between our neural cells' assemblies, behaviours and emotions. This is not to suggests that neural circuitries and triggers can be expunged, for they can't, and they will stay in place even if they are inactive. This is important because these circuitries and triggers evince lived experiences that future generations can benefit from as a legacy.

Our legacy is a reliable record of our history that we can explore to learn about ourselves. It is a gift we should not be encouraged to lose. The object instead is to retire or weaken the connections to maladaptive expressions, to discharge the chaotic energy that sustains them and break them up, in effect. In this way, we can feel ashamed but not descend into a furrow or strike our children; be angry but not attack our friends; be frightened but not flee, fawn, fold or faint. In other words, when we are triggered, we won't act like we are doomed or about to die.

We can also learn to break connections between cell assemblies and trauma triggers so that they don't evoke maladaptive responses in the first place. However, since the assemblies stay in place, there is the risk of reconnection with trauma-based adaptations. This is something to be mindful of and may call for a healing energy that encourages survivors to transcend body and mind in imagination, which not only plays out in the nervous system in much the same way as reality but can also evoke the neurobiology of agency. I shall return to agency in part V in my exploration of psychological well-being SPEARS that are conducive to integration and actualisation of authenticity in the self. It suffices to say here that it is an essential resource along that journey and in the consideration of three important steps:

1. For the survivor, the first step in neuropsychosocial integration is radi-cal acceptance of your whole self in your life story, precisely as you are, with your imperfections, perfections, dissatisfactions, satisfactions and authentic emotions, which can be comforting, upsetting or both. A modest example is gratitude or ambivalence for being alive. There may also be insecurities, depletions and feelings of powerlessness that must be accepted, reflected upon and honoured. As you go along, you may find that this first step involves acceptance of immense loss that evokes sensations of shame, grief and guilt, as well as the features of trauma explored in part II. This is because unmetabolised loss and its attendant emotions—anger, frustration, sadness—embed in the nervous system. *Unmetabolised* is a fancy word for undigested, so it is analogous to hav-ing undigested food resting in your gut. Unlike undigested food, which can be regurgitated, unmetabolised—or more precisely, ungrieved—loss

will protect itself underneath heaps of adaptations. And, before integration can occur, it will need to be surfaced and grieved.

2. The next step involves cultivating capacity to attune inward, to read one's own mind, reach into one's own heart and connect with one's own soul. This is the essence of mindsight, a term Siegel (2010) introduced into the neuropsychology lexicon to speak to the imagining of oneself as one might be without the experiences of which one is aware have contributed to inner disturbance and prejudiced perceptions of the world. This is a cognitive exercise, and it is possible that—as a survivor of psychosocial trauma—access to your cerebral-cognitive self and your capacity to imagine may be disturbed.

3. Now that we are convinced the vagus nerve network plays an important role in our reactions to life events, including adversity and, for my purpose, the preservation, transmission and discharge of psychosocial trauma, we can learn to orient it to work as nature intends. More precisely, we can honour appropriate 'vagal breaks'—to use Porges's phrase—that disrupt maladaptive expressions and reinforce vagal flexibility. For in modulating the organs of the viscera with which the ventral vagal fibres interface, the vagal breaking mechanism enables us to flexibly engage and disengage with life events in order to promote and retain resilient well-being. This is the third step, and it is about orienting to social engagement, the state in which we attune emotionally, self-regulate and co-regulate in ways that are conducive to our well-being and growth. Mind-heart-soulfulness lives here, and so too does gratitude over entitlement, love over hate and forgiveness over bitterness. Setting this up can begin with an appreciation of the dominant sensory systems—auditory, olfactory, visual and so on—through which we experience the world and the vagal state in which we present ourselves. Psychotherapists Deb Dana's (2020) Flip Chart and Babette Rothchild's (2017) ANS Table are two practical resources that can be helpful in this task. They each explicitly encourage the recognition that a story of trauma is typically accompanied by one of adaptation and resilience, and significant relationships are key pieces of these stories. As such, I am most naturally inclined to explore survivors':
    a. Relationships with their whole self and its different configurations.
    b. Relationships with others, the social world and relational demands.
    c. Supraconscious, transpersonal or spiritual self if it is present.

These different types of relationships reflect experiences in different ways that contribute to a fuller picture of a life lived. More precisely, the relationship with the self tells me something about the survivor's self-concept, about how the whole self is perceived and—to an extent—in what they believe. With regards to the social world, it is about interpersonal relationships, opportunities, conflicts and fears. When it comes to other selves, it is about capacity for empathy and compassion, as well as for co-regulation. And, ultimately, with regards to the supraconscious or transpersonal, it is about any relationship with the esoteric.

We share a lot about our purpose in the ways we relate and care for ourselves and others. Hence, these relationships—taken together—tell a fuller story about what moves us and gives our life meaning. Our beliefs, Lipton (2015) tells us, are biological properties of our subconscious, extant beneath our conversations. It is at this level that we appreciate the extent to which our whole self is integrated and protected. For instance, we can discern healthy relationships in which our life is affirmed and our body and mind are cared for. In our quest for meaning in our experiences and life more generally, we will be motivated to act in service of our purpose, and this involves a kind of hunger to take responsibility for improving our life and the lives of those we care about as a precondition for neuropsychosocial integration and well-being.

CENTERING THE SURVIVOR FOR NEUROPSYCHOSOCIAL INTEGRATION

With essential processes and steps in neuropsychosocial integration in hand, the next imperative on this journey is reconciling another crucial piece of the survivor's story: the default autonomic state through which the survivor moves through life and navigates the social world. This may be maladaptive fight, flight, fold, float or furrow that inevitably projects to chaos and inflexibility in relationships. This could manifest, for instance, intrarelationally as inadequate self-care; interrelationally as disagreeableness, ragefulness, suspiciousness and other 'crazy-making' impulses that are associated with relational abuse and adrenalised ways of moving through life that lean towards stuckness in a state of emotional dysregulation and sympathetic chain activation.

At the other end is the survivor who self-negates, self-abandons or neglects their needs in attending to the demands of others. Or who dissociates socio-emotionally, appearing hypo-emotional, folded into themselves as if to avoid being known, or altogether withdrawn socially, floating in time and space like my volleyball adrift in the ocean. These quiet ways of being in the world, with which I am often met in psychosocial trauma survivors, fall on a discernible sympathetic-parasympathetic spectrum.

In her conceptualisation of autonomic anchorage, Dana (2021) demonstrates how, at one end, sympathetic activation involves mobilisation in which being in the world is contingent on some kind of action. Parasympathetic depression, on the other end, calls for hypomobilisation. Surviving in the world is contingent on being inactive, inoffensive, hidden—as with social withdrawal. In previous chapters, I talked about the anciency of these adaptive states and how they entertain chronic dis-ease in the body and mind that characterise neurosis. Conclusively:

- in sympathetic activation, neurosis provokes sensations of insecurity and confusion that characterise anxiety, impulsivity, hypervigilance and hypermobilisation to survive under conditions of privation
- in a parasympathetic depression, neurosis proliferates sensations of hopelessness, helplessness and worthlessness that characterise anergia, social isolation, depression, fatigue and suicidality

In states of chronicity, sympathetic and parasympathetic activation disrupt integration and promote addictions, violence, loneliness, abandonment, social isolation and incompetency in building close and trusting relationships that proffer pathology and premature death, in spite of which the survivor stays alive. How? This happens to be another of my pet questions in neurophysiology, as I can practically reduce it to our protective will to live and heal when we are wounded, which is supported by our native gifts of immunity, neurogenesis and neuroplasticity.

In centring the survivor for neuropsychosocial integration, immunity ensures that inflammation is available to heal injuries in the body and mind. This is sperate from the chronic inflammation and autoimmunity that bear harmful consequences. For instance, recall from part II that chronic neuro-inflammation—or emotional inflammation when it is caused by emotional injuries such as shame, grief and guilt—can give rise to a range of mental and behavioural problems that are features of psychosocial trauma. Think of obsessive thoughts, irritability and the many proliferations of compulsions that satisfy diagnostic criteria in the *DSM* and ICD. Examples include attention deficit disorder (ADD), hyperactive disorder (HD) and behaviour disorders that are differentiated as oppositional defiant disorder (ODD) and conduct disorder (CD), which are core features of antisocial personalities (ASPD). Given these diagnoses' association with morbidity and premature mortality, interrupting their incidence is best treated as a social-health imperative, one that must be understood in terms of how diagnoses derive from inadequate psychosocial conditions that give rise to pathologies in affected people groups. As this consequence cannot be good, I am compelled to adjust my impression of inflammation to consider it necessarily restorative.

Inflammation is good when is works as nature intends. In the face of an acute injury, it is the immune system's property that protects bodily tissues and initiates healing. This extends to all injuries, whether emotional, psychological or physical, although it is more readily perceived in a physical sense by the redness, swelling and mucus procured by immune cells acting to prevent decay and infection from, say, toxins from a bug's bite. This is trickier when the injury is emotional or psychological, or protracted, as is the case with psychosocial trauma. The healing process, however, is very much the same, in that injuries will feel and look worse as the body and mind undertake to self-serve and heal, enlisting the immune system in this task.

Naturally, this will surface defences that derive from the subconscious, that vast database of our life experiences—both lived and inherited—and evolutionarily derived survival mechanisms that are concerned with environmental signals and engaging in expressions of stimulus-driven behaviour without prejudice. So the varying degree of resistance is natural as the nervous system is at the mercy of its historical programs and legacy. Recall that defences—other references include 'protective reflexes', 'immune response' and 'adaptations'—are both necessarily protective and vital to recovering authenticity suppressed in the subconscious. Hence, tension between the conscious desire to change and the subconscious impulse to protect one's legacy can result in neuropsychosocial injury momentarily.

I have mentioned neurogenesis and neuroplasticity as features of this process. Neurogenesis involves neuronal healthcare (Alshebib et al., 2003), neural cells restoring their capabilities where possible, given adequate nourishment. An important paper that was published in the journal *Nutrients* (Balan et al., 2018) looked at depletion, death and senescence in neural cells that are consequent of psychosocial stress. The researchers argued, convincingly, that these incidents can be reversed with physical exercise, good nutrition and a positive outlook that promotes not only a long and healthy life but also new neural connections that are important for healthy expressions in the body and mind and integration across different survival states, specifically between the parasympathetics and sympathetics.

We understand this success in terms of neuroplasticity, the nervous system's native ability to grow, change and self-heal. As we are exposed to life events, including ALEs and the mundane events of ordinary life, energised neurons across the entire nervous system signal for action, establishing patterns of signalling together that, when strong enough, create memories. With recurrence, these patterns strengthen and stabilise, becoming second nature. This is learning. In constantly learning and changing, the big brain, in particular, establishes patterns in networks across its continents and substructures that it will remember with little stimulation and even without stimulation. Like that sticky song, dance move or curse word that keeps popping up in 'your head' without conscious recall. The patterns we entertain will become stronger and install as prevalent memories as they are a marked as desirable and rewarded by our dopamine reward system. Those patterns we do not entertain will weaken as the neurons involved are denied energy and in turn decrease their signalling, causing the patterns to wither away or become inactive. The brain thrives on these events—the patterns it establishes and rewards reflect its dynamism, and when those patterns are expressed in cognitions, emotions and behaviours, we know that resilient change has occurred. This is how we learned our alphabet, how to count and how to climb trees without falling in childhood. It is also how we learned to drive, to protect ourselves and to raise our children in adulthood. And, ultimately, how we will learn to cultivate well-being and discharge chaotic energies of trauma to bring integration to our nervous system.

Understanding this is a nod to therapy's promise of improving survivors' life outcomes. For instance, in becoming an active operator of their nervous system, survivors are encouraged in the therapeutic space to cultivate neuroplasticity resourcefully and resiliently. Part V explores therapeutic SPEARS that can are deployed in this space. It suffices here to say that this is a relationship in which the therapist brings a restorative presence to empower the survivor to rewrite their life story to promote well-being through empathy, hopefulness and imagination, and to contextualise any stuckness in sympathetic activation or parasympathetic depression. In the therapeutic relationship, the survivor is nourished and empowered to tap into their inner resources to foster a deep connection with themselves and others within a circle of influence. Getting to this circle, however, involves enlisting the neurobiology of motivation to reach out and connect, sequestered in the basal ganglia in a substructure called the nucleus accumbens, where our likes and desires are regulated. These distinct sensations coincide when what we desire is what we actually like and are adrenalised to pursue in order to achieve. This is motivation, our brain-based mechanism for getting our needs met. So pursuing desires and cultivating resources are sometimes necessary, but these comes with the costs of wear and tear in our mind, body and relationships that can be mitigated by inner strength and resilience.

This appeals to the dopaminergic pleasure-reward circuitry that encodes our likes, desires and goals (see figure 8.1). Recall this circuitry derives from the instinctive brain ventral-tegmental area and extends to the dorsolateral prefrontal cortex, the part of our cerebral-cognitive brain where cognitive empathy and exercise of compassion—including self-compassion—are regulated and our efforts and achievements are rewarded. These events, however, begin with neuroceptions reaching the cortices, affirming safety and fulfilment, thus moving us to deploy intelligence, resilience and well-being (see part V) SPEARS and act with authenticity, generosity and gentleness in our relationships. The stages and considerations are explored in the next chapter.

Chapter 11

Neuropsychosocial Integration

Stages and Considerations

In theory, therapy brings a wholesome state of integration for the trauma survivor. But it is much more than that. It is also a structured healing space in which the survivor shows up, typically in a state of vulnerability or disintegration or in some way lost. The attuned therapist brings a restorative presence to establish, first, a relationship of resonance. From this point of view, the therapeutic space, the relationship it gives rise to and the interventions it promotes are interdependent. In other words, if the relationship is restorative, so too will be the space and practical intervention. As for intervention, a good way to think of it is as a kind of a noninvasive neurosurgery for integration across the body and mind.

This comes from the conceptualisation of the nervous system as the host of the body and mind in society (Vygotsky, 1978), and where intervention to promote integration must begin. I consider this a core condition of neuropsychosocial therapy that centres integration in the nervous system along with authentic self-discovery, self-development and self-transformation. I am compelled to stress here that this is not an alternative for psychiatric intervention, which may be necessary to manage troublesome clinical diseases and disorders, such as schizophrenia, resistant mood disorders and personality disorders. Rather, neuropsychosocial therapy is about interrogating the body, mind, ancestry and wider social history to contextualise and discharge the chaotic energy of psychosocial trauma, restore authenticity in the self and equip the authentic self to serve the evolutionary imperative of preserving life and well-being.

Guiding the survivor on this path is a vital role a therapist plays, one that calls for the therapist to have some awareness of psychosocial trauma carried by populations of which the survivor is a member. To take an example, I have discussed the history of economic marginalisation, social exclusion and exploitation in medical research that connects black and indigenous peoples of the Americas to intergenerational trauma from chattel slavery, which may show up in the therapeutic space. This level of awareness, however, although helpful, may not be necessary. A way forward may be to organise the therapeutic work around change-oriented story-retelling. I tend to put it to my therapy students as 'we are working on your quiver of SPEARS, to shape and strengthen them, and this involves cultivating your inner capacities'.

Recall from chapters 1 and 2 that our first lot of SPEARS is somato-psycho-emotional attunement and relational security (see figure 2.1). When bent by psychosocial trauma and neuropsychosocial disintegration, these SPEARS are liable to manifest as somato-psycho-emotional misattunement and relational insecurity. Questions 12 and 19 on the ALEs survey are designed to surface this situation. In a clinical sense, however, the survivor will complain of relational anxiety, emotional confusion, spiritual vacancy, psychological rigidity, social apathy and mind-body dissociation that reflects a distorted sense of safety.

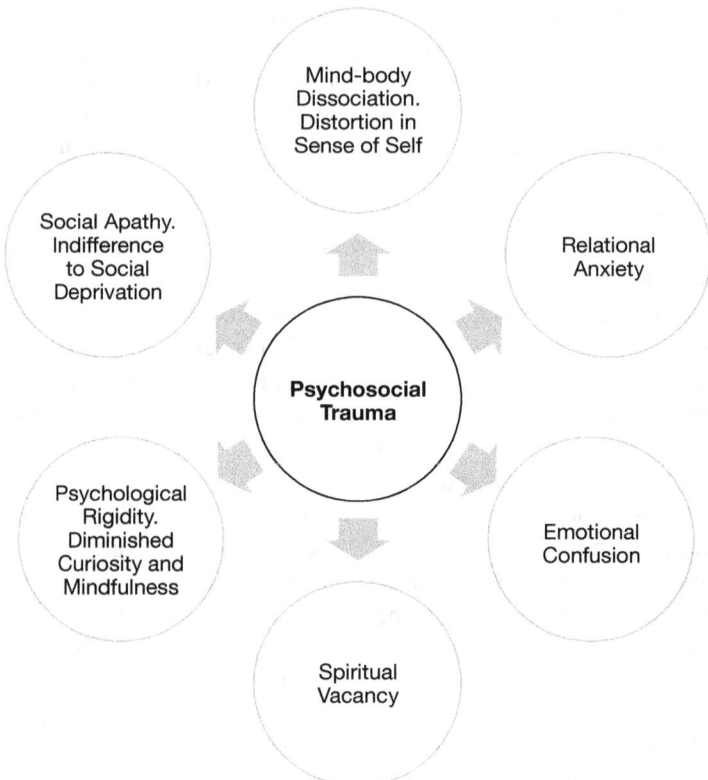

Figure 11.1. Psychosocial Trauma Clinical Expression

Within the context of the therapeutic relationship, the survivor is not only encouraged to revisit their social history, interrogate their ancestry, descend into their body and mind, and discharge the energy of psychosocial trauma that expresses itself in these maladaptations, but also to cultivate inner resources to flourish in wellness. There may be the experience of transcendence, that transpersonal trip my grandmother would tell me about and which I now understand involves a level of consciousness one can arrive at after freeing oneself from deep psychosocial trauma and when the psyche, soma and soul are engaged in a synchronous dance with each other and with the social world. This dance metaphor speaks to the steps, patterns, boundaries and continuity that characterise a dance as orderly, soothing and restorative. Healing, in a word.

In this dance, the psyche, soma and soul are not merely nourishing each other but also entertaining the inflow of virtuous information, including the awe inspiring and magical. Such information may be for the benefit of one's own self, as in a righteous revelation about one's loving-kindness arriving in a dream, or a state of mindfulness when attention influences brain activity and establishes links across its continents, thereby shaping its structure. It could be for the benefit of others, such as a cure for a disease afflicting kin, a friend or even a stranger. What is important is that the nervous system is integrated, the mind is present, the heart is open and the soul is free, so this kind of information—ordered and bounded—flows uninterrupted. This may also mean that it comes in suddenly without warning, or after a period of preparation and expectation. I consider this state one of neuropsychosocial integration, which involves three key stages.

NEUROPSYCHOSOCIAL INTEGRATION CORE STAGES

Stage I

At Stage I, the survivor becomes aware of their nervous system playing host to historical trauma in their psychosomatic subconscious. This may occur gradually through interrogation of social history and interpretation of their reactions to life events. That trauma might be conspicuous or less so. It may be ancestral, derived from a forgotten lived experience; it could be prenatal; or it could otherwise be embedded in early life before the development of the survivor's declarative memory system. Recall from part III that trauma can embed in the developing nervous system in utero and create vulnerabilities for which the survivor will compensate—psychologically, emotionally and behaviourally.

Surfacing this trauma and the adaptions behind which it preserves itself in therapy, and within the restorative relationship, can prove troublesome.

My example of a progressive approach is to begin with a conversation in which the survivor is invited to talk about how adverse as well as restorative experiences are processed and reacted upon in their nervous system, learning that this is part of the therapeutic process. The idea is that, as the survivor becomes aware of what might be going on in their body when they are exposed to certain life event, it should become easier to make sense of their thoughts, feelings and behaviours and to act with intention to improve their well-being by changing the story of what serves and does not serve them. Since this is a stage of awareness and relationship building, it may not involve practical therapeutic intervention, although the survivor will be aware that intervention involves working at the neural level.

Stage II

The second stage involves contextualizing, discharging and grieving traumas and trauma-based responses. Contextualising is about confronting active traumas; executing therapeutic intervention is an extension to this. I tend to begin this stage working backward, by 'naming to tame' and micro-restructuring narratives surrounding cognitive, emotional and relational maladaptations. And, only if necessary, I might employ operant conditioning techniques, where positive feedback rewards desired neural activities and psychosomatic expressions and negative feedback discourages undesirable neural activity. Whatever the technique used, the objective must be that maladaptive trauma responses become dissociated from traumatic wounds and active traumas lose their charge. Much like with any loss, these traumas must be grieved in stages.

First, like a child who loses its mother, the sensation of that lost is instinctive and emotional, overwhelming and inconceivable. And then, like a mother who loses a child, the sensation is upsetting, but then moves upwards to cognition, where it is rationalised and accepted as a new reality. Therapy is effective and neuropsychosocial integration is in progress when this level of emotional regulation becomes normative. At this stage, the survivor can feel disrespected as an authentic emotional sensation, but not inclined reactively to reach for a weapon to hurt the person who is disrespecting; the survivor can feel ashamed, but won't reactively say yes to a proposition they should say no to; they can be assaulted, but not feel it is their fault or that they are responsible for other people's bad behaviour. This is truly a phenomenal stage of change and endless possibilities for new neural patterns to be established and normalized using techniques to improve resourcefulness, reflectiveness, regulation and resilience—with which we shall become familiar by the end of this book.

Stage III

At Stage III, traumatic wounds are contextualised and integration begins to settle. This is where the survivor can also safely travel into the transpersonal state, to seek guidance—perhaps from ancestral wisdom—and return to the conscious unperturbed, with answers and solutions to sometimes very complex problems. This is also the stage at which the survivor is competent in introducing hormetic stress to build resilient capacities and cognitive reserve.

We evoke hormetic—virtuous—stress when we undertake challenges to exercise and strengthen our body and mind, to prevent our muscles and brain power from wasting away and to help us to build resilience against traumatic stress. It is by using our cognitive and physical muscles in a controlled and safe way that the memory and muscle cells will stay nourished and enable us to weather the stress of ALEs with resilience and to heal and reintegrate more quickly when traumatic cleavages occur. Before we can explore this in practice, we must be acquainted with considerations for neuropsychosocial integration.

NEUROPSYCHOSOCIAL INTEGRATION CORE CONSIDERATIONS

I mentioned earlier that the psyche, soma and soul are in synch with each other and the social world in a state of neuropsychosocial integration. This is a feature of well-being and the object of neuropsychosocial therapy, which I will now refer to as NPS-T for short, that incorporates relational, psychological, emotional and somatic considerations in liberating the survivor's instincts and capacities to self-heal.

We have learned throughout the chapters that people who move through life with psychosocial trauma are incredibly creative and adaptive, including in how they survive ALEs. An important aim of NPS-T is, therefore, to free up the survivor's inner creativity with attention, insight and inspiration. This work must begin in a space safe enough to be authentic, set boundaries and pursue wellness, as opposed to one in which the survivor is told what to do or how to be, to fit into a way of life and mimic a personality structure that they did not participate in designing.

This is achievable with resilient psychosocial resources that can be cultivated in the therapeutic space around core considerations, the first of which is neuroplasticity, the nervous system's mechanisms for learning and adapting to new experiences, which can be suppressed by disintegration. This can reflect in loss of authenticity, vulnerability, purpose and so on, which needs

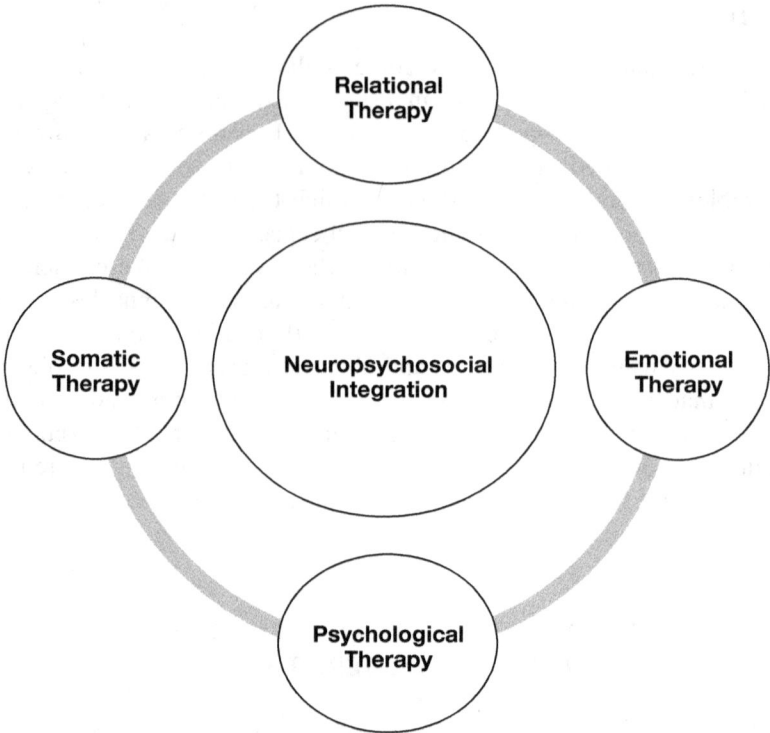

Figure 11.2. Neuropsychosocial Therapy and Resourcing

to be processed to completion but for which the capacity to do so is inaccessible or absent.

Neuroplasticity is an eternal gift that allows for learning new ways, discovering how these ways might work for the survivor, and installing these ways in personality, even in the most limiting of circumstances, say an injury or mutation in the nervous system that compromises its structural integrity and impairs its ability to carry out certain functions. In fact, the old equipotentiality hypothesis holds that the nervous system is disposed to redirect the potential and role of parts that are absent, damaged or inaccessible to other parts that are intact. This is how people who are born without arms learn to use their feet to do things—such as eat, take care of their bodies and care for their babies—that arms are usually used to do. Another good example is the recovery of losses that can occur after accidents. A person who loses a finger in an accident may find that the area of their sensory cortex that received information from the missing finger receives input from the adjacent fingers, causing their remaining digits to become more sensitive to touch.

Our nervous system, however, is the most plastic in childhood, as it is rapidly developing. It is also during this time that we learn the most about our environment and our ability to control specific bodily functions, such as movement, vision and hearing, that are regulated in specific areas—such as the parietal, occipital and temporal lobes—in the cerebral cortex. Damage or disorders in these areas, say by a physical injury, may mean we lose the ability to perform certain functions. For instance, an infant who suffers damage to facial recognition areas in the temporal lobe may never be able to recognise faces (Farah et al., 2000). However, the nervous system is not divided up in an entirely rigid way. Neurons have a remarkable capacity to reorganize and extend themselves in response to stimulation and injury. Furthermore, although specialist neurons generally cannot repair or regenerate themselves, as skin cells can, the nervous system can generate new neurons from stem cells in very specific and deep areas (Lieberwirth & Wang, 2012) that migrate to other brain areas to join networks or form new connections with other neurons. This remarkable feat enables the nervous system to grow, change and adjust to new experiences. Or, more precisely, allow the nervous system to change its structure and adapt in response to experience and injury.

And because changes to the nervous system occur continuously, when a traumatic memory is recalled in a safe context, we are forcing the memory to be stored differently in the body and mind by creating new pathways through which it travels to consciousness and recall. It is by this mechanism that new response patterns are created to compete with old, unuseful and undesirable ones. As this is encouraged, the more new appropriate adaptive response patterns that are created, the greater the chance one will be chosen over a maladaptive one. Practice will bring stability in appropriate response patterns, which will become default as the chaotic energy depletes in undesirable ones, which then retire away as legacy.

Obviously, reprocessing traumatic memory of any kind can be challenging for the best among us. The vulnerable edge in us, however, is liable to respond to compassion. This is especially true when working through cumulative traumas, such as abuse and neglect in childhood, where the presence of a compassionate therapist can help the survivor to confront and process painful sensations and memories in a safe and validating relationship. We established from the outset that survivors need a safe space in which to explore how trauma shows up in their body and make sense of neuroceptions.

It also helps that recalling traumatic events or details is not necessary in order to discharge the chaotic energy that sustains trauma. Once survivors discover they are custodian to a legacy of trauma, they can choose how that story ends, say by committing to letting go of burdens of the past and creating a future in which they can experience a fulfilling life, as their ancestors would have wanted. Recovery of that self—deserving of the best experience in life—can then begin with contextualising behaviours and sensations through which old trauma manifests. Where there is dissociation, survivors may use terms like *intolerance, fatigue* and *numbness* to bring character to the trauma and create some separateness from it. The goal is to identify traumas as belonging in the past and to reconcile them by focusing on choices available in the present. This work can be difficult and may be best accomplished in a functional therapeutic relationship.

Part V

NEUROPSYCHOSOCIAL
INTEGRATION IN THERAPY

Chapter 12

Neurorelational Integration

Throughout this book, I have pointed to the necessity of functional relationships in neuropsychosocial integration and leading a life of authenticity and fulfilment. This is based on the assumption that authenticity and fulfilment in the self can be achieved in relationships and spaces that are well-being affirming, wherein we share our gifts and losses and are encouraged to open up—not only to heal when we are wounded but also to receive virtuous blessings, co-regulation and social affirmation.

The obverse is the chokedness we can experience from being filled with the gifts of love but with no one to share it with; fascinating stories, but no one to tell them to; wealth, but no one to enjoy it with. Or depletion from neuroses, but no one from whom to receive compassion, or any other disturbance to our well-being or that of our generations to come.

An important component of integration, hence, is coming to terms with this native vulnerability. This task requires that we are intentional in our building and nurturing of functional relationships and relational resiliency, and in promoting the same in our families and communities. Relationships, however, take on lives of their own and can function in very different ways. Our interest here is the therapeutic function and the corresponding well-being SPEAR through which this function can be actualised, not only to procure integration but also to promote well-being.

NEURORELATIONAL WELL-BEING

In a practical sense, neurorelational well-being is our goal when we undertake to relate engagingly, communicate meaningfully, think creatively and live purposefully. Preceding this goal is a healing experience centred around 'secure attachments' that can be cultivated for the purpose of well-being. It is helpful to mention that secure attachment is a pattern of relating first observed by the American psychologist Mary Ainsworth among mothers and children who participated in her seminal research on caregiving relationships in early life. However, before it is a pattern of relating, it is a relational disposition with which we can be primed before birth (Bowlby, 1982), deriving from the native need for intimacy that persists throughout the life cycle, shielding us from the forsaken feelings of irrelevance and alienation.

My goal here is to emphasise that secure attachment is much more than a human capacity and pattern of relating. It is a fundamental human need that is promoted by neural substructures in the socioemotional-brain limbic system, which become active in the first trimester of gestation, to a greater extent in the right cerebral hemisphere (Schore, 2019). This occurs through a neurobiological process that begins in the brainstem, from where self-preservation circuitries work to distinguish whether a relationship is safe, chancy or life-threatening and to select for opportunities to connect in safe relationships. Stress regulatory catecholamines and cortisol, for instance, will warn against relationships that are chancy or life-threatening, whilst prosocial oxytocin and dopamine will reward safety in resonant relationships (Schore, 2015).

Before the oxytocin and dopamine circuitries, however, ancient wisdom submits that a crude attachment system through which the infant survives in the uterine environment favours and promotes safe connections. This begins at conception, following the zygote implanting in mother's womb and the creating of the cord that binds mother and child. It is first a system through which the child receives nourishment and information about the world. But quickly it becomes a mechanism through which the child—and the adult the child becomes—learns to relate competently. This going wrong can have catastrophic consequences.

Case Study: Misinterpreting and Mishandling Relational Trauma

Millions of people around the world are ordinarily diagnosed with relational disorders—such as pathological disagreeableness, defiance and oppositionality—that are controlled with a range of therapies, including psychostimulants and antipsychotic drugs. For children who behave in ways that are inconsistent with our expectations, the message is that the behaviour should be controlled, and we can do that easily although not always effectively with drugs and violence. The experience of six-year-old Kaia Rolle, who was arrested in 2019 at school in Florida, speaks to this reality.

The distressing images from the arrest showed armed police officers leading the young child with her hands zip-tied while she wailed and pleaded for her 'grandma' to be called. The child seemed to know she needed attunement to a nurturing caregiver, a parent, a teacher or a child therapist who could co-regulate her internal chaos. This is precisely what the children I work with, who have difficulty with relating, seem to want and with whom attunement and co-regulation almost always work in returning them to relational competency. This was not Rolle's experience, and it is not isolated.

Crime statistics in the United States show that between 2013 and 2018 at least 296,000 children under age twelve were arrested. In England and Wales, this number was 71,885 in 2019. Offences for which children are commonly arrested include assaults, prostitution and truancy. And, in addition to these ALEs, an arrest has the potential to derail a child's future. For the neuropsychosocial therapist, behaviours have relational input, and when behaviours do not serve the patient, we want to ask what is happening relationally, whether a relational trauma might be affecting the survivor's capacity to relate appropriately.

In the absence of disorder, we begin life with an advanced capacity to relate, and we will swiftly begin to demonstrate this—upon our arrival in the social world—to smiling faces and soothing voices signalling to us that we are welcomed, belong and are supported in our need for relationship and safety. Naturally, we will not yet have the cognitive facility that allows us to respond with any degree of hindsight, insight or foresight, to help us to make sense of this experience and the neural activities surrounding it. However, when the pangs of our first hunger are quickly met with warm breast milk; the unfamiliar air on our skin tempered with warmth from mother's bosom; and the crude oxygen making its way through our lungs is flavoured with the familiar smell of mother, we are learning that life is good, we belong in this world and we are safe enough. Such a welcome to social life is ideally met with optimal mitochondrial function, a brain anointed in dopamine and oxytocin, a gut lined with lactase and serotonin, the cells in our body sufficiently supplied with growth hormones, and our ventral vagal fibres sufficiently myelinated and interconnected with the other cranial nerves.

This is the neurobiology of social engagement, and neuroscience submits that it sets us up for optimal development and functioning in a relational world that can be unpredictable, tumultuous and at times downright unsafe. In childhood, it signals to us that we are in attunement with a caregiver to whom we will turn when we are confused, distressed or otherwise need guidance to make sense of adverse life events. These include events that may arise inside of our own body, such as a tightening in the chest, or from outside of our body, as in an act of nature, such as a hurricane, or in an act of inhumanity, as in a civil war. This kind of attunement is a condition for optimal learning, growth and character building. However, research tells us, ALEs included, we do not all come into the world so prepared.

Many of us are here because our innocence, small bodies and inability to prevent our exploitation in childhood were useful on a farm or on social media, our parents did not act to prevent an unwanted pregnancy or the abortion that was meant to terminate our existence failed. In all these circumstances, and the many variants one can imagine, life chose us and biology equipped us to survive, overcome our adverse reality and even thrive in spite of them. Often, however, those for whom these ALEs have warped their sense of self and promoted self-destructive impulses—whether that is to self-loath, self-negate, self-sacrifice or entertain a negative self-image—can find recovery difficult and distant. And by recovery, I mean healing their wounded self and surfacing their authenticity to lead a life free from the chaos of trauma that derives from a history of harmful relationships. This recovery is to be actualised within the context of more relationship—safe, healing and nurturing relationships—which can seem unfathomable. But within the therapeutic space, these relationships can be cultivated as the survivor undertakes to integrate their wounded selves with deserved attention and compassion and in so doing reorient their perception of the world as one in which kindness and belonging exist in abundance and are available to them.

This is possible because the need to feel cared about and protected in our relationships is eternal. The British psychiatrist John Bowlby, who acquainted the world of attachment psychology with this need, argued persuasively that it can be activated at any time throughout the life cycle (Bowlby, 1990), a saving grace from which we can begin to make sense of relational injuries that feature in adverse life outcomes. Consider, for instance, socioeconomic privation, psychosomatic maladies and premature death that deplete our capacity to weather relational stress in ordinary life, even when anticipated.

I am here compelled to share an unfortunate incident that occurred during the pandemic. A friend's ninety-six-year-old grandmother transitioned to rest in peace, and within days of her passing, her lifelong spouse succumbed to a 'broken heart', an unconventional term for distress-induced cardiomyopathy that can be caused by overwhelming relational loss, such as the loss of a loved one, whereupon the heart cannot recover from its lost resonance with the other heart it holds dear. Symptomatically, the increased activity of stress-regulatory chemistry in the cardiac arteries results in overwhelming enlargements and constrictions that cause the muscles to fail, fatally, as the blood flow becomes disorganised. Whilst beginning in the heart, this kind of death manifests symptomatically as extreme apathy, hopelessness and desertion of the will to live, the first purpose of life itself. The psyche is then forced to disconnect from the body's perception of its needs and retire itself. This psychogenic death is followed by a somatic death to affirm that traumatic stress arising from deep relational injury can be consequential in the severest of ways.

The loss of significant relationships in which we enjoy security—food, affection and intimacy—can cause indeterminable suffering. Beyond the individual, this is known to undermine safety and progress across generations at group and community levels. I can speak to the experience in black communities in the Americas, including the Caribbean, where childhood has an upward of 70 percent chance of being lived in socioeconomically vulnerable lone-parent and grandparent households, alongside an elevated risk of premature death from intimate partner violence among black women (Beckett & Clayton, 2022), the high incidence of premature death reflecting a prevalence of relational crises that are overwhelming and too traumatic to endure.

Preceding this crisis, however, is chronic helplessness and hopelessness in boys and girls arriving in adult life wounded, disintegrated and desperate to rein in pains of neglect, abandonment and often battery inflicted by moms, dads, grandparents and other caregivers possessed by a perverse spirit, typically of community, education, religion or a combination. With little or even a deficit in relational resources to protect themselves from these pains, survivors move through life with maladaptations in personality, neurobiology and defences that typically do not serve them, nor anyone in a relationship with them.

Think of sequestering their pain in an inauthentic self, dampening it with drugs and projecting it onto intimate partners. Or, at the level of the neurobiological, an altered hypothalamic-pituitary-adrenal axis (HPAA) that leaves them vulnerable to stunted psychosocial development and neurosis. Since Felitti's ACE study, premature separation from caregivers has been a better understood relational trauma that informs these adaptations in children. Premature separation can come because of death, divorce or a parent not wanting to be a parent anymore and leaving, maybe going to the shop and never coming back, which is my first memory of my mother when I was about age six. It may also be factors in the caregiver's life—such as abuse, addictions and mental illness—that can cause relational trauma that transcends childhood, influencing confidence, self-esteem and choices of intimate partners as well as how relational needs are met. Thanks to ACE, we have learned that these events in early life are inimical to a child's somato-psycho-emotional attunement and relational security, and in fact promote relational insecurity.

Insecure patterns of relating can result in behavioural issues and emotional challenges. For example, uncertainty about a caregiver's availability can trigger incessant crying and clinginess in a child and may show up in adult life as insecurities that drive relentless attention seeking and stalking in relationships. A participant in my research, whom I shall call Aaron and whose consent I have to share his experience, likened this insecurity to the daemon that occupies a child's mind when the lone parent (his mother) is out working, but he doesn't know where she works, what work she does and when she will come home with whatever she finds to eat or rage about.

This kind of unknowing or uncertainty in attachment relationships is a source of relational anxiety for the children who arrive in adulthood withdrawn from their relational need and bereft of a relational SPEAR. They may perceive their lack, but this awareness alone is of little value given how they were treated by the people who were meant to care for them. Here we are forced to imagine how these lives emerged despite not being sufficiently held, spoken to and reassured as a child. They lack the common childhood experiences of being held physically and rhythmically, cuddled, read to, lovingly tossed in the air, held upside down for a bouncy moment, or engaged in rough-and-tumble play in a way that makes children feel at home in their own skin and safe in their relationships. However such individuals adapt to cope with these unfulfilled relational needs—the pangs of abandonment, neglect and other traumatic separation from caregivers—in the long run they are liable to be vulnerable to dysautonomia, traumatic stress disorders and developmental problem that can last a lifetime.

The therapeutic relationship will encourage them to remember what might have happened to them whilst at the same time reflecting on how they carry themselves—in how they stand, speak and react to other people's invitations and demands on them and on their emotions when they are invited to touch, laugh or engage in play. Recognising these patterns is a step towards discharging the chaotic energy that sustains them, as the trauma-informed therapist creates the conditions for activating the fibres of the social engagement nerve, so that the renewal cycle can begin and integration in the nervous system can be achieved. In surrendering to the therapeutic relationship, the survivor is encouraged to redirect their relational story. The first task in this process is to acknowledge the trauma, a task for which the ALEs questionnaire can be helpful, as the survivor gets to label and score their ALEs and create some distance between particular events and their whole self. The next task involves cultivating a relational SPEAR.

NEURORELATIONAL SPEAR

Relational therapy allows us to safely confront relational injuries and express relational needs within the context of a relationship. This is an empowering experience that is facilitated in a space of optimism wherein we can explore our story about who and how we are, as well as the impact of social history, beliefs and behaviours on our relationships, and retire maladaptive patterns that are expressions of psychosocial trauma. At the neurorelational level, the energy that fuels these patterns may come from past generations who passed on to us biology and cultures to survive in our relational world, and it flows freely in our autonomic nervous system, from where our navigation of this world begins. This includes the chaotic energies of self-destructiveness, absence, confusion, selfishness and dissonance that characterise dysfunctional relationships in which we suffer, and which can be overcome with the healing energies of self-compassion, presence, equanimity, altruism and resonance that together constitute our neurorelational SPEAR.

Self-Compassion

Self-compassion is a prosocial emotion that entails sensations of connectedness and fulfilment in the self and is a psychosocial resource at the heart of neuropsychosocial integration. It is the capacity to act in service to one's own well-being, and it cannot coexist with the chaotic energy that sustains self-destructiveness. Self-compassion involves turning inward, to view the self from the mind's eye and be disposed not only to self-preserve but also to self-promote and fully self-actualise. It is not uncommon to find that people who move through life besieged by psychosocial trauma—say the cycle

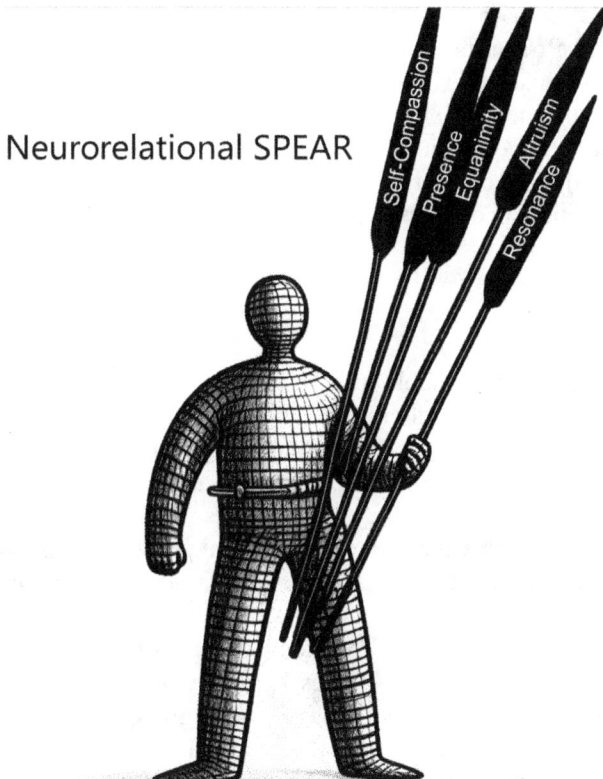

Figure 12.1. Neurorelational SPEAR—Therapeutic Resources. *Figure courtesy of Dagmar Roelfsema.*

of shame, grief and guilt or a sense of being lost—will have difficulties in accessing this healing energy, for the capacity for self-compassion is often impaired by trauma.

> **Task:** Interrogate your relational story to establish whether you can recognise deficits and fractures in your relationship with yourself. This may be from having compromised your moral boundary. In your changing story, commit to having moral boundaries that you honour and reinforce with consequences, and to fully accepting and forgiving yourself for taking on responsibilities that are not your own and which deplete you. Freely ask for forgiveness and accept consequences for having caused others in relationships with you to suffer, intentionally or unintentionally. Can you commit to this change? The idea is that relational boundaries informed by your morals and values represent a secure base from which to engage relationally, without becoming burdened with self-compassion fatigue.

In cultivating self-compassion, the survivor is encouraged in the therapeutic space to reach inside their body and mind and acknowledge any deficit in how they relate with themselves and others. They must accept fully any disposition to self-sacrifice or self-abandon in service of relationship and bring it to consciousness. This is an important stage in assessing the potential for relational fulfilment where the nervous system, led by the brain, scans for resonance and trust, conditions the therapist brings to the relationship and, when registered by the survivor's nervous system, will activate the secure attachment circuitry and respond to invitations to connect through the compassion neural pathway.

Presence

Presence means being available in body and mind for connection and well-being in relationship. Throughout this book, I have talked about survivors of trauma who present themselves in relationships physically but not psychically or authentically. The cultivation of presence is about closing this gap so that when they are present in body they are also present in mind and with authenticity. We appreciate this through our autonomic processes that reflect what is going on inside us and around us and in our intrapersonal and interpersonal relationships.

Our own breath, for instance, which carries out its tasks without us having to think about it, is one of those processes we can use to measure the health of our relationships. For instance, our breath might speed up or slow down when we bring our self to a certain relationship. This could be one we desire, one in our past or one that is active in our life, say with a friend, a spouse or our own self. The practice of breath monitoring— paying attention to our breath as it opens up our lungs and brings oxygen into our body to process these sensations—goes against the course of nature. However, intentionally doing it, which could be difficult at first, is known to promote neural signalling pattens that strengthen with practice. The auxiliary effect is that it blocks intrusive self-judgements and transfers to other autonomic processes, such as emotional reactions and impulse awareness.

> **Task:** Interrogate your relationships of significance that have endured fracture over time as a result of your relational temperature—coldness or absence, whether emotional or physical. This could also be your relationship with yourself, a sibling or a former friend. What is the story? At the point when you recognise a sensation, such as disappointment after constant betrayal or contempt for someone you once loved, stop. Welcome the sensation and study its message. What can it teach you? How can you rework this story to integrate it into the whole and continuing story of your life in a way where it is honoured? Notice how your breath—already inside of you—is responding. Is it shallow, sticking or speeding up as you work on correcting your story of presence and recalibrating your perception of relationships in which you were absent? The aim is to free up tension associated with the sensation of absence and allow it to flow upward from the spinal chain to the cerebral cortex. What is the story of your mood and agency over the sensation? Check that you are present and mindful.

Recall that mindfulness is an ancient practice that involves focusing the mind on internal processes that are innervated by our neural fibres. Mindfulness exercises are empowering in that they can condition the practitioner to interrogate ALEs, act or reflect on them and in so doing bind the free-flowing energy from within their body and mind. In this process, input from external relationships is reduced and the nervous system will recalibrate the social engagement circuit in the hindbrain to invoke a state of openness to learning and curiosity in what is nourishing.

This is a parasympathetic tone in which the amygdala settles down, the mind calms, the body relaxes and neural regeneration gets underway (Eriksson et al., 1998). I appreciate this may be easier said than done for some people who come to the task of life with relational traumas, who might find it easier to do it whilst sitting at home with little to distract them. It can be much harder in the throes of dysautonomia and relational anxiety, when reacting to life events from a place of fear, frustration and woundedness. There, mindfulness and presence can feel out of reach when most needed.

Equanimity

This is the capacity to stay present and composed in one's true self as one navigates the rises and falls that are ordinarily experienced in relationships—and life more generally—which is necessary before integration can be achieved and well-being sustained. Equanimity, at the heart of which lies elasticity in self-control, can become depleted or lost due to psychosocial trauma, especially the kind we inherit from ancestry and family history, in which our capacity to nurture fulfilling relationships in the wilds of life depletes across multiple generations. In *Becoming a Better You*, life coach Peter Vajda (2013) encourages us to cultivate equanimity—the capacity to confront adversity and be at peace—as a foundation for self-compassion and relational freedom, that is, without getting derailed by confrontations or caught up in drama—either our own or that of others. With this freedom, we can allow ourselves to participate in relationships with empathy. And as we agree, disagree or remain impartial in our relating, little is internally dysregulated, as we freely separate people from external actions.

> **Task:** What is the story of your role in the fractures, challenges and fulfilment you experience in relationships? Can you accept that people create the reality through which they respond to pain and suffering? Interrogate how you might improve your reality so that it is not laden with conflicts and crises. In improving your story, commit to being the director of your life outcomes, a role you undertake with courage and confidence in your native and resilience SPEARS, in spite of the challenges of ordinary life.

Courage and confidence at the heart of equanimity promote our integration as we experience and respond to adversity that would otherwise stoke confusion. This could look like interpersonal conflict, in which we may be inclined to project our pain onto others with whom we are related or relating, but will not do so because we are present and rational. In this spirit, equanimity is promoting relational integrity, which helps us to stay courageous and confident in our response to life events without the need to fault, blame or project. Thus, survivors begin to cultivate this resource with faith. Not necessarily religiosity, but faith in the native intelligence and wisdom through which we meet challenges without the fear of sacrificing our self or important relationships.

Cultivating equanimity involves treating reality and its characteristic dynamism as features of life and being okay with rejecting and releasing relational burdens that do not serve us. This is also about balancing our social-emotionality with the power to stay engaged, both of which promote mindfulness. In being mindful, we improve our ability to stay integrated and response-able as we navigate the rough waters of adversity and surf the waves of relational trauma. As we develop this practice, we will experience deeper states of equanimity, which we will recognise as we respond with empathic matter-of-factness to people, events and circumstances that once caused us to be reactive. These will no longer hold any 'charge'. In a word, we will suffer less and respond more effectively to adversity. Our responses will occur in the context of authenticity, through which we are encouraged to experience well-being irrespective of external circumstances. Equanimity opens us up to this, and to being fully present and engaged in our relationships, to speak truth from a place of authenticity and to be both trusting and trustworthy. We can give freely and generously because we do so without losing ourselves.

Altruism

There is a lot that goes on inside of us, in a good way, that we are biologically inclined to share with others generously. This is what altruism is about, that abundance of goodwill and sense of fullness that connect us with others when we give without expecting anything in return. This may not make sense from a rational or even socioeconomic point of view, from which altruism can be seen as unwise in nonreciprocal relationships. However, I am talking about relational resources—like love, encouragement and mindful recognition—that can be shared without oneself becoming depleted. From the point of view of neuropsychosocial integration, this involves giving that does not deplete the giver nor the source of what is given. Nor is it lessened by what is not given.

> **Task:** Interrogate how much of your resources you share with others in a way that depletes you or does not deplete you. How is this story unfolding, from volunteering your time to being fully present in conversations? You might think of yourself as generous and giving in this sense. How about sharing your life experience with others in a way that leaves you feeling vulnerable and exasperated, but also empowered and protective? What is the message and how does it alter your story? There could be an opening of your heart, a sense of purpose or of connection. The goal is to promote the prosocial neurobiology of altruism in your relationships, including with yourself—the most important relationship you have.

It is December 2023 as I write this chapter, and I feel compelled to notice the season's giving spirit. The world is still recovering from the woes of the COVID-19 pandemic through which an inestimable number of people lost their lives and livelihoods. However, the many in need of basic necessities—of food, clothing and shelter—are being reached by the charitable hands of many who are contributing the same, because it is the right thing to do. Why? Not merely because the act of charity promotes our humanity, but more so because neurorelationally it staves of the quiet sadness we experience from having enough to share but being unable to share.

Working virtually with therapists throughout the pandemic, I sensed a quiet sadness alongside a desperation to alleviate it and the available 'enough' to share that was coming from a place of abundance. There was, for instance, an abundance of kindness, but no one to express it to; time, but no one to spend it with; talent, but no place to use it. People's need for relational satisfaction was unfulfilled as their gifts could not flow.

Nowhere was this more palpable than in the emotionally charged streets of Manhattan, New York, where I attended a call for action march against George Floyd's murder in 2020. For me, privately, it was about solidarity, much like for the many millions of souls around the world. Beyond solidarity, however, was my processing of the public execution of Floyd's black life—as a black woman of the Americas—stoking my sense of a particular vulnerability to dehumanisation and premature death that black life bears. Alongside this was my observation of a profound upset and desperation for social engagement and relatedness among people of all kinds—all who were forced to witness the demise of Floyd, identified by his superficial demographics: vulnerably black, under-resourced, harmfully stereotyped. Aha!

I realised that, as we were forced to isolate in our homes, the pandemic exposed us to the disabling relational dis-ease of being out of synch with others' suffering, but Floyd's offered us the opportunity to alleviate this predicament by confronting our authentic need to relate and share our own suffering and in so doing ignite a sense of fulfilment in our own lives. This is to suggest that altruism is not only about having enough to share but also about having others to share with, and sharing freely—of expectation, judgement and shame—in order to protect ourselves from relational dis-ease.

Resonance

The capacity to connect and influence others at the level of the native instincts in known as resonance, wherein resides the need to be connected to others and engaged meaningfully with the social world. Relational resonance—the root meaning of which is to connect intimately—is an output of the instinctive self. Thus, it is safe to say we are wired for resonance, even if to varying degrees. There is resonance with the familiar dog walker that is different from what one experiences in a marriage of twenty years. The latter orients to intimacy, which is necessary to cultivate before the survivor can accept their pleasant and unpleasant experiences and authentic and inauthentic parts. This is a journey, and it is not a particularly easy one for the many of us whose ancestors were treated as less than the humans they were and limited in their ability to pass on resonance to us, to help us to navigate life with a sense of ancestral connection.

Genetic science offers a place from where we might begin this journey, and this is good for those who find satisfaction in discovering their ancestry in their DNA and interrogating their social history to establish resonance with ancestors. This approach, however, may not be good for everyone. My own findings on my ancestors, scattered among peoples of West Africa, Scotland, Wales and Greco-Albania, left me less than satisfied in my quest for ancestral resonance, for I had questions that have stayed unanswered. These are important questions about how my ancestors had enough food, warmth and resonant relationships and were able to keep their selves, babies and elders safe. Whilst the DNA I inherited from them cannot yet answer these questions, I have learned that talking with my elders is a good solution, to find out how my parents, grandparents and great-grandparents lived their lives, what mattered to them, how they overcame adversities and how they envisaged life for their children.

A significant discovery for me in my relational therapy was that my mother's father, my grandfather, was her first love, and until his death when she was nine years old, he ensured she felt safe enough and sufficiently provided for within his means. He didn't have a chance at formal education or a stable first family. His mother passed away when he was small, and from then on he survived with the help of older siblings. In spite of his harsh beginning, he wanted to be married to my grandmother, be the father of her babies and keep her safe. In confronting my own abandonment by my father, I found relief in knowing my grandfather would not want this experience for me and did the best he knew to ensure I would be okay, even if only in imagining he would be present and active in shaping my expectations in relationship. Part of this imagined story is who I am in the absence of parents who showed they wanted me, and neurorelational therapy acquainted me with this version of me, so that when I am wounded in my relationships, when I am stretched out of shape and feel frazzled, I know this is not all of me; there is more.

> **Task:** Interrogate relationships in your life that are characterised by resonance you know to be true, even if you may not really know. This may be your relationship with the divine, your ancestors, parents or your own gut instincts. What is the story of these relationships? How are they different from nonresonant relationships that impact your relational well-being? Is there openness, compassion and congruence that buffer you against relational trauma? If not, how can your story of relationship be altered to include these and show that resonance intersects with compassion and altruism? The greater the resonance, the greater the chance of increasing self-compassion and altruism. And that comes with greater risks too. As you open yourself up to resonant relationships with others, you also become more exposed and vulnerable, since these others can more easily upset and hurt you.

Finding who we are despite chronic relational trauma is an important stage in neuropsychosocial integration, and this can be difficult to accept. Consider the catastrophic relational traumas of intimate partner violence and sexual violence in childhood that are prevalent in our society and perhaps too easily tolerated.

My finding is that the child molester who discovers or senses his father and grandfather were child molesters is unlikely to perceive sexual violence in childhood as a catastrophe that derails survivors' well-being. Similarly, the girl whose father habitually assaults her mother may not perceive assaults at the hands of a spouse in adulthood as a source of dis-ease. The literature in fact affirms this to be true. Girls of violent fathers are disposed to find themselves and stay in intimate relationship with violent spouses. Relational therapy is about confronting these truths and adapting beliefs and behaviours to promote integration, well-being and growth. Recall that disintegration is a chronic cleavage in the body, mind and self that embeds in and dysregulates the nervous system. The resonant therapeutic relationship creates the conditions for reintegrating the fragments, building relational authenticity and flourishing in healthy relationships—say with one's self, spouse, family or divinity—that alter biology.

The therapist's role in this relationship is to facilitate the survivor's exploration and experience of relational safety, authenticity and personal growth. This may involve creating the resonance for letting go of rituals and relationships with social history that do not promote integration and creating or adopting ones that promote emotional attunement through compassion. In addition to the healing energy it brings to the therapeutic relationship, this kind of relational resonance—originating in a ventral vagal chiasma—acts to improve immune system functioning and cardiovascular health, as well as strengthen the protective genetic features at the end of our chromosomes that are vulnerable to traumatic stress, which causes it to unravel.

NEURORELATIONAL THERAPY IN REFLECTION

We have learned that well-being can be difficult to achieve and sustain in the absence of a stable resonant relationship, and this includes the relationship one has with one's own self. The relational SPEAR, which features self-compassion, presence, equanimity, altruism and resonance, is important in structuring and sustaining this relationship, but also in reversing pathologies that derive from psychosocial trauma. For the survivor, a therapeutic relationship is a space to act out the need for integration and to flourish in well-being. But this begins with being cared for by a co-regulator; a therapist may assume that role, nervous system to nervous system, with the goal to resource the survivor so they can recover from relational trauma and build resilience through neuropsychosocial integration. Before we can get to integration, it must be clear how the survivor functions in important relationships, with their self, family and the social world, as well as how relational traumas feature in their life, in behaviour, personality or emotional problems.

In chapter 10, I mentioned different kinds of relationships I am inclined to explore within a therapeutic context, along with a mapping of the vagal state in which the survivor presents him- or herself. This mapping involves measures. Ten is my golden number, by which I mean that I seek to know on a scale of 0 to 10 how functional and satisfied the survivor is in relationships, with 10 being very satisfied and aspirational and 0 being very dysfunctional and dissatisfied. At 0, we may be confronting stubborn maladaptations and disorders—such as oppositional defiant disorder, borderline personality disorder and narcissistic personality disorder—that manifest within the context of dysfunctional relationships.

The survivor may rate their relationship with their self a meagre 2 of 10 to reveal a particularly poor relationship. Interrogation of that relationship may reveal sexual violence in childhood that left the survivor feeling dirty, ashamed or self-loathing. They may award the relationship with their mother a conservative 7 of 10 to reflect fracture and distance in childhood but repair and closeness that developed in adulthood. With the social world, they may award their relationship a moderate 4 of 10 to reflect fear of becoming a victim of social hostility and anxiety about harmful stereotypes. These are significant scores that point to urgency for relational therapy and resources. Relational therapy is where this relational need is explored in a sensitive and supportive way. Hence, a positive appraisal of the therapist's sensibility surrounding psychosocial trauma is important, for, as we saw with Alex, in the absence of this positive appraisal insecurities with which the survivor shows up to therapy are liable to compound and stay unresolved.

Perhaps the most remarkable benefit of relational therapy is that it can help a survivor at any age to cope with psychosocial trauma and reverse its features. It can also be combined with other therapies, for instance, to help a child or an adult develop mindfulness of their dispositions and behaviours that impact interpersonal relationships. In that sense, the therapy is to help the survivor to contextualise traumatic relational memories and move on from them, to bind and discharge the chaotic energy that sustains them, whilst strengthening their resilience SPEARS to better respond in relationship. An end goal might be learning to remain relatively composed during times of high relational stress, recovering quicker from episodes of relational distress or experiencing more and longer periods of comforting relationships. But treating relational trauma will typically need to be multifaceted. Considering that a life with relational trauma is likely to meet the criteria for other maladies, effective treatment must include care for these maladies as well as the trauma itself. Success can be measurable for those who commit to treatment from this integrative approach.

Chapter 13

Neuro-emotional Integration

There is no end to what can be said about emotions as they pertain to neuropsychosocial integration, considering the immense literature, and this is apparent throughout the chapters of this book. For my purpose here, however, emotions are understood as essential programs for survival behaviour that are encoded in our DNA. So integral are emotions to survival that our capacity to express them begins to develop in our social-emotional memory system in the first trimester of our life in utero, and we are sufficiently equipped to express them even if only in a crude sense by the time we are born.

Hence, upon arrival in the relational world, emotions are one of our first means through which we express our self and communicate our needs. For instance, curiosity in the newborn infant is expressed in openness to be fed, to suckle and to be held, and comfort is expressed through restful sleep. Sadness and fear—on the contrary—are expressed in cries and startles, which are also expressions of uncertainty and frustration. As we grow from infancy into caregiving relationships, emotions such as empathy, love, excitement and remorse emerge to move us to connect, build and protect important relationships. Anger, humiliation, despair and shame inhibit these behaviours. Across the range of emotions that move and inhibit us, these examples, and the experiences they derive from, bear implications for neuro-emotional well-being.

NEURO-EMOTIONAL WELL-BEING

In his exploration of the neurobiology of emotional development, the American neurobiologist Allan Schore (2015) points us to the particular role of the amygdala, our emotional safety monitor, in attaching emotional significance to experiences that embed in memory and, ultimately, as impulse. However,

185

traumatic memories can impair the neural encoding of how we experience and respond to different emotions. For instance, much like my example in the preface of flinching in the dark as a fear response to a stranger's touch, traumatic memories can tell us to appease or resent caregivers who abuse us, attack or recoil from teachers who shame and belittle us and engage or run away from the police, who may or may not want to harm us. These are ordinary life events from which we can infer that emotions are adaptive expressions of the self, which could be authentic or inauthentic, and that emotional dis-ease—or chronic emotional dysregulation—is a valid expression of neuropsychosocial disintegration.

Naturally, emotional dis-ease is averse to emotional security and, in a clinical sense, expresses itself as such. Examples of what I mean are the expression of love, instead of resentment, for people who emotionally injure us; loathing, instead of reverence, for expressions of vulnerability; and disdain, instead of empathy, for rituals that evoke shame. I have discussed the extent to which we do not have neural receptors for these emotions because they are largely instinctual, much like the mammalian instinct to protect and nurture children and to derive pleasure from doing so, for these behaviours are rewarded in the social-emotional circuitries.

Turning to the social-emotional system to cultivate emotional well-being involves the capacity to regulate our emotional state and use cognition to address questions of chronic emotional dysregulation. I have talked about the prefrontal cortex and the insula, which when impacted by trauma are not able to identify and regulate emotions and instead activate maladaptive trauma responses. The neuroceptions coming up from the unmyelinated dorsal vagal fibres are slow. In promoting synchronicity across these structure, emotional therapy gets them to work better and promotes flexibility in responses to traumatic stress.

In other words, when faced with ALEs that activate maladaptive responses, the prefrontal cortex can override this circuitry and allow the survivor to be sensible about what is happening. This is a bottom-up approach to integration that starts in the instinctive brain and journeys to the cognitive brain and back, and it may involve intellectual input to contextualise the trauma and retire maladaptive emotional patterns. The objective is to equip the survivor to move through life with wisdom and creative flexibility—the antidote to emotional dysregulation.

At this stage, we could undertake to mitigate environmental influences that are not conducive to optimal interaction between the social-emotional brain and the prefrontal circuits, These include not only inadequate provision in families and education or poor-quality food, but emotionally disruptive influences in the social environment. And this is important because our emotional circuitry adapts to environmental demands, which influence the circuits that develop, whether they develop and how they develop. Traumatic stress that targets these circuits will lead to adaptations necessary for survival, but at a significant cost to long-term emotional well-being.

The role of the emotionally attuned therapist is, therefore, to respond reliably to the survivor's need for emotional attunement and regulation, and to aid in the development of an emotional well-being SPEAR with which to instil emotional security until it becomes a comfortable state as well as a template for emotional intelligence and resilience. This may include mindfulness exercises in managing upsetting emotions as well as how to evoke comforting ones that shift the nervous system out of the maladaptive rigidity and reactivity that are features of psychosocial trauma and into the flexibility and receptivity that are characteristic of social engagement. It is in this state that the survivor is able to perceive accurate neuroceptions about emotional processes in the body and mind and respond to emotional demands in ways that promote well-being.

NEURO-EMOTIONAL SPEAR

In becoming emotionally flexible and receptive, the survivor is working to create connections across vast areas of the nervous system that strengthen with practice, as, according to the Canadian neuropsychologist Donald Hebb (1949), groups of neurons are repeatedly activated at the same time and become associated in neural networks. In other words, neurons receiving oxygen-rich blood that activate simultaneously also synchronise in networks through which emotionally protective experiences—such as self-love, friendship and mindful parenting—are filtered. From the point of view of neurochemistry, this is a state of social engagement in which acetylcholine and dopamine are released in the synaptic cleft and pleasure-reward neurocircuitry in response to prosocial, life-affirming experiences. Acetylcholine acts to keep the synapses strong and active, whilst dopamine rewards pleasure, meaning and value. This is an important goal for neuro-emotional therapy, through which chaotic energies of self-alienation, pessimism, disempathy, misattunement and recklessness are discharged by healing the energies of self-regulation, positiveness, empathy, attunement and reflectiveness that promote well-being and fend off emotional inflammation, neurochemical dysregulation and neurodegeneration.

Self-Regulation

Beginning in early life, emotional resonance in healthy caregiving relationships creates templates for self-regulation (Feldman, 2015). This is the

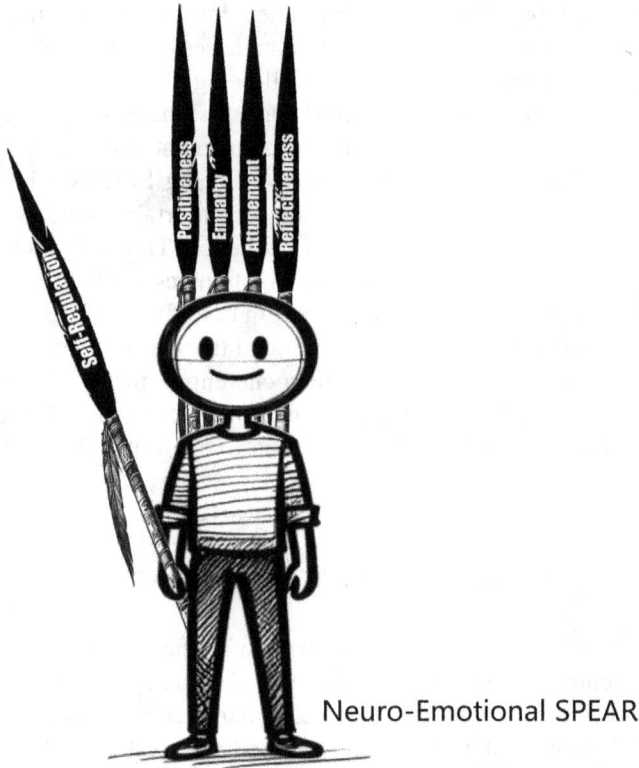

Neuro-Emotional SPEAR

Figure 13.1. Neuro-emotional SPEAR—Therapeutic Resources. *Figure courtesy of Dagmar Roelfsema.*

internal capacity to direct our emotions and regulate our emotional states, which are informed by sensations of safety and danger. When this does not happen and we do not develop a template for safety regulation, tension abounds in our emotional narrative, and the chaotic energy of this tension will inhibit our psychosocial development.

Thus, developmental trauma shows up across our life cycle as a deficit in our capacity to bring our self out of emotional chaos or paralysis. It may be that we feel too little or too much, and this gives rise to self-alienation and reactions that betray well-being. Think of addictive and compulsive behaviours that are features of obsessive-compulsive disorders and the emotional content of these behaviours. What do they tell us about how we are equipped to experience life?

Task: What stories do you tell yourself and others about the dominant emotional state in which you move through life? Is it anger, frustration and bitterness that derive from an early life that was insufferable and emotionally depleting? Or are your dominant emotions less externalising, such as dread, shame and guilt that are less relationally threatening but no less self-depletive? What about joy, passion and gratitude? Collect your stories about these distinct emotions and reflect on how they function in your life. What might you change, want more or less of, and how might you actualise this change as you are empowered?

In accepting that emotions are messages of how we are experiencing life events, we can learn to interrogate them to appreciate the message they bring and to determine whether those messages are true, false, good for us or not good for us. This is about cultivating flexibility to oscillate between emotional states, identify and honour their appropriateness and undertake and become better at self-regulation, competently binding the chaotic energy of self-alienation and reactive impulses. This emotional elasticity is at the heart of integration and is an important goal in neuro-emotional therapy that empowers survivors to take care of themselves and their most cherished in ways that reduce self-destructive thoughts and behaviours that are sustained by chaotic energy—such as thoughts of unworthiness, as well as the emotions that drive problem drinking, smoking and disordered eating.

Positiveness

Openness to engage the big emotions that show up in our ordinary life and relationships demands positiveness. Big emotions can be frightening, especially when they are bigger than they should be. Positiveness is about being able to engage with them with curiosity so that they can be interrogated and contextualised. The objective in emotional therapy is to cut big emotions down to size, and this begins naturally with a positive frame of mind within which they are not to be feared but rather to be understood, welcomed and integrated into their rightful experiential context. However, access to the positive emotional state (PES) through which curiosity is encouraged can be cut off by psychosocial trauma. Thus, the survivor who moves through life in a vacant or pessimistic emotional state may present to the task of life as asocial, folded and closed off to the relational world that—an aching body will indicate—feels unsafe and threatening.

Task: What can you share about strong feelings, say of shame and disgust, and how can you build a narrative around them that can be incorporated into a bigger story about emotions fuelled by unbounded energy? What hopes and fears do you wish to deconstruct, honour and show gratitude for because of the messages they bring? Notice that by these interrogations you are not less positive but are getting more confident, which is better than being less positive because there are tangible things to be positive about and express gratitude for. Bring this together in an emotional dialogue, or a diary, that includes reflections on emotional and physiological expressions such as an increased heart rate, as well as the inability to think clearly that may be less discernible.

The idea of cultivating positiveness is that by leaning into, identifying and bringing positive energy to what we are feeling, and entertaining the attendant neuroceptions, we promote our capacity to respond flexibly to emotional demands, manage our responses and identify how others are experiencing and responding to us emotionally, allowing us to respond appropriately. When we interrogate emotions within a positive frame of mind—in other words, give names and context to them—we are identifying them as real things. This top-down input is to help bind the chaotic energy that sustains negative emotional states.

Empathy

We met empathy in earlier chapters in one of its two configurations, cognitive and emotional. Together, these empathies are necessarily a feature of the neuro-emotional SPEAR that we cultivate when we connect with another sentient in a way that is authentic. This capacity to tune into our own and other sentient's emotional sensations without becoming emotionally stuck is facilitated by our mirror neuron system, through which we perceive ourselves and others. In social psychology, when we mimic others' behaviour, even unconsciously, our mirror neurons spike up to register our empathy.

In a mutual relationship, we know we are empathic when energic boundaries break down momentarily in a shared body-mind state in which synchrony and compassion abound, for we are neural via our mirror neurons, physiological via our heart rate and vagal breaks, hormonal via oxytocin and behavioural via mimicry. In this state, oxytocin cross-talks with other neuromodulatory systems, such as the dopaminergic pleasure-reward system and the corticoid fear-stress response system, allowing us to feel without becoming overwhelmed by what is felt. Within the therapeutic relationship, this may look like the therapist tuning into the survivor's emotional state in order to acknowledge and nurture this capacity.

Task: Reflect on your strengths and vulnerabilities that promote emotional well-being or wear you down emotionally. Interrogate whether you can be honest about what you can and cannot do or give. This is about firm boundaries within which you can respond to emotional demands with flexibility. Your power of no is an important asset that must serve you in this regard, and you can begin by exploring how you use it. Do you find, for instance, that your use of it is weaponised? Is it ineffective in keeping you safe? Do you use it to manipulate and hurt others, and inadvertently yourself? Do you find that it pops up when you do not intend to use it, say when you might confuse the impulse to love with the dis-ease to please?

Empathy promotes integration between the heart and mind, but in a way that honours our own needs for safety and connection. This intelligence allows us to interact with others effectively and safely—not only in being safe physically but in feeling safe emotionally too. And this is important as we move through life, seeking connections and opportunities to work with others in ways that do not diminish or negatively impact them or our own well-being.

Attunement

Our capacity to register and respond appropriately to the rhythm of our body and mind as well as the bodies and minds of others with whom we are connected—engaging the empathy circuitries that intersect the social-emotional brain and cerebral cortex—is called emotional attunement. In theory, it is a connection at the level of the heart-gut-soul axis, which allows us to create a mutual field of resonance. This could be with our self but also with others, such as our ancestors, with whom we are connected biologically, psychosocially and even spiritually.

> **Task:** Explore how much you are able and available to host within you your own emotional demands as well as the emotional demands of others you care about, without becoming overwhelmed or stuck. Can you sense your ancestry? The emotional wounds of your parents, grandparents and great-grandparent you hold in you? Can you feel any profound terror, grief or loss they endured or perpetrated, reminding you that the past is not past, that it is alive in you? What is the story you feel bound to tell yourself and others about this superpower, or the lack thereof? How would you want this piece of your story to show up as you move through life? How would you want it to feature in the whole of your life story?

In cultivating attunement, the survivor is training their body and mind to be receptive and accepting of the healing energies of openness and presence. Thus, presence is important for attunement, because if we are stuffed with chaotic energies of misattunement or any other kind of ALE, our capacity to register and respond to synchroneity in the present, which is the essence of attunement, will be impaired. Cultivating attunement, thus, is contingent on having bounded and discharged chaotic energies of ALEs that occurred in the past but which are held emotionally in the self, creating a space to heal impaired relationships and create new ones. The idea is that, as the survivor becomes more attuned and amenable to regulated synchronicity, they also become better at exploring the relational world with curiosity and resilience.

Reflectiveness

Reflectiveness is the capacity to bring awareness to emotions and emotional states, the origins of such states and what is meaningful in those states. When we reflect, we are paying attention to our impulses and feelings, as well as to how others are feeling. To achieve this within the therapeutic relationship, the survivor is encouraged to focus on inner sensations. The idea is that the more of this they do, the more oxygen and chemistry will be directed to neural assemblies and networks that host the content of their focus. This would be things that are important, nourishing and in line with their well-being—purposeful, in a word. Thus, purpose motivates reflectiveness as reflectiveness motivates purpose, which gives meaning to life events. Events trigger neural activities that strengthen in time as the memory neurons are encouraged to learn and take in new information to enable us to succeed. This is active work that is likely to clash with old patterns.

> **Task:** What is your story about emotionally enriching experiences? This could be volunteering your time and talent to a cause that is emotionally appealing to your, or mentalising true affirmations of self-acceptance and commitment to emotional well-being. How might you alter your story to acknowledge feelings in you, such as hurt, anger, shame and the like, alongside deep and complete acceptance of yourself as resilient with vulnerability, strong with weaknesses, deserving of love, kindness, and good health?

Exposing the nervous system to affirmations that are nourishing and healing promotes neural health and connectivity that buffer against the chaotic energy of recklessness. Affirmations can be adapted in line with the survivor's true sense of self. The key is that affirmations are authentic and reflect truths about the self as they encode in the nervous system. A technique I learned from a practitioner of emotional freedom during my undergraduate study in the Netherlands was to combine emotional-self affirmations with gentle massages of specific areas on the face, neck and upper body that send signals to the ventral vagal fibres—specifically, the orbital oculi muscles that encircle the eyes; the area around the mouth beneath which runs the trigeminal cranial nerve V; the temple area, beneath which runs the facial cranial nerve VII; the sides of the neck, beneath which run the carotid arteries; behind the ears and around the collar bone, beneath which run the glossopharyngeal cranial nerve IX; and under the arm in the direction of the shoulder blade, beneath which run the vagus nerve X. The implication of this gentle massaging is that affirmations combined with ventral stimulation establishes a state of well-being from which emotional growth can be launched.

NEURO-EMOTIONAL THERAPY IN REFLECTION

Self-regulation, positivity, empathy, attunement and reflectiveness together constitute the neuro-emotional SPEAR that can be employed in neuropsychosocial therapy to discharge the chaotic energies of psychosocial trauma and promote well-being. In appreciating the variety of human experiences and cultures with which survivors will show up to the therapeutic relationship, the therapist is tasked to ensure the integrity of this relationship, whilst affirming the realities in which survivors act upon emotions in ways that reflect real as well as imagined life events and emotional dis-ease.

This is distinct from emotionally disordered personalities in which discernible emotions are not experienced (Wink, 1991; Dickinson & Pincus, 2003), as opposed to being dysregulated in the sense that psychosocial trauma implies. One imagines this bears import for how we make sense of actions that are informed by emotion but for which there is an unsettled question of emotional competence.

There is no shortage of insight into this incidence in the literature, and one compelling theory is that a mutation in the monoamine oxidase gene, MAO-A-L, on the X chromosome that codes for degradation of dopamine, noradrenalin and serotonin in the synaptic cleft impairs expression of pro-social emotions, such as compassion, kindness and remorse. Specifically, individuals with a low-activity mutant version of the MAO-A gene have an accumulation of undegraded dopamine, noradrenaline and serotonin in their central nervous system. These neuromodulators, we know, are implicated in mood regulation, impulse control and movement, and as such an excess in the nervous system is linked to emotional lability, difficulty controlling impulses, hypersensitivity to ALEs and a predisposition to a negative bias in the interpretation of social stimuli, which results in a greater propensity for aggressive and impulsive reactions to provocation and psychosocial stress. Put more simply, personalities with an MAO-A-L mutation experience a decrease in emotions that are important for affection and caring behaviours in interpersonal relationships. Genetic mutation—we have learned—is an epigenetic event that can be brought on by methylation, which alters DNA molecules and can switch genes on and off by altering access to their content.

In a nod to Lamarck, the instructions—to switch genes on and off—can be passed from parents to children in DNA transfer. As such, social-emotional pathologies that derive from epigenetics are also inheritable. I might here refer to pathological selfishness, arrogance and the tendency to self-destruct that intersect nature and nurture in narcissistic, histrionic, borderline and antisocial personalities (McWilliams, 2011). However, the field of behavioural epigenetics that is concerned with understanding how nature influences nurture offers a promising literature that suggests mutations generally tend to express only where carriers' social environment promotes expression. And this makes sense when we consider that the behaviours that characterise antisociality are regulated in the prefrontal cortex, the last part of the brain to mature fully, to have its axons myelinated and connection with other neural structures established. This also means it is the part of the brain least influenced by genetics and most structured by lived experiences.

Damage in this part of the brain caused by ALEs, for instance, could mean its capacities are impaired—say the capacity to understand consequences, follow rules or act to mitigate injury to one's self and others. Incidentally, researchers since Bowlby have theorised that features of disempathy (Blair, 2007), especially deficits in sensitivity to remorse, guilt and shame, that characterise disruptive personalities are really expressions of social-emotional injuries that derive from chronic deprivation of parental care in childhood. This theory finds resonance in meta-analyses of the literature on childhood determinants of psychiatric and personality disorders in adulthood (Fryers & Brugha, 2013; Perry & Lee, 2020).

Poor parental care, the literature affirms, leaves children vulnerable not only to stunted growth and neurosis but also to maladaptive personality traits that are persistent. And this happens in part via epigenetic regulations. Take, for instance, the nuclear receptor (NR) genes on chromosome 5 that are involved in inflammatory responses (National Institutes of Health, 2023). The NR3C1 mutant, in particular, links to glucocorticoid resistance that is associated with antisocial behaviour, in addition to depression and anxiety. This lumps the disordered with the dysregulated and grants us leverage to consider survivors' inability to access prosocial emotions as an adaptive defence to psychosocial trauma in early life.

An important task for neuropsychosocial therapy would be to consider a childhood in which parental neglect, sexual abuse and physical violence were extant and the survivor as well as her adaptive defences are operating at a conscious level. This could represent an opening for therapy to improve emotional competency, inner capacity for emotional regulation and the condition for neuropsychosocial integration, starting with contextualising feelings, which can be very complex, and having those feelings recognised and encoded in the nervous system alongside insights into adaptive and healthful emotional states. Such insights would be achieved by turning inwards with self-compassion.

Chapter 14

Neuropsychological Integration

Neuropsychology studies the psyche and its expressions as they are informed by content in the nervous system. Largely, this would be subcerebral emotions and neuroceptions that are expressed in thoughts, judgements, mindsets and ways of making sense of life events. When it comes to the neuropsychosocial, psychic expression—as unique as it is ancient a feature of being human—is informed by both lived experiences and ancestral legacy.

I have talked about ancestral legacy among black populations of the Americas. We might consider, for instance, the hopeless and helpless enslaved black mothers of the Americas, anticipating the violence and forced labour to which their children were to be subjected, preparing them with attitudes and behaviours that would keep them alive under conditions of slavery. Hence, to safeguard intergenerational survival, these mothers needed to internalise racism, vacate their self-esteem and model repressive behaviours that became those of their children, and to this day persist in their descendants (DeGruy, 2017). Essentially, the socialisation of enslaved children involved self-condemnation, which instilled in them a distorted sense of who they were and what they could and could not become because of their blackness. It was an identity in which was stunted the ability to develop and sustain awareness of their psychosocial resources and act to self-preserve or mitigate their own extinction.

NEUROPSYCHOLOGICAL WELL-BEING

Neuropsychological well-being is about bringing awareness to depletion in psychic resources to act in the service of self-preservation, which is the antidote to extinction. It involves interrogating ancestral legacies of neuropsychosocial disintegration, not only to discover how these influence oppressive

195

psychology but also to recover losses that are inherited as psychosocial trauma. On this course, the survivor is undertaking to collect, connect and correct stories from their social history, and to find glimmers in these stories that bring clarity to tension in their psyche. Psychological clarity, however, relies on cognitive information and might not involve consideration for ancestral and preverbal traumas that defy cognition. Translated into the thera-peutic space, the survivor can be encouraged by two important outcomes:

1. Attention is brought to traumatic woundedness, maladaptations and disintegration that disturb the psyche in historical and current scenes.
2. Commitment is made to discharge the chaotic energy of psychogenic tension and reorient subcerebral neural processes that inform the psyche.

In bringing attention to psychological manifestations of psychosocial trauma, the survivor is encouraged to nurture their capacity to direct and redirect the flow of energy that is implicated in both their wounding and healing. And to make as conscious and explicit as possible mindsets and cognition that activate familiar neural patterns, defences and instincts. These are often preserved in stories that acquaint us with the hows and whys of events in our social history, and this can be a helpful place to begin to reconstruct and cor-rect the story of our own life.

An important objective in this exercise is to explore psychologies that are transmitted across generations but which might be inconsistent with sover-eign thoughts and the authentic self. This might include the sense that love and attention are conditional on conceding to one's body being used as an object of violence. For children, this may be experienced as learning from caregivers that they are beaten—even viciously—because they are 'loved' or 'disobedient'; that they are parentified because they are 'good little helpers'; that they are sexualised because they are 'cute' 'obedient' and even 'sexy'. This socialisation results in conditions of worth that masquerade as norms but are characteristically injurious to the survivor's sense of self. They do not merely constitute psychosocial trauma but sustain it.

It is by interrogating these norms and their influence on thoughts, mindsets and judgements that the survivor is encouraged to rescue their own truth, for instance, that they are being assaulted, gaslighted or overworked in their care-giving relationships. The survivor's experience of the social world is, thus, congruent with their cognitive expression. Accurate cognitisation carrying cues of safety, in this sense, is an empowering experience, which activates the social engagement circuitry. And this can be beneficial for a range of maladies that deplete the mind.

Think of morbid ideation, self-harm tendencies and mood disorders that respond to healthful cognitisation (Zuroff & Blatt, 2006). This favourable response, however, is contingent on the capacity for cognition and mindfulness through which the survivor presents psychically and connects with sources of nourishment. In previous chapters, I talked about expression of gratitude addressed to a kind and loving God, a cognitive practice research tells us that induces a vagal tone that promotes peacefulness and neural resilience. Prayer—like cognitive therapy and mentalisation—is a practice through which traumatic memories can be safely confronted and contextualised in the psyche.

It is not uncommon, however, to find that survivors are disposed to quieten their traumatic memories, which makes sense given that the neuro-chemistry of active trauma toxifies neurons and depletes the hippocampal tissues in the declarative memory system (Bremner, 2006). Quieting trau-matic memories, it appears, favours preservation and renewal of neural tissues, the neurogenesis that, incidentally, promotes pruning of unused hippocampal memory.

That the brain alone will grow in mass from 500 to about 1,500 grams between birth and mid-adolescence tells us that neural tissues prune little and grow rapidly in foetuses as they develop and in the still developing brains of children and adolescents. Adaptations to psychosocial trauma at this stage will readily embed in developing circuitries and become a feature of the neu-ral edifice that will present in adulthood. Hence, much of the neurogenesis that occurs in the adult brain involves repair of neural tissues and recon-necting of neural networks. But with toxic levels of stress from exposure to adversity in ordinary life, resources—such as oxygen and nutrients—are shifted from this process to defence, giving rise to cognitive impairments that impact perception, including perception of pain, of value in new ideas and, of course, of people we do not know and people who are different from us and whom we are disposed to reject.

This is because the mind can become closed to the unacquainted, but also to learning, healing and growing, a state in which survivors can stay stuck as they move through life, failing to recall though not necessarily disremem-bering their trauma. The role of the trauma-informed therapist is to offer the right prompts and a safe space within which recall comes naturally. This is something I practice with older people who are engaged socially and—within that context—easily recall events of thirty, fifty or even eighty years ago with clarity as well as rationalisation for their 'forgetting', which is typically that it was an appropriate response. For instance, Nan told me that she had never mentioned her sexual violation at the hands of Fr. Parry for fifty years because she 'didn't have it in mind', even though she acted on the trauma two decades after the incident by disaffiliating from Catholicism. This tells me that traumatic memory is resistant to degradation, even when it is not discernible in a traumatic stress disorder.

Neurodegeneration, on the contrary, is the decay or full-on destruction of neurons in the brain and spine and is commonly associated with degenerative

diseases such as Alzheimer's, Parkinson's and sclerosis. More subtle conditions, such as a negative mental shift, say of perception of the self as undeserving of safety, might look like a psychological defence, a psychology the
survivor adopts to cope with protracted conditions of adversity and that over
time deploys instinctively or somewhat autonomously as if it is genetic.

Healing of these subtle conditions comes from exploring and integrating
defences in their rightful context, and this could begin with an insight into
how they manifest behaviourally. For instance, repression in psychoanalysis
is a behavioural manifestation, a form of relegating traumatic memories to
the subconscious, where they cannot be easily recalled. It is a functional
'forgetting' that blocks conscious recall of experiences that are overwhelming
in a psychological sense and may therefore be a source of pathology (Davis
& Zhong, 2017). These memories, however, are generally unruly and show
up in dreams and free thoughts, through which they can be interrogated.
In surfacing such memories and making them available to cognition—
even if imperfectly—they can be brought to rationalisation and positively
contextualised.

Cognitisation, however, is an executive function that is incredibly vulnerable to psychosocial trauma in early life, so much so that its faculty could fail
to develop. For instance, children who are little spoken to or little exposed
to language in early life could as a result fail to develop the capacity to
express themselves fully using formal language, irrespective of how good
their language centres are or how sufficient for language development are the
genes they were born with. The unfortunate lived experiences of Victor of
Aveyron (Harlan, 1977) and Genie Wiley (Curtiss, 2014)—both victims of
severe neglect and social isolation in childhood who would never learn to use
language competently—suggest cognitive deficits deriving in psychosocial
trauma cannot always be recovered from, even with the best of therapy. The
development of cognitive circuitries requires input, such as sounds, from the
environment, in the absence of which the related neurons will prune and the
neural circuitries will fail to develop. Thus, deficit in cognition reflects deficit
in the environment. But, more precisely, studies have suggested this deficit
derives from the trauma of inadequate sociality. And, as with any psychosomatic wound, such a deficit demands attention, which can be met with a
neuropsychological SPEAR developed in therapy.

NEUROPSYCHOLOGICAL SPEAR

Neuropsychological therapy works to encourage the survivor to cultivate an
inner capacity to regulate matters of the mind in ways that promote well-
being. In a practical sense, this involves creating the space to explore ways

of being in the world, responding appropriately to life events and making true sense of lived and inherited experiences, which is the essence of psychological intelligence. In the face of cognitive incompetency, however, an appeal to adaptive, emotional and social intelligences can be as effective as psychological intelligence in this task. As the survivor moves through life, they must employ smart emotions and social sense to perceive clearly and act with appreciation and good judgment of consequences. This is psychological integrity, which, accordingly, the survivor can be encouraged to cultivate by interrogating what of themselves may be hidden, disrupted or uninvited to belong—consciously or unconsciously—that is, what needs to be reconciled with their authentic self. Their psyche can be equipped for active imagination as its central process in discharging the chaotic energies of self-invalidation, purposelessness, privation and pathological dependency, irresponsibility and immorality, which characterise psychological ill-fatedness. The objective is to cultivate and nourish self-esteem, purposefulness, enterprise, agency and righteousness to bring healing energy to the psyche, and these constitute the neuropsychological SPEAR.

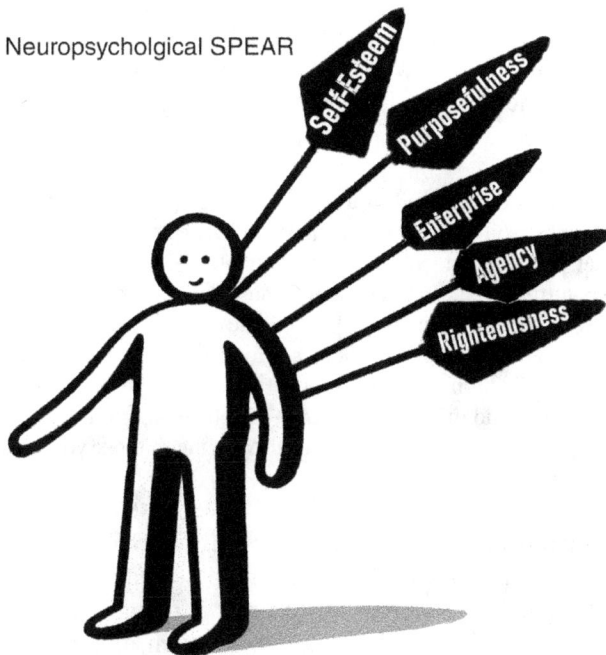

Figure 14.1. Neuropsychological SPEAR—Therapeutic Resources. *Figure courtesy of Dagmar Roelfsema.*

Self-Esteem

From the Latin verb *aestimare*, which translates to 'value', the nineteenth-century American psychologist William James derived the concept of self-esteem, which he defined as perceivable worthiness in the self that results from consistently meeting expectations for personally valued activities. Essentially, self-esteem emerges from successes relative to expectations. For instance, how successful we are in relationships relative to our relational needs and expectations. The smaller the gap between the two, the higher our esteem. The wider the gap, the lower our esteem. Self-esteem, thus, on a continuum from high to low, is vulnerable to psychosocial trauma that can alter the gap between what we want or need and what we get. Neuropsychological therapy works to distinguish between the configuration of the self that suffers in service of a trauma that we get and the configuration of the self that yearns for the safety and authenticity we need.

This safety and authenticity in the self, we have learned, is promoted by the psychological integrity in our resilience SPEAR, which is a feature of a mind that reflects stability and strength. We develop such a mind through conscious and consistent practice of openness, honesty and equanimity that keeps us from being blown away by winds of confusion, conflict and insults. For this mind knows worth, promotes well-being and growth, and reconciles biological instructions to self-preserve and bind contradictory instructions to self-sacrifice that derive from a state of dysautonomia. The goal is to bring order to the nervous system by interrogating and contextualising the contradictions.

> **Task:** What stories do you tell yourself and others, explicitly and implicitly, about your values, self-respect and self-worth? About your competencies and virtues? What thoughts and ideas about yourself show up in your consciousness, at times intrusive and unwelcomed? Interrogate these thoughts and ideas to establish whether they are true. How do they serve you? Would you want people you care about to believe them as you do? Posing these questions to yourself invites reflection—the awareness that every person, including you, has vulnerabilities—and the healing energy of self-expression, whether through talking, writing, drawing or praying about life events that tax your sense of self and your psychology.

Within the therapeutic space, this is an occasion to contextualise trauma-based perceptions about the self and promote self-talk that is nourishing, dialogues that begin with awareness of a specific thought, end with a reflection and are intentionally transformational. As such, this must not only be intentional but also nontriggering or 'nonviolent'—to use the American psychologist Marshall Rosenberg's (2015) concept.

According to Rosenberg, the capacity to identify a specific feeling that surrounds a specific thought, which is associated with a specific life event, is a good indicator of psychological integrity. This is contingent on the thought being true, the feeling being the actual internal experience of the thought, and the emotion the thought arouses and the life event that underlies the feeling being real. It is when we can do this that we can begin to train our mind to calibrate our thoughts in ways that are nonviolent. For example, 'I think I am a bad friend because I am unreliable' can become 'I feel more valued as a friend when I can rely on people I care about, as they can rely on me in times of need'.

Naturally, relationships involve concession, but the key objective is the same: to get relational—and by extension psychosocial—needs fulfilled in a way that matches expectations and promotes self-esteem. This comes with knowing what your needs are, what you truly want to achieve (say, friendship, intimacy, etc.) and what you can do to promote your success. There is the auxiliary benefit to be enjoyed in mindfully interrogating needs and attendant thoughts that preserve psychological health, by binding the free-flowing energy of negative thoughts and beliefs. Often, we will find that free-flowing energy derives from a legacy of trauma that gives rise to untetheredness, the sense that we don't belong (say among those who are celebrated), that we don't deserve kindness, peace and respect and shouldn't thrive in success because this is not our legacy.

In restructuring our thought process and learning to assert our truth, we also promote our boundaries that trauma impacts. But as we grow and strengthen in character, our boundaries will shift to reflect our resourcefulness and tolerance for adversity, keeping us safe and promoting authenticity in our self, which in itself is transformational. As we become more accepting, that there is a real benefit in pursuing or restoring authenticity, we will note gaps between our successes and our goals as well as the parts of ourselves that we want to keep and nurture and the parts we want to let go off and grieve. As we move through life, mindfulness will help us to reduce the tension in our consciousness, as hidden contents of our unconscious surface and are less frightening, and unhelpful autoresponses in the subconscious are retired.

Purposefulness

In chapter 2, we were acquainted with purpose as a neuropsychological phenomenon that moves and motivates our organism. In that sense, we could think of purposefulness as a goal-driven impulse. But it is much more than that, a commission at the John Templeton Foundation agreed, defining it as 'a stable and generalized intention to accomplish something that is at once personally meaningful and at the same time leads to productive engagement with some aspect of the world beyond the self' (Adolescent Moral Development Lab, 2018, p. 4). This would be our 'why' to live that allows us to endure almost any 'how', as the German philosopher Friedrich Nietzsche famously put it.

However, much like love and kindness, we do not have receptors for purposefulness in any particular neural structure to which we can point, but our nervous system knows when it is in deficit. And, as the Austrian psychiatrist Victor Frankl (2008), who survived the Holocaust, points out in his seminal exploration *Man's Search for Meaning*, it will express this deficit in our response to adversity, whether we fight or do not fight for our survival, which is determined at the level of our neurochemistry.

Neurochemically, purposefulness motivates us. When our purpose is resilient, it is something we are biologically inclined to fight for. Beyond neurobiology and personality, purposefulness also directs our life, and having a sense of direction in our life informs our sense of well-being. We may even say our sense of well-being reflects our sense of what we live for or might die for, a sentiment that finds resonance in a study published in the *American Journal of Privative Medicine* in 2021 that pointed to a resilient sense of purpose as a protective force against all-cause mortality, regardless of socioeconomic status. Not only was purposefulness inversely related to premature death, it also corelated strongly with favourable health outcomes and longevity in senior citizens (Shiba et al., 2021).

> **Task:** What stories do you tell yourself about the reason for which you live your life? What is your reason for rising in the morning that shakes you to act, even if it conflicts with your attitude? Do you tell yourself it is important to provide for your family, but your attitude is such that 'society provides for its children'? Interrogate your attitude about your purpose, where it comes from and whether it aligns with your authentic self. Is it even your own, or is it a legacy you are holding on to because you have not known otherwise? If that is the case, rework your story about your purpose to include that a legacy you no longer want to hold on to has betrayed it. This may not be easy. People hold on to unuseful things for many reasons. Examples include to dampen the pangs of shame or to placate the dread of deception and aloneness in a dysfunctional relationship. Explore how your story might change once you are not being alienated from your true purpose and experiencing the fulfilment that comes from self-expansion and growth. This is about leading a fulfilling life and pursuing what is meaningful to you, even in the face of ALEs. You are able to do things that are beneficial to you, to stop doing things that are harmful and to keep going without becoming overwhelmed by the challenges of ordinary life.

In the absence of purpose, we are disposed to float through life untethered and undirected, much like the nomadic floater who wanders the plains of nowhere, or my childhood ball in chapter 7, adrift on the ocean, where no one will come to our aid should we find ourselves in distress or lost to our true self, to which we would be vulnerable. Purpose is the neural compass that orients us towards our authenticity, anchors us in our social environment and directs us to what fills our life with meaning—to what we are responsible for and which makes our life worth living and preserving.

Enterprise

Enterprise is the audacity to undertake and promote craft and craftmanship as a mechanism of safety and survival. Maslow's hierarchy of developmental needs encourages us to think of this as an impulse to pursue socioeconomic mastery in service of survival. Socioeconomic mastery, however, is a cognitive task that employs the settler's impulse to establish structures—family, community, religion and so on—in service of security. And, as the Irish psychologist Peter Dempsey's (1982) old insight on 'the psychology of enterprise' suggests, this impulse underpins the human will to solve complex social—and by extension economic—problems and make progress in spite of ALEs, such as poverty and marginalisation, that give rise to trauma. Incidentally, this impulse is also incredibly vulnerable to conditions of psychosocial trauma, under the weight of which it can be crushed, but nonetheless it can be recovered with neuropsychological therapy.

> **Task:** Curate a story about a project that could eventuate personal reverence and relief in a social and economic sense. Imagine how this project would affect your life and the life of people it reaches. What benefit would it offer, what drawbacks, and what resources are needed to bring it to fruition? A bakery, for instance, would involve producing baked bread and cakes that satisfy hunger, a condition of being human. Bread is also a staple people enjoy, find nourishing and can easily afford. But it doesn't have to be bread, it could be an undertaking to self-rescue.

Neuropsychological therapy seeks to recover and nourish the impulse for enterprise, which subverts in the subconscious under conditions of psychosocial trauma, engaging in this task the intelligence SPEARS that promote our survival and growth by opening us up to opportunities and challenges in our cnvironment. We might think of this as the spirit of enterprise, or the 'hustler spirit' of which Lloyd speaks in chapter 7, which is understood as an impulse to safeguard against privation. Enterprise, thus, is therapeutic not only in a neuropsychological sense but also in a socioeconomic one.

Agency

Good things in life—we could think of reverence, respectability, relationality—that coalesce around a sense of fulfilment require agency, the native drive that combines with responsibility to self-preserve and self-actualise. As such, agency is a psychological imperative not only to keep the self safe but also to explore possibilities beyond what is obvious and convenient. This is the essence of self-actualisation, and its circuits are primed to become active in early life, before the age of three, when we learn we can do things to and for ourselves and undertake to do these things freely, and when our counterwill emerges in our defence arsenal to protect us from others' will and coercive control. Hence, we have agency over our life or to influence a life event—our own body, an achievement or the protection of our family—when three things are true: we have the freedom that allows us to be responsible for it, we accept this responsibility belongs to us and not to anyone else, and we have access to resources with which to act upon this responsibility.

I have talked about responsibility as the ability to respond to life events with competency, but beyond this it is a condition of being human that is vulnerable to trauma. Short of responsibility for our well-being, which is a reliable feature of psychosocial trauma, we cannot be said to have agency. The goal of neuropsychological therapy is to recover and preserve this ability, which is necessary in our role as steward on the journey to our authentic self-discovery and finding fulfilment in our life—as a woman, a man, a black person, a child of God or any other identity.

> **Task:** What stories do you tell yourself about what you can and cannot do? Reimagine dreams resting somewhere inside of you that you may have dismissed or deferred. There might be good reasons they were set aside, or perhaps no concreate reason at all. Interrogate these reasons and reconcile their meaning. Bring your awareness to a person in your life, say a friend, parent or teacher, who has encouraged or helped you to achieve something important to you. What stories do you tell yourself about this achievement? Collect those stories and reflect on what you would change, if anything, and what you might want more of. Check in with the sensations in your body that this mentalisation evokes. Name your sensations: for example, are you grateful, thankful, proud? How could you alter your story to experience more of these sensations?

In cultivating agency, which may have been vacant or eroded by trauma, the survivor is encouraged to lead with responsibility and resourcefulness in their recovery from loss and response to conflict. This is the antidote to helplessness that is fuelled by a bounded energy, but in a way that leaves us paralysed in a psychosocial sense, where we cannot seem to move or act to help ourselves or all our attempts seem to fail. It is with the help of predictable input from a nourishing relationship that we can learn to differentiate what comes from us, our own self, from what comes from others. And this differentiation initiates a sense of agency and resilient selfhood.

Recovering and integrating agency in the self is about promoting faith in our own ability and never losing hope, even when the world appears to offer little more than protracted misery. Another word for hopefulness is optimism, which may be more emotive in promoting perseverance, achievement and well-being. For, it turns out, optimistic people, who retain agency over their lives, tend to lead more fulfilled lives, with better health that translates to longer life (Peterson, 2000).

Righteousness

The compass of morality that directs truth, uprightness and our evolutionary imperative to preserve life and to grow virtuously into our full humanness— this is the essence of righteousness, what we are when we are congruent with the sacredness of life and our impulse not only to preserve it but to experience it fully. This requires us to be evangelical about preserving life, nurturing well-being and growing in virtuous relationships, including with ourself and with the divine. Righteousness, thus, encourages in us an appreciation of self-awareness, self-healing and self-development. For the spiritually inclined, this may involve exercises in accepting spirituality as a source of meaning that permits a reconceptualisation of suffering as a sacrifice for a greater good, a benevolence. This can be achieved in a real or imagined relationship with a loving and forgiving God, who represents a source of comfort and safety and a guide to being empathic and nurturing. The more of these virtues we embody, the more likely we will be attentive in our relationships and to our children and will confer on to them a sense of belonging, worth and connectedness.

> **Task:** Explore your relationship with universal truths. In the patchwork of your mind and personality, what virtues have you been unable to express with authenticity—say intelligence, wisdom or conscientiousness? These must be virtues you want to reconcile and strengthen—to help you to show up and move through life with resilient capacities to overcome adversity, effectively express your needs and fulfil those needs. Reflect on how you experienced the inability to express these virtues and how you could expand your story to include your commitment to nurture them. What thoughts are associated with them, and how are they helpful or unhelpful?

This righteous way of being in the world encourages us to rise above primitive tendencies to act in ways to protect our self from feeling unsafe, but at the expense of important relationships and global peace, for instance, the tendency to lead with ingroup-outgroup distinctions that allowed our ancestors to survive in ancient times. When our warrior ancestors in cave X took without permission from ancestors in cave Y, they would kill them or be killed by them. Therein lies the origin of the distinction between us and them that gets simplified by the nervous system as us against them and that gives rise to hostility. The survivors of these ingroup-outgroup distinctions and hostilities are our ancestors, so we cannot help that they have passed on to us genetic information to allow us to survive in archaic conditions of hostility. Today, whether we call ourselves Israelis or Palestinians, brown or white, Democrat or Republican, this is our legacy—we are disposed to treat people like us with empathy and kindness and others with antipathy. Antipathy can be triggered when we feel wronged, and the adrenaline rush of righteous anger will ring up our defensive dragon, which can feel appropriate as it is empowering, making it extremely difficult to perceive the high cost of the negative emotional state in which we are acting and can stay stuck. Everything and everyone is a potential threat, and the nervous system is hijacked by a powerful negativity bias that fuels hostility and literal war. Whilst we are not at fault for our ancestral heritage or this primitive instinct, we are responsible for rising above it. Neuropsychosocial integration is about discharging its chaotic energy and bringing the rational mind in line with the needs of the body and soul.

NEUROPSYCHOLOGICAL THERAPY IN REFLECTION

The neuropsychological SPEAR with which we are now acquainted is essential for restoring integration to the body and mind affected by psychosocial trauma. The complexity and long incubation of this trauma, especially in how it develops, means it is not necessarily easy to contextualise, for it could mean little connection is made between adverse life events and psychological dis-ease or psychiatric diagnoses in the survivor's life. As such, it is not uncommon to find among survivors a calculated 'forgetting' of cruelty that represents an adaptative response to cruelty, such as that caused by neglect or sexual violence that was prevalent in childhood.

Complex psychosocial trauma in early life demands such adaptations alongside the normal development of the nervous system, thereby initiating a pathway to pathology that can have a hidden or delayed expression later in life, when it is liable to be attributed to psychological problems, neurodegeneration or neurochemical dysregulation that mimics or expresses itself as a pathological forgetting. This kind of forgetting helps explain the impulse and attendant compulsion to self-medicate to ward off psychological distress from memories that evoke deleterious emotions, such as guilt, grief and shame. As such, pathological forgetting has useful implications for neuropsychosocial integration when it implies a provisional disruption in the healthy functioning of the declarative memory system. That the memories are not only intact but also retrievable is important for integration.

This model of therapy does not consider the challenging disease states that destroy memory and may not respond to psychosocial intervention. However, it can be complemented with more technical intervention, such as biofeedback, wherein the survivor is connected to sensors that monitor inner physiological processes, such as breath, heart rate and muscle contractions. This is to provide feedback about how the body is functioning and to allow the survivor to make changes to improve their health. This is a fairly non-invasive approach to therapy that may be ideal for people who do not feel safe with other people, and to increase its efficacy, it can be combined with other modalities such as art therapy (AT) and animal assisted therapy (AAT) to treat psychophysiological symptoms, such as social anxiety and hypertension. The objective, still, is to establish a relationship with an emotionally available sentient, such as a dog, horse or image that is dependable, validating and available to create a neurocircuitry of safety.

For more troublesome psychosocial and developmental traumas in the nervous system, a revolutionary biofeedback technique known as neurofeedback can be employed in therapy (Cohen, 2020). It is a technique that involves recording neural activities that can be collected via sensors placed on the scalp. The display of neuronal activities in the brain is possible through smart imaging technology—such as electroencephalography (EEG), which records electrical activity among neurons in the brain; positron emission tomography (PET), which measures levels of oxygen and glucose in the brain; and magnetic resonance imaging (MRI), which highlights neural structures. The goal is to establish and strengthen patterns of neural activity that promote well-being, to which the brain is inclined naturally. The survivor is encouraged to carry out practical or mental task in a specific way, and when success is achieved, the brain receives (visual or auditory) reinforcement through a stimulus presented onto a screen and is encouraged with focus to do more of what is rewarded. By localizing deviant brain areas and activities and stimulating those areas to progress more towards the norm, pathological symptoms can be improved or alleviated. This is possible because, with persistence and practice, neural circuitries of healing thoughts and activities that are rewarded get stronger and more resilient and compete for energy with old patterns that are not rewarded. Bounded energy flows in the direction of focus, motivation and action, which establish and strengthen synaptic communication and neural networks based on repeated practice and, in so doing, improve neural function and psychological well-being.

This system utilizes operant conditioning to teach the brain to function more efficiently and to treat psychological disorders that derive from trauma. Addiction, for instance, is an example of a diseased state in which the motivation system has become chronically disordered by the incitement of a stimulant, whether a chemical, such as alcohol, or an experience, such as childhood sexual assault. The nervous system has adapted to a heightened state of stimulation, and to achieve a similar sense of stimulation, more of the stimulant is needed over time. In the absence of influence from the stimulant, unpleasant withdrawal symptoms set in. This is first a state of dependency, which may be tolerable. However, when a chronic preoccupation with the heightened state of stimulation persists and motivates behaviour to seek out the stimulant at the exclusion of what is truly good for the body and mind— say resting, eating and love making—this becomes a diseased state in the reward-motivation system that has a precise neuropathophysiology.

Neurofeedback can target this neuropathophysiology for reversal by combining neural activity reorienting and behaviour activation. In practice, the therapist is employing the basic principles of positive psychology—positive emotion, engagement, relationships, meaning and accomplishment—in the approach to treating trauma. The objective is largely to guide the survivor to recognise how positive thoughts and feelings translate into actions that improve well-being by improving capacity to integrate the nervous system. This integration occurs at the intersection of the big brain, the body and the whole self, as positive and nourishing thoughts, emotions and bodily sensations integrate in a synchrony to transcend the trauma state.

Importantly, the survivor receives cues and feedback on how managing emotions and executing suitable behaviours help them to stay in control of their impulses. In other words, the survivor develops a sense of agency over their cognitive psychology and is encouraged to retire maladaptive thoughts and behaviours that are not conducive to their well-being and growth.

Unfortunately, for those who have suffered severe cortical damage or live with cognitive deficits and struggle with learning, psychological therapy may not be ideal. However, much like with acquired blindness that is a consequence of loss of vision, or the loss of the ability to talk, other neural circuitries are enhanced to compensate for lost functions and to allow survivors to benefit from the healing power of another therapy. A helpful example is that of the increased sensitivity to touch, which could be channelled in somatic therapy, the focus in the next chapter.

Chapter 15

Neurosomatic Integration

In this final chapter of part V, I explore the role of the body in neuropsycho-social integration. I begin with the wisdom of the physical body and its bid to do what comes to it naturally, and that is to protect itself from injury and heal when it is wounded. This is ordinarily a perceptible woundedness, which expresses itself differently from the relational, emotional and psychological woundedness I explored in the previous chapters.

In her work *The Body Remembers*, the American somatic therapist Babette Rothschild (2000) encourages us to think of this woundedness as the body's travail, which is a source of memory and evidence of protracted suffering the mind may doubt or forget to remember.

NEUROSOMATIC WELL-BEING

The ways through which the body expresses its woundedness are endless. I have talked about asthma, allergies, cancers and diabetes that intersect multiple bodily systems. On the skin, one can think of the less virulent dermatitis, eczema and rosacea. In reproductive health, this could be the paralysing erectile dysfunction, infertility and uterine diseases, and in the endocrine system this could by histamine intolerance, hypercortisolaemia or insulin resistance. Chronic fatigue, gut dysbiosis, restless legs and tremors are also discernible ways through which the body protests, seemingly autonomously, when it is stuck in its woundedness, ailing and unable to heal itself. Much like the symptoms of relational, emotional and psychological dis-ease, these bodily protests are fuelled by unbounded energy that sustains trauma and disintegration in the body and undermines its health.

Unbounded energy in the body derives from lived experiences, which influence neurochemistry, epigenetic regulations and protective defences. Naturally, the body does not function in isolation of the mind, but here we are concerned with the massive amount of information it receives from the environment—via the senses of smell, taste, touch, sight and hearing—and must process in the half second before about sixteen bits of that information make their way to consciousness to be processed every given second (Norretranders, 1996). By this, we are confronted with the body's dynamism, its expansive memory, and the mechanism through which it undertakes to protect itself. All of which points to neuroplasticity, upon which neurons that fire and wire together depend to encode new and different responses to trauma.

For instance, neuroplasticity allows for opening up communication streams across and between neural and visceral structures that are disconnected by trauma and letting sensory information flow uninterrupted inside the body, but also between bodies that are engaged in the dance of life. Another way to think about this is as a bodily awareness that is congruent and reflects sensations in other similarly present and integrated bodies. It is what we mean when we say we can feel someone or an experience in our body. One might say, 'I feel safe, I am safe, and others around me feel safe'. This is an output of a neuroception of safety reaching the social-emotional brain from the social engagement nerve, which interfaces with parasympathetic control of organs in the viscera—the heart, lungs and gut, for instance. This neuro-psychosocial phenomenon eventuates naturally in a state of somatic safety that can be reinforced with a well-being SPEAR, to safeguard against ALEs.

NEUROSOMATIC SPEAR

The chaotic energy of ALEs, like that of the psychosocial trauma to which they give rise, retains in somatic memories and will fuel the adaptive responses. This emerges from how the survivor responded as well as how they would have responded instead but failed. In the neural tissues, this memory will associate the adaptive trauma response with ALEs, both real and imagined. And, like a sculpted antibody tasked with latching onto a detectible pathogen, deactivating it and marking it for destruction, this memory will be tasked with swatting detectible sensations of future ALEs, marking them for repression or dissociation in a bid to protect the body from imminent peril. In parts II and III, I explored how children inherit this memory type from parents and examined some adaptive responses to psychosocial stress different personalities are disposed to employ in this task, with each disposition bearing its own neurobiology and embedding in personalities that are persistent, unless intentionally restructured and released of the chaotic energies they accrue.

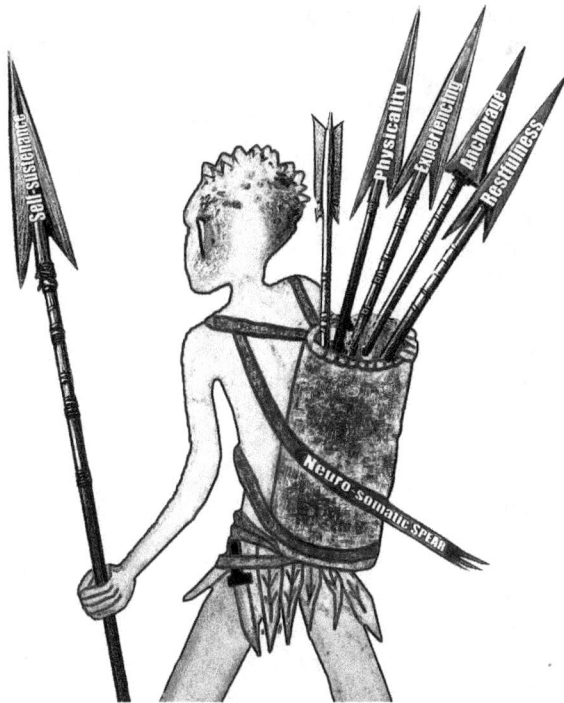

Figure 15.1. Neurosomatic SPEAR—Therapeutic Resources. *Figure courtesy of Dagmar Roelfsema.*

This is the goal of neurosomatic therapy: to bind and discharge the energies of self-sacrifice, stuckness, numbness, homelessness and restlessness that sustain disintegration, and invite the healing energies of self-sustenance, physicality, experiencing, anchorage and restfulness that bring integration to the body and together constitute the neurosomatic SPEAR.

Self-Sustenance

From old French *soustenance*, translating to 'source of health', sustenance meets the body's need to be nourished in a way that sustains well-being. Naturally, this excludes a bad diet, one that functions to inhibit as opposed to promote health and well-being. I could point to excessively processed sugars, unhealthy fats and foods laden with additives and allergens that dysregulate our immune and neural systems and undermine our body's ability to heal itself as examples of such a diet.

A dysregulated immune system, we know, procures chronic inflammation and autoimmunity that wrecks bodily tissues. The American nutritionist Dean

Ornish (2019), at the Preventive Medicine Research Institute in Sausalito, California, encourages us to prevent or undo this consequence with appropriate nutrition that promotes cardiovascular and neural health and sustains somatic health. This begins with anti-inflammatory diets, consisting of foods in their natural state: green vegetables rich in chlorophyl, minerals and vitamins that nourish neural tissue; fruits that provide natural sugars the mitochondria convert into energy; nuts and seeds with essential fats that promote neuronal myelination and communication; and wild fungi that provide rare vitamins and promote BDNF (brain-derived neurotrophic factor) synthesis, neuronal growth, repair and resilience. Beyond nutrition, however, sustenance is also about preserving the instinct to protect bodily systems from the psychosocial trauma that signals self-neglect, self-sacrifice, body mutilation and suicidality.

> **Task:** Explore your body as your source of wisdom. To what extent do you own and nourish it because you care about its health? Does your agency over it involve protecting it from the injury and depletion that exposure to toxins causes? How to you present it to the world? For instance, small, slouched or morbidly large? Or open, proud and strong? What does it mean to present your body in this way? Is it sufficiently nourished with life-affirming nutrients that are derived organically in nature? Or is it under siege by synthetic nutrients it cannot digest, and which keep its immune system chronically activated, defending it from what it perceives as alien and so diverting energy away from its growth? How about your relationship with food and where it comes from? How might you alter your food story to transform your relationship and heath.

Our relationship with food reflects our relationship with our body, as our body reflects its relationship with nutrition. Psychosocial trauma in our food story could manifest in many ways, from eating to soothe emotional pain to the sense that we do not have access to clean, nourishing food. In exploring our food story, we are encouraged to correct it in line with our body's need for sustenance and to honour our body as a source of wisdom, to retire its role as a trauma trough, starved, overwhelmed with the demands of toxins and disconnected from the mind that it is tasked to carry. The demands of carrying, in this sense, point to the extent to which the body is engaged physically in the task of life as a vessel for somatic substructures and systems, but also to protect itself.

Physicality

Our body is physical in a way that our relationships, psychology and emotions are not. Its most basic needs are the food, water and warmth that sustain life, and the lack of these it will express through physical pain, the body's language when its needs are unfulfilled. This includes the need to appropriately process the inflow of information from the senses without becoming overwhelmed, and to physically move out of harm's way without becoming stuck when this is the appropriate course of action. The nature of psychosocial trauma is such that these capacities are depleted, dysregulated or may have failed to develop, and the body can be held in a physical pain state out of which it is unable to move.

As much as it is physical, this stuckness can also be emotional, psychological or relational. Examples of what I mean include the emotional pain of depression and shame, the relational pain of loneliness and rejection, and the psychological pain of inadequateness and unworthiness—all states of suffering that are fuelled by unbounded energy the survivor is unable to discharge on their own, because they are not in control of their body's defence or their somatic narrative expressed in their gait, posture and even body shape. In a real-world sense, this might look like hyperphysicality and defensive posturing in the warrier who moves through life with a curled fist, hypermobility in the nomad who moves through life without a home address, and hypoactivity in the settler who moves through life bent at the cervical spine, clinically obese or in a state of drunkenness. It is like being unhelpful to one's own self, which may be a manifestation of having lost the will to act in service of well-being or ask for help.

Understanding that the survivor has been, for example, neglected as a child or batted as a wife makes sense of why they are vacant of confidence to reach out for help or have given up after having learned from experience that help—however badly needed—will not be forthcoming from the people who cared for them. This trauma-based adaptation may also be connected to ALEs for which the survivor does not have a declarative memory, but the memory, nonetheless, is held implicitly in the body. It is not uncommon to find that such memories express themselves in compulsions and sensory fragments of smells, tastes and sounds that are disconnected from explicit experiences, which is a feature of neuropsychosocial disintegration.

The therapeutic space is one in which the survivor is encouraged to cultivate self-compassion in order to move out of this state of helplessness and into one of helpful protectiveness, to collect and interrogate the stories their body holds in its trillions of cells, connect those stories in a hybrid state wherein they are resourced to act in service of their well-being, and correct their story of survival to include mobilisation to act for themselves.

Task: Explore your relationship with your body to establish where its care and protection fit in your priorities. This is to determine whether it feels alien and unloved or appreciated and cared for in a way that aligns with its needs. What affirmations does it receive from your senses, say from the orbital areas that travel with the optic nerve (CN11), which innervates the eyes and informs vision and imagination; from the mouth area that travel with the trigeminal nerve (CNV), which connects to the torso via its bid to ensure food reaching the gut is chewed and travels down the throat; or from the collar bone area that travels with the accessory nerve (CNXI), which moves the neck and head? The idea is to acquaint yourself with the neural fibres that transport healing energy to your viscera and establish how you may alter your life story with commitment to increase the flows of this energy, which also fuels its impulse to move in service of its safety.

Recall from part II that a mobilised state is activated by stress and that there are different kinds of stress, including the baseline stress that moves us to find food, warmth and friendship and the hormetic stress we cultivate when we exercise, which helps us to build physical strength and resilience. The endorphins and dopamine of hormetic stress, deriving from physical movement, counteract the corticosteroids of traumatic stress that—in a chronic state—poison neural cells and weaken neural circuitries, leading to shrinkage, memory loss and cognitive impairment, and, equally importantly, increasing the level of calcium in the body that when transported to the brain increases syntheses of dopamine, noradrenaline and endorphins that are important for learning, complex problems-solving and working memory. There is also the corollary increase in the release of BDNF that stimulates growth of new cells in neurogenesis, as well as the neural cells' capacity to recycle and eliminate waste that is associated with neurodegenerative disease—such as Alzheimer's, dementia and Parkinson's. By these quantifiable benefits, the intentional movement of our body functions as a buffer again symptoms of psychosocial trauma that manifest somatically.

We are inclined to move with intention in our ordinary life, from undertaking personal care that soothes our muscles to the curated movement of our body out of harm's way, as opposed to engaging with danger. In her exploration of how the body heals itself, somatic therapist Emily Francis (2018) charts how this impulse informs our psoas nerve, which encircles our reproductive area and is tasked with moving us physically. When it fails in the face of trauma, say to move our body away from sexual abuse or other things happening to us without our consent and which we are not proud to share, it also retains that memory. In that way, the psoas nerve protects our secrets and yearnings, including for safety and connection, in which our body is protected from assault. This is not actively thinking, for instance, 'I could get hurt by a specific person, and how can I prevent this?', but rather it is living life in a way that feels courageous and powerful, whilst at the same time strengthening our survival instincts.

This is the neural state we evoke with mindful movement and rhythms that have been used in ancient traditions to heal the body and help it to reconnect with the mind when this connection is disrupted by trauma. We can identify this disruption in a body that feels numb, homeless or alien and which the survivor is averse to protect. Neurosomatic therapy can encourage the survivor to reconnect with their body by experiencing it in a physical way, for instance, through the power of touch and physical posturing through the art of tai chi, swimming or kickboxing, under the guidance of a trauma-informed therapist.

The uninterrupted flow of healing energy throughout the body is at the heart of well-being that begins in the cell with mitochondrial health. We learned in part III that mitochondrial energy fuels every cell in our body, except the red blood cells that transport the oxygen the mitochondria need to generate energy. As such, mitochondrial health reflects in our body's ability to use energy, including for physical movement that takes us out of stagnant and sluggish life states and into active consciousness that stimulates us to experience connections and restrictions without the fear of stuckness or paralysis. For instance, gently massaging and stretching the body—things we are inclined to do naturally to release muscle tension—is about the survivor engaging the healing power of their bounded energy, over which they have a degree of sovereignty, and so is less led by the chaotic energy that governs the body in a state of disease and disintegration.

This is also about the power of touch in soothing the self and healing the body. I am here referring to gentle touch and other low-intensity stimulation of the skin that is associated with trust and relationship building and is affirmed by neurochemistry, especially the increase in oxytocin secretion that supresses cortisol. It is through this effect that oxytocin functions to promote healing connections that counteract the effect of traumatic stress's cortisol. By this, our reach for connection and attunement that is welcomed and met with empathy creates in us a sense of well-being that is selected for and rewarded. This curves back to ancestral bases and psychosocial resources that function to ensure we belong, say in a family, tribe or society, and inform our nervous system, which has evolved to rely on interaction with sentients who necessarily co-regulate our somatic states, through which we experience both suffering and well-being.

Experiencing

This is the capacity to sense and respond to our body and its messages in a way that promotes resilient well-being above vulnerability to psychosocial trauma. This capacity is often inhibited in survivors, who tend to move through life in a state of numbness or one of dysregulating anxiety, in which they are unable to bind and discharge the chaotic energy of somatic symptoms. Examples of what I mean include the hypertension and restlessness that indicate one is not okay. Or the ability to be okay is disrupted by a traumatic wound in bodily tissues that expresses itself in a crummy feeling, which warns of a disturbance in the body that cannot be put into words. This is cognitive disconnect—when the central nervous system fragments to protect itself. The sensation from the body it too painful to process, and to bring it back naturally is to bring the mind, emotions and gut in synch with each other using the body's own survival force.

> **Task:** Interrogate how your body experiences and responds to different seasons, different temperatures or even different stressors. For instance, how does it respond to hot water or cold wind? These are physical experiences that rev up the sympathetic nerves and can force the body and mind to connect, for the body's very survival under such conditions is contingent on this connection. The quick, successive and deep breaths that are associated with being hot or cold open up your lungs to take in oxygen to the organs in your viscera, and in so doing energise and connect your gut with the rest of your nervous system. Subsequent lengthened exhales will activate the parasympathetic nerves, but gradually. This is the state in which you are able to perceive butterflies, hunger and bowel movement, which tells you that your mind and body are synched. How would you alter your life story to experience more of this synchronicity?

Collecting somatic narratives about how your body experiences life events forces you to consider what is it not telling you too. The rhythm of the breath, for instance, is a metaphysical barometer of how the body is functioning. The rhythmic breathing that takes clean oxygen deep into your belly's cavity—free of fumes and other toxins that disrupt your nerves—offers you the chance to observe your somatic response to the healing power of oxygen that moves your body. By bringing your focus to this rhythm, you can learn to listen to your body and interpret and honour its messages, even those messages that are not of adequate strength to reach perception.

For example, this could address a neuroception about another person's hurtful intention that enters the gut and causes a rattle but stays there. This is what we call a gut feeling or gut instinct, which is based on more information than is available to cognition. As such, honouring intuition at the gut level is a marker of somatic intelligence that not only complements cognition but also compensates for cognitive impairment. Hence, gut intuition is as valid as cognition in allowing us to engage with life in an intelligent way.

By honouring this somatic wisdom and experiencing it with gentleness, we can isolate and discharge the chaotic energy of traumatic memories, even those we do not have the language to express but which nonetheless show up in our body and health outcomes, such as in mysterious gnashing of teeth, restless legs, hypertension and histamine intolerance. Healing comes with experiencing the body as strong, erected and present. Incidentally, the neurochemistry of strength, erection and presence involves an increase in testosterone and decrease in cortisol. Oxytocin and the healing power of the vagus nerves can be invited with gentle massage to the temple or back of the neck, bringing regulation to the emotional limbic brain and the more ancient instinctive brain from where maladaptive defences are reinforced and the chaotic energy of trauma-based responses derive. Engaging with this part of the nervous system is about gently guiding it to experience safety whilst creating anticipation for its homecoming.

Anchorage

From old French *ancrer*, 'anchorage' translates to a sense of resilient rootedness—or, more literally, a firm foundation to and from which we can safely retreat as we move through life. As Dana (2021) puts it, when we are anchored, 'we have a sense of being safely held, so we can venture out into the world, and explore its opportunities for growth and face its adversities without becoming adrift.' We might think of this anchorage as a safe place, a home of sorts, to which the nourished, physical and experienced body retreats to rest and heal when it is tired and wounded. But anchorage is also a symbolic state, as in the autonomic state in which we experience connection and integration, fall in love with life, entertain authenticity in our self and reflect on our life challenges without becoming overwhelmed. And this is because the neuroceptions of safety that are characteristic of anchorage are functioning to downregulate our adaptive defences and upregulate the conditions for social engagement and growth.

> **Task:** What stories does your body hold about where it belongs and who owns it? What is your story about where you belong, the place you tell yourself and others? Where is it located; how does it look, sound, smell, feel to be there, and who else is present? This could be an actual or imagined place where you connect with your true self or even nature. Smell the aroma of maturing herbs and ripening berries. Hear the sound of birds' cries and the wind whistling through the trees. Feel the breeze on your skin, touch the stumps of dead trees and taste clean air. Where are your senses engaged naturally, and where can you be fully present with your true self and engage the energies of different autonomic states in an enlivening experience? This is a home.

Knowing we are home is also knowing when we are not home. For home is where the heart is, goes the old adage. Being away from home, thus, is a somatic state of either being lost and adrift or of mobilisation to find our way home. Your home could be in nature, as in the above exercise, but for some people this could be a mountain, seaside or a garden in their own mind. It may even be a spiritual state. My grandmother reminds me at every opportunity that this world is not her 'home', and she has been forever preparing to go home in the spiritual realm where God lives, the God to whom she prays and appeals for guidance in times of need.

By this conceptualisation, home is our own creation, where we experience peace, acceptance and fulfilment, and which we can take with us wherever we go. It is also where our capacity to engage and move with flexibility in and between different autonomic states is resilient, where we can identity and bind chaotic energies in our body and mind and co-opt the healing energies of integration. This is also the home of homeostasis—a concept of home that invites the need for boundaries within which the body and mind are held safe and can be safety stretched. It is where we can safely interrogate different sensations inside our body, such as whether we are fulfilling our purpose and honouring our yes and no within appropriate survival states, for instance, when we are activated or engaged and our affirmations and rejections reflect what is good for us. Here our maybes appropriately indicate curiosity about possibilities and uncertainties.

Restfulness

We can begin here with the restlessness associated with psychosocial trauma that prevents the body from getting the necessary rest it needs to replenish its resources. Restfulness, in this sense, promotes restoration. We have already learned that restlessness is a mobilised state fuelled by corticosteroids, which incidentally suppress the GABA and serotonin that promote restfulness, the capacity for the body and mind to just be, whilst wounds are encouraged to heal, resources replenish and reserves restore.

Needless to say, these events are characteristically disrupted by psychosocial trauma, and cultivating restfulness is about bringing regulation to the body's natural rhythms that govern them. I have mentioned the rhythm of heart, lungs and blood flow throughout the chapters of this book, but there is also the rhythm of sleep that, when disrupted, skews the experience of wakefulness and well-being. This is because a disrupted sleep rhythm, which is also known as the circadian rhythm, points to dysregulation in neurochemistry—in serotonin, dopamin and GABA circuitries—that regulates the healing energy upon which sociality and nourishing relationships depend.

Thankfully, the neurotransmission literature affirms what our body and nature know: We can upregulate this neurochemistry through our diet. More precisely, a paper published in the journal *Nutrients* (Briguglio et al., 2018) identified organic pineapples, oranges and bananas as nutrient-dense foods that increase by up to 200 percent the levels of serotonin the body can convert into melatonin, the sleep regulatory hormone. These natural foods, it turned out, are also rich in vitamins that keep anxiety in check and promote sensations of fulfilment and relaxation. As the researcher Saundra Dalton-Smith (2019) found, this is the necessary physiological quietness that exerts little demand on sympathetic activities and tunes down the demand for energy, including that of chaotic energy that sustains trauma and restlessness.

Naturally, our physiology is informed by our emotions and psychology, so restfulness is about emotional and psychological quietness too, a quietness that appeals to the healing energy of restfulness and parasympathetic activities through which the body heals itself at the cellular level. For instance, low demand for energy in the digestive and immune systems during a period of fasting—whether lengthy, short or intermittent—means the gut and immune cells are allowed to rest and renew themselves. The immune system, in particular, on a break from its lookout for pathogens entering the gut, redirects its focus to breaking down its own cells for energy, using first older, damaged ones, which are replaced by new healthy ones. The parallel decrease in digestive activity will also lead to an increase in the level of pro-gut biome and chemicals that cross the blood-brain barrier to promote BDNF synthesis and—in effect—regeneration of dopaminergic, cholinergic and serotonergic neurons in the mood and motivation circuitries.

This is a task the body undertakes naturally when we sleep well. The altered state of consciousness and near paralysis that characterizes sleep is one in which both sensory and muscular activities are inhibited, stress-related neurochemistry is suppressed and the body builds up and restores the immune, nervous, skeletal and muscular systems. There are different phases of sleep through which the body carries out these activities. The fifth and final stage of sleep, in particular, is a somatic state in which noradrenaline synthesis in the brain is turned off and the nervous system surfaces and processes its unconscious psychological and emotional contents, which is what Freud (1997) called dreams.

In his thesis on why we sleep, the British neuropsychologist Matthew Walker (2017) describes this state as 'overnight therapy' through which broken neural circuits reconnect to promote integration. This is the healing power of sleep, he agreed with Washington University's psychiatrist Murray Raskind, who affirmed his patients with traumatic stress disorders had reported lower blood pressure, fewer nightmares and longer sleep, through which sleep had a chance to take effect as a 'healing balm', after they were treated with psychotropics to mimic the effect of rapid eye movement (REM) that is characteristic of deep sleep. This is because REM, whilst occurring in a state of altered consciousness, activates the occipital lobe and suboccipital muscles in the brainstem, from where the vagus nerve initiates its activities. By this activation, the ventral fibres are stimulated in a state of restfulness, which is the natural condition for social engagement and connection. Hence, good sleep is a state in which the nervous system experiences restfulness and the chaotic energy of social disengagement and disconnection is bounded.

> **Task:** What is your sleep story, your relationship with sleep? Commonly, this is broadcasted to the world by the orbicularis oculi that encircles the eyes and retains the stress of inadequate restfulness. In massaging this muscle, can you sense that it promotes calm and authentic expressions, or a release of tension that announces itself, say, in a yawn or sigh that takes oxygen into or out of the body and resets the autonomic nerves? How about a facial massage to stimulate cranial nerve V and mirror neurons to invoke the neurobiology of self-compassion that can be enhanced with a dot of calming castor oil applied behind the ear lobe on the mastoid bone, to stimulate the release of anti-inflammatory acetylcholine? The idea is to get a sense of how your nervous system behaves in a state of restfulness, and rework your life story with a commitment to promoting this sensation.

The benefits of restfulness that can be cultivated within the therapeutic space are endless, including ritualistic, religious and ethical ones. The role of the neurosomatic therapist in guiding this intervention is also to consider that certain modalities of rest, such as fasting, can be harmful when inadequately considered. For instance, excess fasting can evoke the consequence of famine, which include chronic elevated stress levels that accelerate wear and tear on the body. This goes against the goal of neurosomatic therapy, which centres the ancient wisdom of the body, honouring its biological imperative to heal, and this occurs in the course of resonating with other bodies. Moreover, a specific trauma in the body that manifests in destructive sensations, such as helplessness and suicidality—which are unlikely to respond with necessary urgency in the therapeutic space—may call for a more clinical approach to process or reprocess this specific trauma before the nervous system can be freed for integration. Another way to understand this is as an injury in somatic integrity, in the body's natural ability to heal itself.

NEUROSOMATIC THERAPY IN REFLECTION

Neurosomatic therapy that address psychosocial trauma works to restore somatic integrity. However, by itself, it may not be completely healing, and clinical intervention may be necessary to manage or reverse diseases in the body occasioned by traumatic stress, or even adverse epigenetic modification in neural structures. Researchers at Mount Sinai Hospital in New York discovered that traumatic stress in early life that resulted in epigenetic modification can be countered with psychotropics that mitigate the attendant vulnerability to severe disease (Kronman et al., 2021). The study, which involved animal models, found that exposure to stress in early life that gave rise to genetic modification in the nucleus accumbens, a critical structure in the basal forebrain that is involved with reward, motivation and pleasure-seeking behaviour, responded to oncogenic drugs that inhibited the protein responsible for the modification and decreased the effect of trauma on stress response later in life. In the field of oncology, psychotropics that treat some cancers by epigenetic mechanisms are already in clinical use. So time will tell if psychotropics that modify epigenetics will become a bigger part of the treatment arsenal in neuropsychology and to prevent transmission of vulner-abilities across generations that deplete the body's capacity to heal itself.

Naturally, this would be revolutionary in the treatment of transgenerational trauma and neuropsychosocial disintegration. Until then, we can be satisfied with the hope that other revolutionary approaches in the treatment of trauma are available. A good example is the healing effect of REM sleep that we can already replicate with EMDR therapy, which brings calm to the nervous system by evoking rapid, rhythmic eye movements to dislodge and reprocess traumatic memories (Shapiro, 2017), shifting traumatic memories from the social-emotional brain to the rational brain, where these memories are ration-alised and released of chaotic energy.

In practice, this involves the patient's eyes following the therapist's finger movements in order to loosen connections in neural structures that allow people to access injurious memories from the past, memories from specific adverse life events. It would not be that you were neglected as a child, but that being neglected as a child has led you to dissociate from your body, discon-nect from your caregivers, isolate from your tribe and feel redundant in your community. EMDR can help to reverse this state by connecting the body with the mind and reestablishing equilibrium in the nervous system. The activation of neurogenesis is about the nervous system healing itself and rebuilding lost connections, particularly in the insula and limbic structures, to keep them regulated and resilient so they do not misinterpret or exaggerate memories.

I say this is 'revolutionary', but working with the eyes in somatic therapy is as ancient as the eye itself. Beginning life as neural structures that are extruded during the course of foetal development, the eyes retain power as windows to the nervous system. We can interpret this literally, for we use our eyes to express our inner world—our joys, fears, pains—and to inform others of how we are receiving them, including that we may not be receiving them empathically.

In my clinical experience, this latter expression is one I perceive often in eyes that are adapted to having seen incredible suffering. And one may say that to protect itself from the incoming dysregulating sensation of such suffering, the nervous system severs its connection with the eyes—hence eyes that don't cry to express pain or gaze to express empathy. Think of the blank, rigid, even hostile eyes of infamous serial killers Harold Shipman (1946–2004), Eileen Wournos (1956–2002) and Samuel Little (1940–2020) that tell stories of exposure—particularly in childhood—to ALEs that were awfully painful to see, and for which protection might have come in closing their eyes physically and themselves emotionally.

Such experiences effectively deactivate the orbicularis oculi that encircles the eyes and comes into play by the sweet emotions of the soul, not for instance by deceitful laughs or fake joy. As the French neurologist G.-B. Duchenne de Boulogne (2008) put it, the eye-orbiting muscle tightening the lids and skin directly below it, lifting the cheekbones and expressing signals from a regulated nervous system, 'does not obey will; it is only brought into play by true feelings, by agreeable emotions' that are actual or recalled. A happily married couple's smile as they reconnect after being away from each other, a baby's coo at the sight of an emotionally attuned parent after a day in kinder school, my grandmother's squinting eyes and mutters of 'pretty gal' when she sees me after a long time—all originate from this instinctive subconscious process at play when we engage empathically. However, when people are long stuck in a state of distress, the muscles in and around the eyes adapt to reflect that chronic distress. Gently massaging these muscles could bring relief, which can be extended to the face and the entire body. This is possible because the face is innervated by fibres of cranial nerves V and VII that are liable to respond to comforting massage reaching into tissues beneath the skin, and relay this comfort to the vagus nerve for cascade.

Part VI

EMBRACING NEUROPSYCHOSOCIAL INTEGRATION IN WELL-BEING

Chapter 16

A Survivor's Guide to Neuropsychosocial Integration

This final part of my exploration of neuropsychosocial integration for well-being brings focus to the body and mind in the experience of life—from birth to adolescence, adulthood and elderhood—throughout which we suffer and entertain disintegration, desire and pursue integration, bind and discharge the chaotic energy of psychosocial trauma, and seek and recover authenticity in our self. And we do these things with the help of our inheritance, such as our generic memory; possessions we cultivate within ourselves, such as mind-heart-soulfulness; and metaphorical spears that promote our survival, well-being and resilience.

We also learn through what we care about that the first purpose of life is the preservation of life itself, and this involves pursuing and preserving wellness. This wellness may differ in interpretation, but it is generally that state in which the nervous system in its relationships with the internal and external worlds is functioning optimally—in a word, as nature intends, keeping us safe and healthful. In acknowledging and preserving this state as we move flexibly in and out of stimulation and rest and repair, we promote integration in our body and mind.

NEUROPSYCHOSOCIAL INTEGRATION AS PURPOSE

From the outset, I introduced neuropsychosocial integration as an approach to rescuing the authentic self from psychosocial trauma that leaves survivors vulnerable to peritraumatic disintegration and maladies. This rescue is about freedom to be in charge of one's own body and mind, and it is precisely what is achieved when trauma that carves up the body and mind is surfaced, discharged of its energy and contextualised as legacy. Contextualisation promotes stability in neural processes that underpin well-being and chemistry that fuels passion, perseverance and purpose, the three important Ps of a fulfilling life that, incidentally, sustained me throughout my research and exploration that culminate in this book.

Along with safety and secure attachment, these necessary features of a fulfilled life, although interlinked, are cultivated and regulated in different areas in the nervous system, and this is precisely how they become vulnerable to traumatic wounds that embed in the nervous system. For instance, purposefulness, a uniquely human psychological feature, is cultivated in a neural substructure called the orbitofrontal cortex in the cerebrum, which is roughly 80 percent of the entire brain. This is also known as the cognitive brain system, where we make sense of life events—the positive, negative and neutral—and understand and negotiate consequences. It is also where our passion and perseverance are selected for and rewarded, in the parking lots of our dopaminergic pleasure-reward circuitry that encodes our goals. All these important conditions of being human, under conditions of psychosocial trauma, are liable to disintegrate, and naturally this has implications for how we confront adversity that—beyond early childhood—impacts our ability not only to solve complex problems but also to preserve life.

In establishing a resilient state for learning and well-being, neuropsychosocial integration is protective against this vulnerability, promoting connection and resilience across the billions of neural circuitries that process inner experiences and complex sensations about our task of life, such as who we are in the world and how we respond to adversities and opportunities to socialise and build relationships. This comes together in our life stories. Those we appropriate, those we imagine—beginning in childhood—about who we are, and those we create as we move through life, experiencing, learning and solving problems—ranging from the simple personal, such as foraging for wild berries to satisfy a nomadic hunger for sweet adventure, to the complex relational, such as peer pressure and coercive control that engage our protective defences.

These impulses and capacities—where inhibited or obliterated by psychosocial trauma—can be recovered with the help of well-being SPEARS that evoke 'outside-the-box' and lateral realities that enrich our life stories. By any measure, this is an artistic and creative approach to improving our life outcomes, one that finds resonance in the teaching of the Maltese psychologist Edward de Bono (2015), who coined the phrase *lateral thinking* to encourage artistry and creativity in our approach to solving complex psychosocial problems.

A good example we are confronted with in ordinary life is the use of art in family planning and population management, rather than banning abortions and enforcing sterilisations that cause futile suffering and should impel us to consider psychosocial solutions for such deeply psychosocial issues. Within a therapeutic context, this involves designing a life that differs from a trauma-suffused one and acting to create that different life, free from the chaotic energy that sustains trauma.

At the level of the individual, consider, for instance, the chaotic energy of sexual violence in childhood that is held in place by dissociation. As one survivor put it, 'while it was happening, I would imagine I was somewhere else; I would leave my body'. This is a psychosocial trauma for which a solution might involve affixing this adaption to its originating event in the past in which it occurred, so that the need for dissociation from the body loses its bearing in the here and now. The new story might include an authentic appreciation of the survivor's body in the here and now as their own to love, care about and create a safe home for. This is relational self-compassion, psychological agency and somatic anchorage brought together in a perhaps more exciting story that integrates the psyche and soma in a relationship that is nourishing and safe.

An image I encountered endlessly on my long drives throughout the United States and in particular the state of Connecticut, where I stayed during the COVID-19 pandemic, brings this idea to life. It is the sight of a family of two adults, two small children and a pet feasting in the beautifully manicured garden of a lush suburban home. Despite betraying representativeness and the dynamics in family life that can look very different across cultures and nations, in the middle of what was arguably our time's most catastrophic human disaster, it was an impressive image that conveyed a powerful message. For my objective in this book, it is about how we can engage our imagination, creativity and the neurobiology of relationship and belonging to serve us in our quest for integration and well-being.

Beginning in this example, with the visual cortex in the occipital lobe that sits atop the brainstem, from where it interfaces with the vagus nerve, notice that I used the adjectives *beautiful* and *lush* to describe the environment in which the family is relating and also to guide your visualisation. My intention is to bring alive in your nervous system an experience that is acceptable and desirable in contemporary life—American democratic life, to be specific.

To do this, the image activates the suboccipital muscles, which evoke the social complex of the vagus nerve and the secretion of dopamine from the ventral tegmental area (VTA) in the social-emotional midbrain, which will travel to the prefrontal cortex to reward a positive perception, hopefully one of intimate relationship. This is a higher mental process that intersects cognition, emotion and instinct in the creation of a new and nourishing story, for it includes mindfulness, use of imagery and language and abstract neuroceptions, such as freedom and happiness, that are real and virtuous, even if indefinable as far as our perception may be concerned. But this is okay; our system of perception is an imperfect one, and the reality of delusions is a consistent reminder of that.

NEUROPSYCHOSOCIAL INTEGRATION: A CLINICAL APPROACH

An integrative approach encourages us to pay attention to this condition of being human, especially as it is vulnerable to trauma, to consider perception and neuroception as psychosocial phenomena that inform the way we understand and treat psychosocial trauma, where we are treating the relational, emotional, psychological and somatic manifestations as one condition.

With an integrative approach, we are looking for features that show up across different complaints or diagnoses. For instance, where depression coexists with obesity, we would be looking at environmental factors, lifestyle factors and genetic and neurobiological vulnerabilities in the diagnosis of depression but also in the diagnosis of obesity. And, remarkably, when we look at the neurobiological factors, the same neural structures and chemistry show up. That is, along with dysregulated levels of corticosteroids that inhibit prosocial neurochemistry, deficits and inflammation in the amygdala, hippocampus, hypothalamus, insula, thalamus and frontal cortex are implicated in these diagnoses, as well as many other psychosomatic maladies. And the main complaint is almost always a psychosocial pathology—social disease, relational anxiety, problems with mood regulation, rational decision-making, impulse control, thought processes and so on.

This makes sense when we consider that the social-emotional brain is connected with the cognitive-rational brain, so when the emotional brain is dysregulated, so too will be the cognitive-rational brain. Emotions inform behaviour, so whether we feel loved, safe or lonely will feature in behaviours such as eating, stalking and rage, but also whether we fight, flee or fold in the face of adversity. Integration gets us to think about these adaptations as expressions of disintegration rather than features of distinct diagnoses. The overlapping features are then reclassified as expressions of a neuropsychosocial condition that can be treated in an integrative way. An integrative approach towards a healthful mind might consider, for example:

- The survivor's psychosocial strengths, deficits and vulnerabilities
- The survivor's dominant emotions and how they are regulated
- Behaviour activation to address resistance and other maladaptations
- Mental activation to address unhelpful thoughts, memories and images
- Strategy for promoting intelligence, well-being and resilience SPEARS

An appeal to the survivor's strengths is important in the therapeutic space, particularly where they are showing up with complaints that cut across multiple diagnoses—in our example, we are looking at depression, obesity and an endocrine disease. These comorbidities are classically treated separately, but we now know they overlap in neuropsychosocial disintegration and might respond to neuropsychosocial therapy. And this would involve identifying the maladaptive psychological, behavioural and somatic processes that intersect and give rise to the depression, obesity and endocrine disease with which the survivor will be suffering, and addressing the expressions and aetiologies of these maladies in an integrative therapy.

An aetiology of ALEs and psychosocial trauma will require a strategy for promoting intelligence, well-being and resilience SPEARS. This will also invite a nuanced consideration of the timing of the ALEs, the nature of the trauma and the adaptations in a conversation about the variety of responses that people have to a wide range of circumstances in their lives. This is where we accept that psychosocial trauma and the attendant neuropsychosocial disintegration can intersect with different clinical diagnoses. To take an example, an impaired perception of risk and safety that originates in an altered nervous system after exposure to domestic violence is a feature of depression. Similarly, an impaired perception of risk and safety is a feature of attachment disorders that originate in childhood, and also of physiological trauma that originates in brain injuries. A survivor may show up to the task of life or a therapeutic relationship with an impaired perception of risk and safety and all three of these ALEs.

Embedded in the nervous system—these wounds will demand attention at some point along the life cycle in a range of diseases and disorders. Recall my mention in earlier chapters of inflammation and the random pain in our body we experience as spasms and restlessness, unregulated growth in our cellular tissues that metastasize into tumours and cancers, and dysregulation in our vascular system we experience as hypertension. All these maladies will respond to binding and discharging the chaotic energy that fuels the state of disintegration in which they develop and thrive. And this is important because the disintegrated state is the opposite of where we need to be for healing to begin.

The disintegrated state is highly perceptible—we feel the expressions in our bodies long before they are diagnosed as diseases and disorders. This might be felt as fatigue, insecurity in our body or a fright we cannot discharge. Or we may have issues with rest. This might look like difficulty getting to sleep or staying asleep, indicating that a perception of our social world as a dangerous place, and we have trouble feeling safe enough to sleep. When we bring regulation to this perception with the neurosomatic SPEAR, the body's wisdom and capacity to heal itself surface naturally.

But, foremost, the survivor must be empowered to embrace virtue, including attention, peace and nourishing relationships, in all areas of life, to experience and integrate the varied and complex pieces of past, present and future stories that bring clarity to troublesome thoughts, feelings and behaviours that impact health. The goal is to transform this outcome, rather than merely changing thoughts or behaviour patterns that correspond to specific complaints. For the therapist, the goal is to guide the survivor to a state of well-being in which they are functioning to their fullest potential and can respond with flexibility to difficult experiences. This outcome begins with a story of well-being, of what it looks and feels like, and deploying well-being SPEARS to break down experiences that undermine well-being into chunks that can be more easily metabolised.

Adverse experiences may be painful and can at times be difficult to delineate and pose a challenge in this regard. Or the challenge may be one of organising the nervous system and reintegrating the wounded body and mind, so that they promote and reinforce each other. Naturally, in this process, an important step is to acknowledge that the autonomic nerves, like the body and mind, are infirmed by trauma, and this trauma expresses itself in specific and nonspecific ways, such as in a pervasive sense of helplessness, hopelessness, powerlessness and isolation, which can be reversed by the rediscovery of help, hope, power and connection. This speaks to the ability to present oneself relationally without being overwhelmed by sensations and neuroceptions of woundedness, a state wherein safety and control are restored in the survivor's life story, their sympathetic and parasympathetic nerves are homeostatic and their body heals and renews itself.

Following this step is the actual healing of traumatic wounds, which happens when the trauma is discharged of energy. This might look and feel different for different survivors. For instance, in part I we were introduced to Dr. Felitti's patient, who had quickly regained lost weight as a way of covering up traumatic wounds of sexual abuse and betrayed innocence at the hands of her grandfather in childhood. To this survivor, healing was in effectively treating her underlying trauma of sexual violence and betrayed innocence, which expressed itself in her lingering psychalgia, anxiety and fear. Dr. Felitti was to discover by accident that it was not in eliminating her obesity, which helped her to cope, and the problem he was trying to treat was in fact a solution to a different kind of problem.

Similarly, Alex, who suffered with poor mental health throughout the pandemic, could not be helped by his therapist, who failed to recognise the deep injury to his purpose that caused him to suffer. It was in turning to alcoholism that he was able to separate himself from the sensation of this suffering. Much like overeating, it turns out that this behaviour, however injurious, effectively hid his more severe injury. To him, healing was in effectively treating his underlying trauma of forced isolation from his purpose, which manifested in a lingering sense of worthlessness.

This disparity in perceptions of well-being is among a myriad of factors that can impact the therapeutic experience. Another and perhaps worse factor is experienced among people groups where the psychosocial and socioeconomic determine access to healthcare. For instance, socioeconomically disadvantaged children who suffer with traumatic stress are many times more likely than their affluent peers to be treated with antipsychotic medications. And they will often miss the opportunity to build metaphorical spears and develop into competent personalities with capacities to imagine, play, plan, build meaningful relationships and monitor their psychological, physiological and social transformation.

This is the definition of psychosocial deficits and developmental stuckness, so when survivors say they have benefited from therapy, it is not only about less painful symptoms but that they are equipped to unstick themselves in situations that could prevent them from moving forward in a positive way, say to build a good relationship or pursue something they enjoy whilst not feeling ashamed of their history of trauma or guilty that they survived. This goes beyond less anger, less tightness in the chest and fewer knots in the stomach, although these improvements are important. It is about nurturing authenticity in the self and altering their life story to include pieces about falling in love with life and well-being. And, according to Richard Davidson (2023) of the Centre for Healthy Minds at the University of Wisconsin–Madison, it involves cultivating awareness, connection, insight and purpose to promote adaptations in the nervous system in ways that improve health and well-being.

Self-awareness encourages us to pay attention to what is going on in our body and mind as well as in our environment. For it is in being introspective that we mitigate the toll on well-being that distraction exacts. Connection encompasses the ability to pick up on the mindsets and emotions of others in bidirectional relationships held intact by prosocial virtues, such as kindness and empathy. Insight speaks to wisdom derived from experience that can be used to reconcile false narratives, much like purpose—the resilient sense that life has meaning—which has been linked with faster recovery from ALEs and even with longer life.

Summarily, in this state of recovery, the survivor is nurturing inner strengths, developing values, forming resonant relationships, discovering meaning and altering their life to include new paths and opportunities. In this story, trauma does not persist throughout the life cycle but is a wound from which survivors heal, learn and move forward with resilience and a focus on experiences that make life worth living. In imagination, this may be a life enthused with joy, humility and well-being, informed by a positive psychology, and outside of memory and folklore, it can be recorded for reflection in a private journal of self-discovery.

JOURNALING OUR INTEGRATION AND AUTHENTIC SELF-DISCOVERY

The survivor is now a hero in their life story of tribulation and triumph, having been called to venture into dark and dangerous places—at times in the recesses of their own mind—to slay a dragon and bring fulfilment to their life. In this story, pure authenticity is discovered and reconciled in the self, before which the unbounded energy of psychosocial trauma will have been discharged. By implication, this is also a heroic journey of authentic self-discovery that begins from a place of vulnerability and ever-present danger. For the American mythologist Joseph Campbell, the most well-known chronicler of the hero's journey, this danger was the fiery dragon, which is a metaphor for hardship.

In the story of this book and the survivors for whom it is written, the dragon is psychosocial trauma and attendant neuropsychosocial disintegration, which can be slayed with carefully crafted metaphorical spears, beginning with the native, intelligence and resilience SPEARS and continuing with the well-being SPEARS, with which survivors can reach into their body and mind to bind the chaotic energy of trauma and return stability to the nervous system, synchronicity to the body and mind, and authenticity, strength and wisdom to the self.

This is difficult work best accomplished in a compassionate therapeutic space in which the therapist guides the survivor. The survivor, nonetheless, is the curator of their life's story, which might look like a storybook in which they are encouraged to write thoughtfully about their lived experiences, personalities, aspiration and yearnings, and in so doing bring structure to the information held about these in their nervous system. As structured information is fuelled by bounded energy, the practice of revisiting lived experiences, adverse ones in particular, in a structured way competes with the chaotic energy of the trauma they installed in the nervous system and, in this way, can be healing as opposed to distressing. The storylike structure, which is ordered and free of distress, invoking energy that underpins imagination, creativity and foresight, will also serve to open up the survivor to articulating a vision of the future.

Whilst this kind of journaling is healing in the sense that I have explained, it is unlike others kinds, say gratitude journaling, in which survivors are encouraged to write about being grateful and things they are grateful for. Here, the survivor, in writing about adverse lived experiences, deepens emotions and thoughts around these experiences that show up at specific times in their life or ancestry and reflections on how these experiences shape who they are, were or can become.

There is also auxiliary benefits of tracking their progress, as well as expressing gratitude, speaking kindly to themselves, interrogating thoughts and challenges, and reflecting on opportunities to try new things and to learn and grow from mistakes. They also benefit from protecting themselves and honouring their boundaries by saying no when needed, as well as trusting their intuition, listening to their inner voice and acting daily in ways that promote their well-being. This is the essence of therapeutic journaling for integration and self-authenticity.

In my own experience, this kind of journaling encourages me to organise my stories in a way that can be helpful in identifying not only why certain episodes occur but also when they are most likely to occur, and to reflect on changes that I can make to react less regretfully and to identify and encourage more successes and lessen failures. In the therapeutic space, this can be helpful in confronting reality with intention, to learn from history but also from lived experience.

This began for me subconsciously, with an appreciation of the information I get from my intuition and lucid dreams, which led me to explore my ancestral healing practices and to seek out my authentic self, the self that I would discover once I had retired many of my protective layers of defences. Journaling was about bringing out that self and increasing my awareness of my belongingness, thoughts, fears and hopes and capturing the changes and growth in this space.

My journal began its life as my private space within which I engaged and reflected upon my feelings, thoughts and images I held in my mind and perceived as important, especially in how they related to other experiences. This included, for instance, an ethnic Caribbean self, a racialised black self and a gendered feminine self that are all complex but nonetheless sit comfortably in me alongside a compassionate self, which, incidentally, allows me to experience my other selves in a way that is not despairing and from which I am not inclined to take flight. In accepting and exploring these different selves of mine, I became competent in presenting them to others when their presence was called upon, say to serve in natural dialogues, to meet another survivor where they are within the therapeutic space or to connect with another person and determine what they want from me. And this ability, of course, comes from a place of awareness of myself and of the workings of my conscious, my subconscious and all that lies in between.

It behoves me to acknowledge that this ability to bring attention to what's going on inside and around you and to write the detail in a journal, or even to have those sensations and observations painted back to you by an attuned therapist, can be validating but also tiring, triggering and stressful. So you will need a self-rescue plan or recovery kit that includes action to build awareness for internal tension and to recover compassion when it is lost or depleted. This might include occasions to forgive and live without grudges. And here I want to emphasise that forgiveness is not the same as forgetting. In her exploration *Forgiving What You Cannot Forget*, author Lysa TerKeurst (2020) reminds us that forgiveness is about freedom from internal suffering. It does not mean the bad stuff that happened was acceptable, nor does it require you to reconcile with or befriend people who caused you to suffer directly or indirectly. Rather, it is about discharging the chaotic energy associated with unresolved pain that hinders nourishing relationships and a fulfilled life, such as with people who demonstrate trustworthiness, kindness and compassion.

Chapter 17

Beyond Psychosocial Trauma and Disintegration

As I come to the end of my exploration into the chasm of the neuropsycho-social and its dynamic structure, chemistry and energy, I am compelled to reflect on its implication for resilience in the body and mind as well as growth in the self that are integrated and unimpaired by trauma. At the heart of this reflection is the resonant relationships we form through our exposure and contacts in social networks, which help us to find our way through life as competent personalities equipped to thrive through opportunities. We begin this journey developing psychosocial resources with which we will move through ordinary life and respond to ALEs. Along the way, we will learn to process to completion the sensations, emotions, memories and adaptations associated with psychosocial traumas, and we will come full circle to well-being, having altered our life story with a commitment to our well-being and growth.

POST-TRAUMATIC GROWTH

I am referring to a pattern of change that involves regression and progression surrounding integration and sustained well-being. With psychosocial trauma as our refence point, growth demands the normalcy of downtime when we do not feel capable, resourceful or resilient, but also looking back on life with insight and coming to see our self as stronger and wiser and with new mean-ingful commitments that lead to a fulfilled life.

Moving between these two states of being cannot be easy; with internal chaos but glimmers of hope that progression brings can motivate survivors to make changes in their life that reflect their strength. It is then that help and encouragement is needed to experience growth as a process that unfolds in time, to build reserves of resourcefulness and resilience by recognising and cultivating the capacity to grow, even through challenges. There is also the pleasant sensation of purposefulness that enlivens the nervous system, and by focusing on it, survivors can strengthen their immune, gut and muscles systems, which are nourished by restfulness, sustenance and physicality. Physical exercise, in particular, is associated with the feel-good effect of noradrenaline and endorphins that are implicated in orientation towards new possibilities, creativity, open-mindedness, bravery, persistence, integrity, kindness, fairness, leadership, humility, forgiveness and gratitude.

Beyond trauma and disintegration, these are virtues we nurture with our native, intelligence and well-being SPEARS, which empower us to live through purpose. Equally important is the piece of our story of having healed our woundedness and reframed it as a legacy that informs our learning, as opposed to one that defines our life, where we accept that the work of discharging the chaotic energy that sustains trauma—however messy and difficult—is rewarding as we orient towards our strengths and a fulfilling life. This new life is one in which we are not merely resourced and encouraged to live well but relish resilience in somatic safety, psychological integrity, emotional attunement and relational satisfaction.

In my experimental work, these achievements tend to coalesce around what can best be described as a post-traumatic growth, which is inversely related to the stuckness and stagnancy that are characteristic of cumulative psychosocial stress and trauma, when adaptive defences require the closing down of growth systems, from which life-promoting energy is redirected to protection. In this sustained state of protective defence, growth is compromised or altogether inhibited.

One observation that emerged from my ALEs research is that psychosocial trauma also leaves the survivor with a toxic script that is readily turned to in the face of adversity. This script might be, for instance, a default to emotional numbness and crazy-making behaviour fuelled by the same energy that sustains the trauma from which it derives. Such scripts, however, are responsive to therapy, through which they can be rewritten to promote the survivor as a master of their resources, and that includes their metaphorical spears. The idea is that the more resourced the survivor becomes, the more they are encouraged to take ownership of their problems, to resolve them, and the less likely they are to project or pass them on to their children through biological, neurobiological and psychosocial maladaptations.

This is a feature of growth, where growth-factor hormones secreted from the pituitary gland in the midbrain suffuse the nervous system and in so doing downregulate the chemistry of trauma. This chemistry, of which cortisol is a main constituent, and growth-factor hormone are anticorrelated, so when one is up the other is down. Its dampening requires compassionate support and intelligent guidance as the survivor orients towards integration and post-traumatic growth. This is not to say the survivor is free of trauma and disintegration, but rather, in the aftermath of an ALE, there will be resources and opportunity to recover. With opportunity and resources to recover, resilience and growth will emerge naturally.

In this state of resourcefulness and growth, we can be competent in our families and communities and approach life events with the orientation that no large part of us could be denied or easily become dysregulated and disintegrated. For our heart-mind-soul axis is active and ensuring our feeling hearts and thinking minds are paying attention to our individual and collective vulnerabilities in a way that we can consistently and consciously respond to adversities and prevent trauma from embedding in our nervous system and being passed on to our children and grandchildren. This is where—in earnest—I want to begin to reflect on transgenerational resilience.

TRANSGENERATIONAL RESILIENCE

Our capacity to recover from ALEs that impact our well-being, some of which we inherit from our ancestry and will pass on to posterity, is transgenerational resilience. In her exploration of how we might 'rise strong' (Brown, 2015) and 'brave the wilderness' of life (Brown, 2017), the American research psychologist Brené Brown inspires us to think of this capacity as the rubber band in our survival, for it speaks to the elasticity in our survival instinct that can be tested in much the same way as a stretched rubber band that comes hurling back. In other words, resilience is elasticity in our ability to bounce back from being stretched by ALEs and attendant trauma, whether lived or inherited, and to transcend and transform this experience into a legacy that is significant only in that it is a piece, not the whole, of our life story. Our resilience SPEAR is an important tool with which this transcendence and transformation can be achieved, for it promotes integration and authenticity in a self that is resourced relationally, emotionally, psychologically and somatically, setting us up to survive and adapt to adverse and traumatic life events with the right mindset, behaviour and physiology as individuals, but also as collectives, for we are often survivors of collective traumas that influence how we show up in the world and respond to life events.

For the collective, any common catastrophe can act as a gauge we can use to measure our resilience—as well as to determine the degree and nature of our vulnerabilities. For example, the coronavirus pandemic, the opioid epidemic and the ongoing refugee crises around the world speak to collective traumas that strike at the core of our human vulnerability. They speak not only to our cruelty but also to the chronic and unforgiving pain many of us experience, often vicariously.

The opioid epidemic (NIH, 2021; United Nations Office on Drugs and Crime, 2019), in particular, which is indicative of a great deal of pain as survivors are inclined to self-medicate, is a clear marker of the problem we face as a collective, because its origin can be traced to psychosocial traumas more easily than the coronavirus pandemic or refugee crises, which are relatively peculiar anomalies psychologically. The traumas to which ALEs give rise, nonetheless, however identified, are cumulative in our bodies, minds and shared humanity. Succeeding generations will enter the world bearing adaptations to these traumas, and it will be their task to bind and discharge the dysregulating and disintegrating energies as they undertake to heal themselves and build resilience in their own bodies, minds and collectives.

In part, this will involve correcting of their life stories to reflect their orienting towards preserving life and promoting well-being, and the growth that comes as a reward. But, foremost, this will be a task in self-discovery, in how these generations' ancestral stories combine with their own reality to shape their view of the world and how their senses and stories of how they are and where they belong will show up in the legacy they pass on to their children and grandchildren, whether genetically or psychosocially.

At this level, we might think of the psychosocial as a vector of genetic legacies, as we fall in line with science's contention that our organism transmits hereditary information via two mechanisms, nature (or genetics) and nurture (or epigenetics, which reflects the influence of the environment), which shape neural structures and activities that are expressed in personality. For instance, a personality who experiences social isolation in childhood may have broken neural circuitries or inadequately myelinated connections in the social-emotional brain system that express themselves as social deficits the nervous system compensates for with an increased sensitivity to noise, sounds and light. Neurogenesis and neuroplasticity encourage us to feel confident that survivors can go on to lead a fulfilling life given the right intervention, the kind that stimulates changes in neural structures and chemistry to offset the impact of trauma and promote resilience. This has been evident in the life stories of survivors of collective traumas, which are never uniform in how suffering and healing from trauma unfold. Consider, for instance, survivors of the Holocaust (Fňašková et al., 2019) and the orphaned children of Ceausescu's Romania (Nelson et al., 2014).

Beginning with the obvious fact that these survivors' lived experiences are unique to them, we are then encouraged to honour the collective experience, from which we learn that what is more common is that in adversity and trauma there is almost always a piece, even if only in the incarnation of a lesson, that has utility. The tricky question is mostly whether the utility is worth the suffering, which can be examined in the light of the wisdom it contributes and the benefits it confers to posterity. Specifically, this examination might establish whether, for instance, social engagement and resourcefulness are derived, the capacity to respond to change with flexibility is cultivated or the transformation facilitates individual and collective resilience.

1. Social engagement and resourcefulness point to opportunities for relationships that are formed in social networks to help us to find our way through life, build resilient capacities and succeed as competent personalities. This is where we are when we have a reserve of confidence and determination with which to approach life and to access opportunities for individual and collective well-being.
2. Capacity to embrace change points to support for growth after recovery from trauma, especially in times of disruption when failing to show up as curators in our life story means change is what happens to us, as opposed to experiences we invite and direct in our own life.
3. Transformation facilitates resilience in the collective space when we are in resonance with the resources of our environment. Depending on how we relate to it, transformation can shape our views of each other and the world in a way that points towards collective resilience.

By these competences, we are equipped to bend with the wind of change that we navigate in different survival states, retaining resilience across generations as a necessity, not only for our growth but also for our existence. It is, however, important that ideas of resilience or even traditions of surviving hardship that are inherited across generations do not inadvertently mask maladaptations we need to retire and penalties we need to overcome. That we have done well surviving hardship across generations shouldn't cause us to lose our way on our path to leading a fulfilling life, or even our capacity to imagine what that life might be in the absence of trauma.

This comes together in the scene of the father who gives his young son a hunting spear for his birthday or teaches his young daughter *sōjutsu*, the 'art of the spear' in Japanese martial arts. In an intellectual sense, this is a terrible gift for a child because the child could inflict a self-injury. But where the family history is one in which ancestors were displaced in war camps or yearned to escape slavery in the wilds of the old American South, where a hunting spear or martial art might make the difference between life and death, it is not such a bad gift.

I appreciate this might be frightening to the conservative mind, but when we talk about adaptations, both psychosocial and epigenetic changes in children of trauma survivors, it is really a conversation about a metaphorical survival spear. We are not necessarily concerned with it serving them in a positive way or causing more vulnerability. This is just a nuanced way to make sense of transgenerational resilience, to allow us to have a useful conversation about what this means and to resist thinking about it in a sense of adaptive versus maladaptive, or a gift versus a penalty. To change and lead a fulfilling life after surviving trauma and to pass on some of the change to our children and grandchildren is in itself evidence of remarkable adaptative intelligence and resilience. In this way do we interrupt the intergenerational transmission of psychosocial trauma and trauma-based adaptations and sustain recovery and post-traumatic growth.

Afterword

Neuropsychosocial Integration in Reflection

Throughout my exploration of neuropsychosocial integration, I have discussed a range of ALEs and psychosocial traumas in contemporary life. Some of these ALEs and traumas were inherited, some were experienced in early life, some later in life, and most affected intrapersonal and interpersonal relationships throughout the survivor's life cycle. My focus expanded to include the impact of ALEs in families and other social settings and recognised the emerging and more expansive discoveries in social history that have brought visibility to trauma in larger fields, such as in ancestry, community and society at large. This is important work, but there are two significant takeaways that I am compelled to reflect on and emphasise.

The first is that over 50 percent of the general population will be exposed—either directly or indirectly—to a significant ALE at some point in their lifetime. As such, it is not hard to find people who assume these events are conditions of being human and should simply be gotten over. The research tells us, unambiguously, that not only are these events not natural conditions of being human, they also exact significant costs upon well-being, and although there is great diversity in reactions to ALEs in children, as in adults, and some survivors appear to survive with little trouble, we do not typically overcome these costs without help. It goes against the course of nature to accept this norm, and I call upon us to mandate a better life for ourselves and our children, and thereby the adults they become.

The second takeaway is that psychosocial trauma—whatever its origin—responds to therapeutic intervention that allows survivors do go on to lead lives infused with meaning and purpose. In fact, 75 percent of trauma survivors who attend therapy will recover a degree of normalcy and go on to lead fuller lives. Some 10 to 15 percent stay the same, and 10 to 15 percent are believed to get worse (Bhatia, 2013). This is to say that—with the right intervention—the majority of trauma survivors engage their body and mind to lead lives that are not besieged by unbounded and chaotic energies of stagnancy, stuckness, irrational fear, loss, insecurity and shame that they may have inherited or acquired in their lifetime.

This is a state of transformation in which pains and frustrations from historical suffering are reflected upon in a contemporary context, a context that intersects past and current states, wherein the past cannot be changed but its impact on the future is contextualised and managed. This may not be easy, but it is part of the healing process, and healing can be tricky, because it confronts forces that can be at odds with each other. For instance, it is common to experience fear and excitement alongside apprehension and aversion during transformation. This is because necessary change is desired strongly but not badly. Much like the caterpillar transforming into a butterfly, you must let go of old forms and enter into the unknown in order to emerge anew. It is through this process that survivors of trauma can learn to recognise the transitional space between their old self and the person they will become. This can feel like an undefined, indeterminate and even unsettling reality, but over time the survivor will become comfortable with letting go and accepting the change. When it is successful, however, it must include the healing of the traumatic injury, as well as strategies for resilience and future orientation.

Winniey E. Maduro
Sale, Cheshire, March 14, 2024

References

Adolescent Moral Development Lab. (2018). *Psychology of purpose.* John Templeton Foundation and Claremont Graduate University.

Adolphs, R. (2013). The biology of fear. *Current Biology, 23*(2), R79–R93.

Ainsworth, M. D. (1979). *Patterns of attachment: A psychological study of the strange situation.* Routledge.

Almaas, A. H. (2000). *Diamond heart book two: The freedom to be.* Shambhala.

Alshebib, Y., Hori, T., Goel, A., Al Fauzi, A., & Kashiwagi, T. (2003). Adult human neurogenesis: A view from two schools of thought. *IBRO Neuroscience Reports, 15*, 342–47.

American Psychiatric Association. (2013). *Diagnostic and statistical manual of mental disorders* (5th ed.). American Psychiatric Association.

American Psychological Association. (2018). Intelligence. In *APA dictionary of psychology.* https://dictionary.apa.org/intelligence

Balan, E., Decottignies, A., & Deldicque, L. (2018). Physical activity and nutrition: Two promising strategies for telomere maintenance? *Nutrients, 10*(12), 1942.

Bandura, A. (2006). Towards a psychology of human agency. *Perspectives on Psychological Science, 1*(2), 164–80.

Beckett, L., & Clayton, A. (2022, June 25). 'An unspoken epidemic': Homicide rate increase for black women rivals that of black men. *Guardian.*

Bergman, K., Sarkar, P., Glover, V., & O'Connor, T. G. (2010). Maternal prenatal cortisol and infant cognitive development: Moderation by infant-mother attachment. *Biological Psychiatry, 67*(11), 1026–32. doi:10.1016/j.biopsych.2010.01.002

Bhatia, R. (2013). *What is psychotherapy?* American Psychiatric Association.

Blair, R. J. R. (2007). Empathic dysfunction in psychopathic individuals. In T. F. D. Farrow & P. W. R. Woodruff (eds.), *Empathy in mental illness* (pp. 3–16). Cambridge University Press.

Blake, A. (2019). *Your body is your brain.* Embright.

Bowlby, J. (1982). *Attachment and loss.* Basic Books.

Bowlby, J. (1990). *A secure base: Parent-child attachment and healthy human development.* Basic Books.

Branco, A., Yoshikawa, F., Pietrobon, A. J., & Sato, M. N. (2018). Role of histamine in modulating the immune response and inflammation. *Mediators of Inflammation, 2018,* 9524075.

Bremner, J. D. (2006). Traumatic stress: Effects on the brain. *Dialogues in Clinical Neuroscience, 8*(4), 445–61.

Briguglio, M., Dell'Osso, B., Panzica, G., Malgaroli, A., Banfi, G., Zanaboni Dina, C., Galentino, R., & Porta, M. (2018). Dietary neurotransmitters: A narrative review on current knowledge. *Nutrients, 10*(5), 591.

Brown, B. (2015). *Rising strong.* Vermilion.

Brown, B. (2017). *Braving the wilderness: The quest for true belonging and the courage to stand alone.* Vermilion.

Buss, C., Poggi Davis, E., Shahbaba, B., Pruessner, J. C., Head, K., & Sandman, C. A. (2012). Maternal cortisol over the course of pregnancy and subsequent child amygdala and hippocampus volumes and affective problems. *Proceedings of the National Academy of Sciences of the United States of America, 109*(2), E1312–19.

Charura, D., & Lago, C. (2021). *Black identities and white therapies: Race, respect and diversity.* PCCS Books.

Clarke, A. C. (2000). *Profiles of the future: An inquiry into the limits of the possible.* Phoenix.

Cloudsley-Thompson, J. (1999). Cannibalism among reptiles. *British Herpetological Society Bulletin, 70,* 11–12.

Cohen, M. P. (2020). *Neurofeedback 101: Rewiring the brain for ADHD, anxiety, depression and beyond (without medication).* Center for Brain Training.

Comer, A. L., Jinadasa, T., Sriram, B., Phadke, R. A., Kretsge, L. N., Nguyen, T. P. H., Antognetti, G., Gilbert, J. P., Lee, J., Newmark, E. R., Hausmann, F. S., Rosenthal, S., Kot, K. L., Liu, Y., Yen, W. W., Dejanovic, B., & Cruz-Martín, A. (2020). Increased expression of schizophrenia-associated gene C4 leads to hypoconnectivity of prefrontal cortex and reduced social interaction. *PLOS Biology, 18.* https://doi.org/10.1371/journal.pbio.3000604

Coussons-Read, M. E. (2013). Effects of prenatal stress on pregnancy and human development: Mechanisms and pathways. *Obstetric Medicine Journal, 6,* 52–57.

Curtiss, S. (2014). *Genie: A psycholinguistic study of a modern-day 'wild child'.* Academic Press.

Dalton-Smith, S. (2019). *Sacred rest: Recover your life, renew your energy, restore your sanity.* FaithWords.

Damasio, A. (2002). *Descartes' error: Emotion, reason, and the human brain.* Penguin.

Damasio, A. (2021). *Feeling and knowing: Making minds conscious.* Pantheon.

Dana, D. (2020). *Poly vagal flip chart: Understanding the science of safety.* W. W. Norton.

Dana, D. (2021). *Anchored.* Sound True.

Dapretto, M., Davies, M. S., Pfeifer, J. H., Scott, A. A., Sigman, M., Bookheimer, S. Y., & Iacoboni, M. (2006). Understanding emotions in others: Mirror neuron dysfunction in children with autism spectrum disorders. *Nature Neuroscience, 9,* 28–30.

Darwin, C. (2019). *On the origin of species.* Natural History Museum.

Davidson, R. (2023). *The four pillars of well-being* [Podcast]. Episode No. 074. Mindfulness Exercises.

Davis, R. L., & Zhong, Y. (2017). The biology of forgetting: A perspective. *Neuron, 95,* 490–503.

De Bono, E. (2015). *Lateral thinking: Creativity step by step* (Reissue Ed.). Harper Colophon.

DeGruy, J. (2017). *Post traumatic slave syndrome: America's legacy of enduring injury and healing.* Joy Degruy Publications.

Dempsey, P. (1982). The psychology of enterprise. *Irish Journal of Psychology, 5*(3), 136–46.

Dempster, E. L., Pidsley, R., Schalkwyk, L. C., Owens, S., Georgiades, A., Kane, F., Kalidindi, S., Picchioni, M., Kravariti, E., Toulopoulou, T., Murray, R. M., & Mill, J. (2011). Disease-associated epigenetic changes in monozygotic twins discordant for schizophrenia and bipolar disorder. *Human Molecular Genetics, 20,* 4786–96.

Dickinson, K. A., & Pincus, A. L. (2003). Interpersonal analysis of grandiose and vulnerable narcissism. *Journal of Personality Disorders, 17,* 188–207.

Du Bois, W. E. B. (2016). *The souls of black folk* (Rev. Ed.) Dover.

Duchenne de Boulogne, G.-B. (2008). *The mechanism of human facial expression* (New Ed.). Cambridge University Press.

Duke University Medical Center. (2003, August 1). Common nutrients fed to pregnant mice altered their offspring's coat color. *ScienceDaily.* https://www.science-daily.com/releases/2003/08/030801081754.htm

Echouffo-Tcheugui, J. B., Conner, S. C., Himali, J. J., Maillard, P., DeCarli, C. S., Beiser, A. S., Vasan, R. S., & Seshadri, S. (2018). Circulating cortisol and cognitive and structural brain measures: The Framingham Heart Study. *Neurology, 91*(21), e1961–70.

Eddo-Lodge, R. (2018). *Why I'm no longer talking to white people about race.* Bloomsbury.

Ekman, P. (2003). *Emotions revealed: Understanding faces and feelings.* Times Books.

Erikson, E. H. (1995). *Childhood and society.* Vintage.

Erikson, E. H. (1998). *The life cycle completed* (Extended ed. with chap. by J. M. Erickson). W. W. Norton.

Eriksson, P. S., Perfilieva, E., Björk-Eriksson, T., Alborn, A.-M., Nordborg, C., Peterson, D. A., & Gage, F. H. (1998). Neurogenesis in the adult human hippocampus. *Nature Medicine, 4,* 1313–17.

Farah, M. J., Rabinowitz, C., Quinn, G. E., & Liu, G. T. (2000). Early commitment of neural substrates for face recognition. *Cognitive Neuropsychology, 17*(1), 117–23.

Fee, E. (1979). Nineteenth-century craniology: The study of the female skull. *Bulletin of the History of Medicine, 53,* 415–33.

Feldman, R. (2015). Mutual influences between child emotion regulation and parent-child reciprocity support development across the first 10 years of life: Implications for developmental psychopathology. *Development and Psychopathology, 27*(4), 1007–23.

Felitti, V. J., Anda, R. F., Nordenberg, D., Williamson, D. F., Spitz, A. M., Edwards, V., Koss, M. P., & Marks, J. S. (1998). Relationship of childhood abuse and household dysfunction to many of the leading causes of death in adults: The Adverse Childhood Experiences (ACE) Study. *American Journal of Preventive Medicine, 14*, 245–58.

Fisher, J. (2017). *Healing the fragmented selves of trauma survivors: Overcoming internal self-alienation*. Routledge.

Fňašková, M., Rektor, I., & Říha, P. (2019). Life-long effects of extreme stress on brain structures: A holocaust survivor MRI study. *Journal of Neural Transmission, 126*(11), 1544.

Francis, E. A. (2018). *The body heals itself: How deeper awareness of your muscles and their emotional connection can help you heal*. Llewellyn.

Frankl, V. E. (2008). *Man's search for meaning: The classic tribute to hope from the Holocaust*. Rider.

Freud, S. (1997). *The interpretation of dreams*. Wordsworth Editions.

Freud, S. (2003). *Beyond the pleasure principle*. Penguin Classic.

Fryers, T., & Brugha, T. (2013). Childhood determinants of adult psychiatric disorder. *Clinical Practice and Epidemiology in Mental Health, 9*, 1–50.

Gilbert, P., N, V., & Coyte, M. E. (2007). *Spirituality, values and mental health: Jewels for the journey*. Jessica Kingsley.

Goleman, D. (1996). *Emotional intelligence*. Bloomsbury.

Goleman, D. (2003). *Healing emotions: Conversations with the Dalai Lama on mindfulness*. Shambhala.

Goleman, D. (2007). *Social intelligence: The new science of human relationships*. Arrow.

Graham, L. (2018). *Bouncing back: Rewiring your brain for maximum resilience and well-being*. New World Library.

Greenspan, S. I., & Wieder, S. (2008). *Engaging autism*. Perseus Books.

Gu, X., Gao, Z., Wang, X., Liu, X. Knight, R. T., Hof, P. R., & Fan, J. (2012). Anterior insular cortex is necessary for empathetic pain perception. *Brain, 135*(9), 2726–35.

Guidi, J., Lucente, M., Sonino, N., & Fave, G. A. (2021). Allostatic load and its impact on health: A systematic review. *Psychotherapy and Psychosomatics, 90*, 11–27.

Hahn, Christopher N, Chong, C.-E., Carmichael, C. L., Wilkins, E. J., Brautigan, P. J., Li, X.-C., Babic, M., Lin, M., Carmagnac, A., Lee, Y. K., Kok, C. H., Gagliardi, L., Friend, K. L., Ekert, P. G., Butcher, C. M., Brown, A. L., Lewis. I. D., To. L. B., Timms, A. E., . . . Scott, H. S. (2011). Heritable GATA2 mutations associated with familial myelodysplastic syndrome and acute myeloid leukemia. *Nature Genetics, 43*, 1012–17.

Halassa, M. M. (2022). *The thalamus*. Cambridge University Press.

Hanson, R. (2018). *Resilient: 12 tools for transforming everyday experiences into lasting happiness*. Rider.

Hashikawa, Y., Hashikawa, K., Falkner, A. L., & Lin, D. (2017). Ventromedial hypothalamus and the generation of aggression. *Frontiers in Systems Neuroscience, 11*, 94.

Hebb, D. O. (1949). *The organization of behavior: A neuropsychological theory.* Psychology Press.

Heijmans, B. T., Tobi, E. W., Stein, A. D., Putter, H., Blauw, G. J., Susser, E. S., Slagboom, P. E., & Lumey, L. H. (2008). Persistent epigenetic differences associated with prenatal exposure to famine in humans. *Proceedings of the National Academy of Sciences of the United States of America, 105*(44), 17046–49.

Heine, S. J. (2017). *DNA is not destiny: The remarkable, completely misunderstood relationship between you and your genes.* W. W. Norton.

Hilker, R., Helenius, D., Fagerlund, B., Skytthe, A., Christensen, K., Werge, T. M., Nordentoft, M., & Glenthøj, B. (2018). Heritability of schizophrenia and schizophrenia spectrum based on the nationwide Danish twin register. *Biological Psychiatry, 86,* 492–98.

Holmes, J. (2020). *The brain has a mind of its own: Attachment, neurobiology, and the new science of psychotherapy.* Confer Books.

Hübl, T. (2020). *Healing collective trauma: A process for integrating our intergenerational and cultural wounds.* Sounds True.

Inaba, D., & Cohen, W. (2007). *Uppers, downers, all arounders: Physical and mental effects of psychoactive drugs.* CNS Productions.

Jablonka, E., & Lamb, M. J. (1995). *Epigenetic inheritance and evolution: The Lamarckian dimension.* Oxford University Press.

Jung, C. (2016). *Psychological types.* Routledge.

Jung, C. G. (1992). *Structure and dynamics of the psyche.* In *Collected Works of C. G. Jung* (Vol. 8; G. Adler, Trans.). Princeton University Press.

Kendi, I. X. (2017). *Stamped from the beginning: The definitive history of racist ideas in America.* Nation Books.

Kernis, M. H. (2009). Toward a conceptualization of optimal self-esteem. *Psychological Inquiry, 14,* 283–357.

Klabunde, M., Weems, C. F., Raman, M., & Carrion, V. G. (2017). The moderating effects of sex on insula subdivision structure in youth with posttraumatic stress symptoms. *Depression and Anxiety, 34*(1), 51–58.

Kouda, K., & Iki, M. (2010). Beneficial effects of mild stress (hormetic effects): Dietary restriction and health. *Journal of Physiological Anthropology, 29,* 127–32.

Kronman, H., Torres-Berrío, A., Sidoli, S., Issler, O., Godino, A., Ramakrishnan, A., Mews, P., Lardner, C. K., Parise, E. M., Walker, D. M., van der Zee, Y. Y., Browne, C. J., Boyce, B. F., Neve, R., Garcia, B. A., Shen, L., Peña, C. J., & Nestler, E. J. (2021). Long-term behavioral and cell-type-specific molecular effects of early life stress are mediated by H3K79me2 dynamics in medium spiny neurons. *Nature Neuroscience, 24*(5), 667–76.

Lane, H. (1977). *The wild boy of Aveyron.* Allen & Unwin.

LeDoux, J. E. (1999). *The emotional brain: The mysterious underpinnings of emotional life.* Weidenfeld & Nicolson.

LeDoux, J. E. (2019). *The deep history of ourselves: The four-billion-year story of how we got conscious brains.* Penguin.

Levine, P. (1997). *Waking the tiger: Healing trauma—the innate capacity to transform overwhelming experiences.* North Atlantic Books.

Lieberwirth, C., & Wang, Z. (2012). The social environment and neurogenesis in the adult mammalian brain. *Frontiers in Human Neuroscience, 6,* 118.

Lipton, B. H. (2015). *The biology of belief.* Hay House.

Maduro, W. E. (2018). *Caribbean achievement in Britain: Psychosocial resources and lived experiences.* Palgrave Macmillan.

Maslow, A. H. (2011). *Hierarchy of needs: A theory of human motivation.* www.all-about-psychology.com.

Maté, G., with Maté, D. (2023). *The myth of normal: Trauma, illness and healing in a toxic culture.* Vermilion.

McEwen, B. S. (2000). Allostasis and allostatic load: Implications for neuropsychopharmacology. *Neuropsychopharmacology, 2*(2), 108–24.

McWilliams, N. (2011). *Psychoanalytic diagnosis: Understanding personality structure in the clinical process* (2nd Ed.). Guilford Press.

Miller, A. (2008). *The drama of being a child: The search for the true self.* Virago.

Muramatsu, Y., Muramatsu, K., Mashima, I., & Gejyo, F. (2003). Bronchial asthma: Psychosomatic aspect. *Journal of the Japan Medical Association, 126*(6), 375–77.

National Institutes of Health. (2023). NR3C1 nuclear receptor subfamily 3 group C member 1 [Homo sapiens (human)]. National Library of Medicine. https://www.ncbi.nlm.nih.gov/gene/2908

Nelson, C. A., Fox, N. A., & Zeanah, C. H. (2014). *Romania's abandoned children: Deprivation, brain development, and the struggle for recovery.* Harvard University Press.

Newlove-Delgado, T., Russell, A. E., Mathews, F., Cross, L., Bryant, E., Gudka, R., Ukoumunne, O. C., & Ford, T. J. (2021). The impact of COVID-19 on psychopathology in children and young people worldwide: Systematic review of studies with pre- and within-pandemic data. *Journal of Child Psychology and Psychiatry, 64*(4), 611–40.

NIH. (2021). *Drug overdose death rates.* National Center for Health Statistics.

Nisar, S., Bhat, A. A., Masoodi, T., Hashem, S., Akhtar, S., Ali, T. A., Amjad, S., Chawla, S., Bagga, P., Frenneaux, M. P., Reddy, R., Fakhro, K., & Haris, M. (2022). Genetics of glutamate and its receptors in autism spectrum disorder. *Molecular Psychiatry, 27,* 2380–92.

Norretranders, T. (1999). *The user illusion: Cutting consciousness down to size.* Penguin.

Nowak, M., & Highfield, R. (2012). *Supercooperators: Altruism, evolution, and why we need each other to succeed.* Free Press.

Ornish, D. (2019). *Undo it! How simple lifestyle changes can reverse most chronic diseases.* Pisces Books.

Perkins, D. (1996). *Outsmarting IQ: The emerging science of learnable intelligence.* Free Press.

Perry, C., & Lee, R. (2020). Childhood trauma and personality disorder. In G. Spallett, D. Janiri, F. Piras & G. Sani (Eds.), *Childhood trauma in mental disorders* (pp. 231–55). Springer.

Peterson, C. (2000). The future of optimism. *American Psychologist, 55,* 44–55.

Piers, G., & Singer, M. (2015). *Shame and guilt: A psychoanalytic and a cultural study.* Martino Fine Books.

Pinto, R., Ashworth, M., & Jones, R. (2008). Schizophrenia in black Caribbeans living in the UK: An exploration of underlying causes of the high incidence rate. *British Journal of General Practice, 58*, 429–34.

Plutchik, R. (1991). *The emotions* (Rev. Ed.). University Press of America.

Porges, S. W. (2020). *The polyvagal theory: Neurophysiological foundations of emotions, attachment, communication, and self-regulation.* Tantor Audio.

Prescott, J. W. (1975). Body pleasure and the origins of violence. *Bulletin of the Atomic Scientists, 31*(9), 10–20.

Rogers, C. (1977). *On becoming a person.* Robinson.

Rogers, C. R. (1995). *A way of being.* Houghton Mifflin.

Rosenberg, M. B. (2015). *Nonviolent communication: A language of life.* Puddle Dancer Press.

Rosenberg, S. (2017). *Accessing the healing power of the vagus nerve: Self-help exercises for anxiety, depression, trauma, and autism.* North Atlantic Books.

Rothschild, B. (2000). *The body remembers: The psychophysiology of trauma and trauma treatment.* W. W. Norton.

Rothschild, B. (2017). *Autonomic nervous system table.* W. W. Norton.

Russell-Brown, P. A., Norville, B., & Griffith, C. (1996). Child shifting: A survival strategy for teenage mothers. In J. L. Roopnarine & J. Brown (Eds.), *Caribbean families: Diversity among ethnic groups* (pp. 224–43). Greenwood.

Salzberg, S., & Kabat-Zinn, J. (2020). Mindfulness as medicine. In D Goleman (Ed.), *Healing emotions* (pp. 107–44). Rupa & Co.

Sapolsky, R. (2004). *Why zebras don't get ulcers: The acclaimed guide to stress, stress-related diseases.* St. Martins Press.

Schore, A. (2015). *Affect regulation and the origin of the self.* Routledge.

Schore, A. N. (2019). *Right brain psychotherapy.* W. W. Norton.

Selye, H. (1974). *Stress without Distress.* Lippincott Williams & Wilkins.

Selye, H. 1978. *The stress of life.* McGraw-Hill.

Shapiro, F. (2017). *Eye movement desensitization and reprocessing (EMDR) therapy* (3rd Ed.). Guilford Press.

Shiba, K., Kubzansky, L. D., Williams, D. R., VanderWeele, T. J., & Kim, E. S. (2021). Associations between purpose in life and mortality by SES. *American Journal of Preventive Medicine, 61*(2), e53–e61.

Shriyan, P., Sudhir, P., van Schayck, O. C. P., & Babu, G. R. (2023). Association of high cortisol levels in pregnancy and altered fetal growth: Results from the MAAS-THI, a prospective cohort study, Bengaluru. *Lancet Regional Health, 14*, 100196.

Siegel, D. J. (2010). *Mindsight: The new science of personal transformation.* Bantam Dell.

Siegel, D. J. (2020). *The developing mind: How relationships and the brain interact to shape who we are* (3rd Ed.). Guilford Press.

Siegel, D. J. (2022). *IntraConnected: MWe (me + we) as the integration of belonging and identity.* W. W. Norton.

Singer, M. (2007). *The untethered soul: The journey beyond yourself.* New Harbinger.

Singh, T., Neale, B. M., & Daly, M. J. (2022). Rare coding variants in ten genes confer substantial risk for schizophrenia. *Nature, 604*, 509–16.

Singletary, W. M. (2015). An integrative model of autism spectrum disorder: ASD as a neurobiological disorder of experienced environmental deprivation, early life stress and allostatic overload. *Neuropsychoanalysis, 17*, 81–119.

Slavery Abolition Act. (1833). https://www.pdavis.nl/Legis_07.htm

Spearman, C. E. (2005). *The abilities of man.* Blackburn Press.

Steele, C. M. (2011). *Whistling Vivaldi: How stereotypes affect us and what we can do.* W. W. Norton.

Stein, M. M. (2021). *Representation of Jews in the media: An analysis of Old Hollywood stereotypes perpetuated in modern television* [Thesis, Florida State University].

Sternberg, R. J. (2021). *Adaptive intelligence: Surviving and thriving in times of uncertainty.* Cambridge University Press.

Stoneking, C. R. (1993). Mitochondrial DNA and human evolution. *Journal of Bioenergetics and Biomembranes, 26*, 251–59.

Sturge, J., & Harvey, T. (2007). *The West Indies in 1837.* Cosimo Classics.

TerKeurst, L. (2020). *Forgiving what you can't forget.* Thomas Nelson.

Thomas, L. (2008). Psychotherapy in the context of race and culture: An inter-cultural therapeutic approach. In S. Fernando (Ed.), *Mental Health in a multi-ethnic society: A multidisciplinary handbook* (pp. 172–89). Routledge.

United Nations Office on Drugs and Crime. (2019). *World drug report.* Report E.19. XI.8.

Vajda, P. (2013). *Becoming a better you.* Infinity.

van der Kolk, B. (2015). *The body keeps the score: Brain, mind, and body in the healing of trauma.* Penguin.

Van Susteren, L., & Colino, S. (2020). *Emotional inflammation: Discover your triggers and reclaim your equilibrium during anxious times.* Sounds True.

Verny, T., & Kelly, J. (1982). *The secret life of the unborn child: A remarkable and controversial look at life before birth.* Sphere.

von Linné, Carl. (2018). *Systema naturae.* Forgotten Books.

Vygotsky, L. S. (1978). *Mind in society: Development of higher psychological processes.* Harvard University Press.

Walker, M. (2017). *Why we sleep: The new science of sleep and dreams.* Penguin.

Walker, P. (2013). *Complex PTSD: From surviving to thriving.* CreateSpace.

Waterland, R. A., & Jirtle, R. L. (2003). Transposable elements: Targets for early nutritional effects on epigenetic gene regulation. *Molecular and Cellular Biology, 15*, 5292–5300.

Watson, J., & Crick, F. (1953). A structure for deoxyribose nucleic acid. *Nature, 171*, 737–38.

Watts, T. (2000). *Warriors, settlers and nomads: Discovering who we are and what we can be.* Bell & Bain.

Wierenga, Lara M., Langen, M., Oranje, B., & Durston, S. (2014). Unique developmental trajectories of cortical thickness and surface area. *Neuroimage, 87*, 120–26.

Wilson, T. D. (2002). *Strangers to ourselves: Discovering the adaptive unconscious.* Harvard University Press.

Wink, P. (1991). Two faces of narcissism. *Journal of Personality and Social Psychology, 61*, 590–97.

Winnicott, D. W. (1984). *Ego distortion in terms of true and false self: The matura-tional processes and the facilitating environment.* Routledge.

Wolynn, M. (2013). *It didn't start with you: How inherited family trauma shapes who we are and how to end the cycle.* Viking.

World Health Organization. (2022). *International classification of diseases* (11th ed.). World Health Organization. https://www.who.int/standards/classifications/classification-of-diseases

Zheng, X., Zheng, P., & Zou, X. (2018). Association between schizophrenia and autism spectrum disorder: A systematic review and meta-analysis. *Meta-analysis, 11*(8), 1110–19.

Zuroff, D. C., & Blatt, S. J. (2006). The therapeutic relationship in the brief treat-ment of depression: Contributions to clinical improvement and enhanced adaptive capacities. *Journal of Consulting and Clinical Psychology, 74*(1), 199–206.

Subject Index

abandonment. *See* self, abandonment
absentmindedness, 71, 131, 146
abundance, 46, 78, 172, 179
abuse. *See* sexual, abuse
acceptance: radical, 120, 140, 152;
    self, 28, 192; social, 63, 104;
    unconditional, 150
accumbens. *See* nucleus, accumbens
ACE, 8, 173
acetylcholine, 130–31, 187, 220
acetyl-group tags, 80
actualisation. *See* self, actualisation
acute myeloid leukaemia (AML). *See*
    AML
acute stress, 47, 100
adrenal cortices, 95
adrenaline, 50, 86–87, 96, 99, 103, 134,
    141, 206
adverse childhood experiences (ACE).
    See ACE
adverse life/lived experiences (ALE).
    See ALE
agency, 19–21, 29, 53–54, 67–69, 92,
    111, 116, 128, 152, 177, 199, 203–5,
    208, 212, 227
aggression, 27, 29, 31, 101, 106, 193
agouti, 82–83
Akan. *See* Ashanti tribe
alcoholism, 105, 110, 115, 230

ALE, 7–8, 10, 13, 17, 19, 35, 60, 72, 76,
    82, 84, 97, 103, 173, 191, 232, 237
alienation, 47, 68, 92, 112, 170, 202
allergies, 86, 211, 209
allostasis, 32, 47
allostatic: burden, 47, 86; overload, 87,
    146
aloneness, 5, 18, 44, 68, 104, 115, 139,
    202
altruism, 23, 35, 41, 56, 69, 175, 179–82
Alzheimer's, 49, 198, 214
AML, 82
amnic fluid, 94–95
amygdala, 34, 95, 99, 145, 177, 185,
    228
analgesia, 50
ancestral: connection, 180; heritage, 81,
    84, 206; legacies, 17, 68, 72, 77–78,
    81, 93–94, 116, 136, 140, 195;
    stories, 77, 121, 123, 238; trauma,
    68, 122; wisdom, 12, 117, 121, 163.
    See also memories, ancestral
anchorage, 61, 118, 155, 211, 217, 227
anosognosia, 62
anterior circular sulcus, 145
anti-body, 86, 210
anti-inflammatory, 46, 212, 220
antipathy, 206
antipsychotic, 170, 231

antisocial: behaviour, 194; personalities, 155, 194
anxiety: chronic, 116–17, 122, 147; relational, 160, 174, 177, 228; social, 160, 207
apathy, 70–71, 102, 117, 120, 131, 160, 172
apoptosis, 51
ashamed. *See* shame
Ashanti tribe, 3
aspiration, 22, 25, 64, 139, 183, 232
asthma, 86–87, 92, 110, 117–19, 122, 138, 147, 209
autism, 86–88, 119, 128, 138
autoimmune diseases, 92, 147
autoimmunity, 36, 49, 86–87, 89, 133, 155, 211
autosomes, 79, 81
axons, 34, 45, 194

basal: forebrain, 221; ganglia, 157
baseline stress, 47, 214
battery, 36, 47, 92–93, 100, 103, 115, 173, 196
belief, 7, 19, 75, 93, 128, 137, 139, 154, 174, 182, 201
belonging: sense of, 91, 109, 205
bias, 87, 193, 206
bidirectional: flow between psyche and society, 44; flow of information, 61, 144; relationships, 231
biofeedback, 11, 207
biological: heritage 76–78, 81; imperative, 35, 43, 220; legacies, 91; vulnerabilities, 134; wisdom, 55
black: communities, 173; people, 104, 195, 204
blood: blood-brain barrier, 133, 219; cells, 82, 215; flow, 12, 32, 81, 119, 172, 218; glucose, 48; pressure, 11–12, 131, 219
bloodstream, 33, 46, 48, 95, 97, 111, 133
bodily: demand, 47; disturbance, 60; functions, 32, 46, 99, 118, 131, 165;

rhythm, 4, 118, 191, 218; sensations, 143, 208–10; systems, 209, 212; tissues, 62, 98, 156, 211, 216. *See also* defences
body-mind-social, 61, 149–50
boundaries, 13, 28–29, 161, 163, 176, 190, 201, 218, 233
bowels, 5–6, 146, 216
brain: areas, 98, 119, 165, 177, 207; derived neurotrophic factor, 212, 214, 219; power, 133, 163; stem, 10, 32, 34, 50, 58, 61–62, 130–31, 141–43, 170, 219, 227; systems, 29, 137, 145–46, 226, 238
breath, 12, 46, 143, 176–77, 207, 216
burden: of the past, 165; relational, 178. *See also* allostatic, burden

C4A. *See* gene, complement component
calcium, 32, 214
calm, 105, 118, 177, 220–21
cancer, 83, 93, 146, 209, 221, 229
cardiopathy, 8, 83–84, 172
catecholamines, 170
cerebral: cognitive, 12, 41, 52, 56, 70, 150, 153, 157; conscious, 71; structures, 49, 53. *See also* cortex, cerebral
cerebrum, 95, 142, 226
charge-and-discharge cycle, 6, 40
chromosome, 79–82, 88, 182, 193–94
cleft. *See* synaptic, cleft
CNV. *See* cranial nerve, trigeminal
CNXI. *See* cranial nerve, accessory
cognitive: brain, 144, 186, 226; circuit, 146, 198; disconnect, 216; disengagement, 137; dissonance, 139; empathy, 157; exercise, 153; impairment, 49, 144–45, 197, 214, 216; incompetency, 198–99; 208
collective resilience. *See* resilience
compassion: bid for, 114; capacity for, 154; cultivate, 99; exercise of, 136, 157, 172, 190, 193; intrapersonal, 29;

receive, 169; recover, 234; virtue of, 35. *See also* self, compassion

complex: malady, 78; neurochemistry, 51; problems, 57, 137, 163, 214, 226; relationships, 8. *See also* language

compulsion, 36, 118, 155, 206, 213

conception, 3, 27, 101, 170

confidence, 9, 55, 138–39, 173, 178, 213, 239

confusion, 5, 22, 55, 105, 112–13, 139, 155, 160, 175, 178, 200

consciousness, 11–12, 34, 57–58, 60, 64, 68, 70–72, 104–5, 129, 131, 138, 150, 161, 165, 176, 200–201, 210, 215, 219

contempt, 36, 63, 177

co-regulate, 7, 29, 117, 128, 153–54, 169, 171, 215

coronavirus. *See* COVID-19

cortex: cerebral, 33, 34, 57, 141–42, 145, 165, 177, 191; dorsolateral prefrontal, 157; orbitofrontal, 226; prefrontal, 60, 78, 88, 105, 137, 157, 186, 194, 227

corticosteroids, 62, 86–87, 94, 120, 214, 218, 228

cortisol, 46–50, 85–87, 95–97, 99, 103, 134, 170, 215, 217, 236

counterintuitive, 9, 50, 136

counterwill, 204

courage, 27, 72, 119, 139, 178

COVID-19, 11, 18–19, 45, 51, 146, 179, 227, 237–38

cranial nerve: accessory 143, 214; glossopharyngeal, 143, 192; optic, 142, 214; trigeminal 42, 192, 214; vagus, 130, 133, 141, 143, 153, 192, 217, 219, 222, 227

crazy-making, 154, 236

culture, 3–4, 30, 68, 81, 104–6, 121, 128, 133, 136, 174, 193, 227

curiosity: approach life with, 100; curtail, 7; lack of, 131; in the newborn, 185; about possibilities, 218; to problem-solve, 116;

surrounding how environmental influence, 83; surrounding trauma, 9; towards future, 150

cutting, 22, 64, 104, 146

cytokines, 132–33

danger: cues of, 36; disposition to underestimate, 145; engaging with 214; escapes from, 133; ever-present, 232; exaggerate 146; experience of, 59; imminent, 50, 56, 103, 143; reactions to 65; real, 40, 100; response to, 34; sensations of, 69, 112, 188

death. *See* premature, death

declarative memory, 60, 161, 197, 207, 213

defences: adaptive, 21, 29, 34, 57–58, 60, 62, 66–67, 96, 98–100, 106–7, 109, 117, 122, 134, 136, 194, 217; protective, 94, 210, 226, 233, 236. *See also* maladaptive, defences

dehumanisation, 36, 68, 93, 103, 115, 120–21, 180

delusions, 150, 228

dendrites, 32–33, 45

deoxyribonucleic acid (DNA). *See* DNA

depression, 8, 46, 49, 65, 105, 110, 155, 157, 194, 213, 228–29

deprivation, 64, 69, 71, 82, 87, 97, 102, 140, 160, 194

diabetes, 8, 34, 48–49, 83–84, 92, 110, 116, 209

diagnostic and statistical manual (DSM). *See* DSM

diet, 34, 80–81, 83–84, 211–12, 218

digest/digestion, 96, 99, 130, 212

discipline, 29, 68, 111

disempathy, 187, 194

dissociation, 66–67, 70, 160, 166, 210, 227

dissonance, 3, 22, 139, 175

distress, 37, 47, 53, 57, 67–69, 71, 85–86, 95, 97, 100, 104–5, 112–14, 117, 183, 203, 206, 222, 232

diversity, 51, 84, 87, 102, 116, 122, 130

divinity, 119, 138, 182
DNA, 77, 78–80, 84, 180–181, 185, 193
dopamine, 42, 45–46, 51, 69, 103, 118, 131, 133, 170–71, 187, 193, 214, 218, 227
dopaminergic pleasure-reward, 157, 190, 226
dragon 29, 31, 35, 94–95, 206, 232
DSM, 43, 155
dynorphins, 50, 103
dysautonomia, 48–49, 66, 100, 147, 174, 177, 200
dysempathy, 135

early: adulthood, 5, 78, 88; childhood, 5–7, 82, 88, 111, 121, 226
early life: demands, 206; neuropsychosocial disintegration in, 21; neuroscience of, 69; relationships, 37, 170; social and cultural in, 8; traumatic stress in, 27, 112, 161, 220–21
education, 65, 92, 111, 114, 116, 173, 181, 186
electroencephalography (EEG), 32, 207
embryo, 80, 82–83, 94
EMDR. *See* eyes, in somatic therapy
emotional: attachment, 28; attunement, 22, 25–26, 41, 51–52, 54, 56, 61, 88, 118, 182, 187, 191, 236; brain, 45, 145, 228; challenges, 173; chaos, 188; competence, 193–94; confusion, 160; connection/disconnection, 112; demands, 187, 190–91; dis-ease, 114, 186, 193; dysregulation, 154, 186; elasticity, 189; empathy, 88, 135; inflammation, 155, 187; intelligence, 54, 187; neglect, 121; numbness, 236; pain, 42, 212–13; reaction, 11, 177; regulation, 57, 162, 194; safety, 185–87; sensation, 45, 162, 190; therapy, 164, 186, 189; well-being, 186–87, 190, 192. *See also* memories
empathy: capacity for, 154, 190; circuitries, 191; expression of, 29,

69, 96, 145, 150, 178, 185–87, 193, 206, 215, 221, 231; integrous135–36. *See also* cognitive; emotional
empower, 121, 157, 179, 189, 230, 236
endocrine: disease, 229; system, 48, 86, 209. *See also* gland
enkephalin, 50, 103
enslaved, 37, 47, 114, 120–21, 134–35, 195
enterprise, 21, 52, 65, 101, 105, 199, 203
environment: external, 12, 50, 83; social, 22, 56, 70, 87, 127–28, 130, 138–39, 143, 186, 194, 203; uterine, 120, 170
environmental: adversity, 87; changes, 55; demands, 80, 84, 186; disasters, 47, 60, 127; influence, 79, 83, 186; stress, 47, 82
envy, 42–43, 64
epidemic. *See* opioid, epidemic
epigenetic: inheritance, 79, 81; modification, 220; profile, 87; regulations, 80–84, 119, 194, 210
equanimity, 175, 177–79, 182, 200
equipotentiality, 164
esoteric, 136, 141, 150, 154
esteem. *See* self, esteem
evolutionary: adaptation, 94–95; biology, 35, 75, 79
expectation, 22, 64, 112–13, 115, 170, 200
exteroceptions, 141, 143
eyes: innervation of the, 142, 96, 214; minds', 135, 175; oculi muscles encircling the, 192, 220, 222; rapid eye movement (REM), 219, 221; in somatic therapy, 221

faint, 104, 134, 152
faith, 56, 63, 85, 114, 178, 205
family: history, 93, 140, 143, 178, 239; life, 56, 65–66, 68–69, 93, 102, 110, 116, 121, 227
famine, 80, 133, 220

fasting, 47, 219–20
father: fatherlessness, 17, 11; relationship with, 19, 98, 114, 181–82, 239
fatigue, 49, 67, 131, 135, 155, 166, 176, 209, 229
fawn, 36, 103, 152
feedback, 3, 71, 103, 208; negative, 133, 162; responsiveness to, 104, 139. *See also* neurofeedback
filicide, 43
fires, 29, 34, 99, 121, 140, 149, 210
flight, 50, 95, 97–98, 100, 107, 154, 131, 233
float, 99–101, 104, 107, 116, 154, 202
flourish, 61, 161, 182
FMR1. See gene, fragile mental retardation
fMRI. *See* neuroimaging
foetus, 81, 128, 197
fold, 34–35, 80, 99, 102–4, 107, 139, 152, 154, 228
forebrain. *See* basal, forebrain
foresight, 55, 171, 232
forget, 85, 197–98, 206, 209, 234
forgiveness, 153, 176, 234, 236
freedom, 119, 121, 178, 192, 204, 225, 227, 234
freeze, 50, 103, 134, 137
friendship, 52, 56, 187, 201, 214
furrow, 19, 99, 104–7, 116, 147, 151–52, 154
future generations, 19, 55, 67, 75–76, 81, 128, 149, 152

gamma-amino-butyric acid (GABA), 46, 50, 146, 218
gene: CEBPA, 82; Complement component, 79; fragile mental retardation (FMR), 88; glutamate ionotropic receptor (GRIA), 78–79; monoamine oxidase (MAO), 193; nuclear receptor (NR), 194; synaptic scaffolding (SHANK), 88
genome, 77, 79, 84, 88

gestation, 53, 94, 97, 170
gland: adrenal, 46, 87, 95; pancreatic, 48; pituitary, 95, 131, 236
glossopharyngeal. *See* cranial nerve
glucocorticoid, 47, 194
glutamate, 46, 78, 87–88, 94
gratitude, 41–42, 46, 128, 152–53, 189, 197, 232–33, 236
GRIA3. *See* gene, glutamate ionotropic receptor
grief, 63–66, 92, 97, 110, 112, 121, 128, 152, 155, 176, 191, 206
GRIN2A. *See* gene, glutamate ionotropic receptor
guilt, 5, 20, 27, 52, 63–66, 92, 112, 128, 152, 155, 176, 189, 194, 206
gut feeling, 144–45, 216. *See also* instincts

happiness, 11, 42, 46, 227
hardship, 114, 138, 232, 239
harmony, 42, 52–54, 88, 118
healthcare, 82, 99, 121, 156, 231
heart: gut-soul axis, 137, 191, 237; rate, 6, 11–12, 32, 97, 131, 141, 190, 207
helplessness, 19, 67, 116, 131, 155, 173, 204, 213, 220, 230
heritage. *See* ancestral, heritage; biological, heritage
hippocampus, 34, 49, 197, 228
histamine, 86, 209, 216
histone, 77, 80
holocaust, 202, 238
homelessness, 72, 94, 98, 144–45, 211, 215
homeostasis, 6, 12, 56, 146, 218, 230
hope, 5, 18, 23, 29, 102, 114, 205, 221, 230, 235
hopefulness, 42, 46, 128, 139, 157, 205
hopelessness, 19, 43, 49, 112, 116, 139, 155, 172–73, 195, 230
hermetic, 47, 163, 214
hormones, 46, 50, 80, 86, 94–95, 98, 120, 170–72, 218, 236

hunger, 4, 6, 44, 46, 68, 80, 97, 141,
    145–46, 154, 171, 203, 216, 226
hustle, 105, 203
hypercortisolaemia, 47, 209
hyperglycaemia, 48
hyperinsulinemia, 48
hyper-mobilisation, 155, 213
hypertension, 8, 49, 92, 110, 116, 143,
    207, 215–16, 229
hypervigilance, 36, 131, 155
hypothalamic-pituitary-adrenal axis
    (HPAA), 62, 173
hypothalamus, 29, 34, 46, 83, 95, 131,
    145, 228

ideation. *See* morbid ideation
imagination, 61, 105, 116, 144, 152,
    157, 199, 214, 227, 231–32
immune: cells, 133, 156, 219; response,
    133, 156; system, 36, 79, 82, 86,
    131–32, 156, 182, 211–12, 219. *See
    also* defences
imprinting, 81–82
impulse, 177, 193, 228
inauthenticity, 14, 21, 37, 39, 67, 102,
    104, 112, 149
incompetency, 36, 66, 143, 155, 199
incongruity, 71, 135, 139
infancy/infant, 3, 5–6, 43, 51, 66, 117,
    165, 170 185
inflammation: chronic, 86, 133, 147,
    155, 211; of the meninges, 33; in the
    psyche, 135, 139; regulate, 99, 131
inflammatory: molecules, 49; response,
    65, 194
injuries. *See* brain injuries; social-
    emotional, injuries; somatic, somatic
    injuries; relational, injuries
insecurities: material, 92; income, 17; in
    our body, 229; social, 68; vulnerable
    to, 139. *See also* emotional,
    insecurity; relational, insecurity
instinctive: brain, 45, 50, 62, 144,
    157, 186, 217; self, 41, 43, 180;
    unconscious, 57, 66, 71

instincts: brute/crude, 52, 56, 206;
    death, 41, 45; gut, 135, 216;
    mammalian, 104, 186; reptilian, 103;
    survival, 32, 36, 49, 61, 106, 128,
    214, 237
institutionalisation, 101
insula, 34, 135–36, 145–47, 186, 221,
    228
insulin, 48, 131, 209
integrity: psychosocial, 138–39;
    somatic, 54, 220. *See also*
    psychological, integrity
intelligence: adaptative, 240; native,
    49, 52, 56, 58–59, 65–66, 92, 178;
    psychological, 54, 199; social, 52,
    118, 199; somatic, 49, 53–54, 97,
    216. *See also* spears, intelligence
    spears
interneurons, 45, 79
interoception, 54, 141
interpersonal: compassion, 29; conflict,
    178; neurobiology, 36, 135;
    relationships, 23, 29, 56, 104, 154,
    176, 183, 193
intimacy: betray, 120; experience, 18,
    42, 173; need for, 52, 170; orients to
    180. *See also* relational, intimacy
intrapersonal, 23, 29, 151, 176
intuition, 55, 61, 216, 233
isolation: forced isolation, 231; self-
    medicating and, 18, 105, 98, 230;
    social, 56, 60, 133, 155, 198, 238

jealousy, 42–43
journaling, 232–33

kidneys, 46, 60, 87, 95–96, 133, 141
kindness, 41–42, 46, 67, 69, 103, 136,
    150, 172, 179, 192–93, 201–2, 206,
    231, 234, 236

language, 12, 60, 88, 104, 198, 213,
    216, 227
legacy. *See* ancestral, legacies;
    biological, legacies; psychosocial,

legacies; psychosocial trauma, as legacy

life: affirming, 72, 137, 151, 187, 212; challenges, 30, 93, 217; experiences, 7, 9, 56, 93, 156, 179; promoting, 82, 236; lifestyle, 13, 80, 228; threatening, 8, 170; time, 19, 75, 115, 122, 174

life stories: alter, 214, 216, 231, 235; beginning of, 77–78; connecting, 57–58; correcting, 72, 238; curation of, 232, 239; hows and whys of, 75, 55, 140; maladies in, 83–84, 98; self as a host of, 40, 43, 152; therapeutic reworking of, 920, 37, 157 220

limbic, 29, 34, 57, 94, 118, 135, 145, 170, 217, 221

loneliness, 143, 155, 213

loss: fear of, 42; lasting, 64; of authenticity, 163; of significant relationships 8, 110, 115, 172, 173; recovery from, 21, 204; ungrieved loss, 62, 152

love: examples of 42, 44, 153, 186; impulse to, 191; parental, 35; perverse, 11, 64, 67 70, 93, 112

maladaptive: defences, 10, 14, 65, 92, 107, 154, 217; expressions, 152–53; impulses, 37, 39; responses, 34, 88, 147, 152, 162, 186

maladies. *See also* life stories, maladies in; psychosomatic maladies/diseases

mammalian instinct. *See* instincts, mammalian

manifestation: of chronic stress, 87, 89. *See also* psychosocial trauma

marginalisation, 63, 75, 116, 122, 139, 159, 203

maternal stress 85, 97

medicine, 86, 110, 117, 119, 121, 202, 212

melatonin, 218

memories, 40; ancestral, 53, 55, 99–100, 102, 106, 114; emotional, 11, 58; somatic, 19, 210. *See also* declarative memory; traumatic, memories

memory systems, 26, 52, 161, 185, 187, 197, 207

meningitis, 33

mental: disorders, 43, 110, 173; health, 99, 114, 150, 230; processes, 54, 144, 227; states, 50, 143;

mentalisation, 197, 204

metaphorical spears, 10, 52, 56–57, 69, 72, 225, 231–32, 236

methylation, 80, 84, 193

microglial cells, 79, 133

midbrain, 32–33, 57, 61–62, 131, 227, 236

mind-body: connection, 145; dissociation, 160

mindfulness, 32, 64, 70, 72, 138, 160–61, 177–78, 183, 187, 197, 201, 227

mind-heart-soulfulness, 136, 153, 225

mindsight, 153

misattunement, 160, 187, 191

misery, 39, 64, 113, 115–16, 136, 205

mitochondria, 77, 81, 128, 171, 215

mood: disorders, 115, 147, 159, 196; regulation, 193, 228

moral: boundaries, 28, 176; compass, 26; development, 202; judgment, 55

morality, 26, 28, 205

morbid ideation, 67, 196

motivation, 28, 42–43, 51, 54, 118, 157, 207–8, 219, 221

movement: neurobiology of, 142–43, 193; physical, 57, 214–15; voluntary, 45, 131

muscle: cells, 163; groups, 98; spasms, 119; tension, 144, 215

myelination, 147, 171, 194, 212, 238

narratives, 63, 65, 71, 127, 150, 162, 188–89, 213, 216, 231

native: needs, 3, 5–7, 14, 20, 23, 52, 56, 111, 118, 150, 170; stress-response, 67; vulnerability, 169

neglect, 8, 22, 35, 103, 114, 117, 121, 165, 173–74, 194, 198, 206

nerve. *See* cranial nerves; psoas nerves
neural resilience. *See* resilience
neuroception, 141–47, 157, 165, 186–87, 190, 195, 210, 216–17, 227–28, 230
neurocircuitry, 87, 187, 207
neurodegeneration, 49, 187, 197, 206
neurodynamics 50–51
neurofeedback, 207–8
neurogenesis, 155–56, 197, 214, 221, 238
neuroimaging, 11, 32, 87
neuroinflammation, 89, 131, 155
neuroplasticity, 47, 155–57, 163–64, 210, 238
neurotransmitters, 31, 46
neuroses, 98, 112–13, 119, 139, 143, 155, 169, 173, 194
nomad, 81, 98, 100–101, 106–7, 129, 202, 213, 226
nonviolent communication, 200–201
noradrenaline, 50, 96, 99, 131, 133, 193, 214, 219, 236
nourishment, 26, 69, 97, 114, 156, 170, 197, 199, 203, 212
nucleus: accumbens, 118, 157, 221; ambiguous, 131
nutrients, 32, 83–84, 95, 133, 156, 197, 212, 218
nutrition, 80, 83, 95, 156, 212

obedience, 103, 111, 116
obesity, 8, 49, 83–84, 213, 228–30
occipital lobe, 165, 219, 227
oculi orbicularis, 192, 220, 222
operant conditioning, 162, 207
opioid: endogenic, 50, 111, 134; epidemic 237–38
optimism, 113, 174, 205
overwhelm: in the absence of, 32, 94, 190–91, 202, 213, 217, 230; by anxiety, 69; experiences, 116, 198, 114; by loss, 172–73; sensations of, 40, 43, 60, 134

oxytocin, 42, 45, 51, 69, 87, 94, 103, 170–71, 190, 215, 217

paralyses, 19, 27, 44, 146, 188, 215, 219
parasitosis, 143–44
parasympathetic: activation, 155–56; calmness, 103; depression, 155, 157; nervous system 130, 150; state, 134, 146
parentification, 146, 196
parietal lobe, 145, 165
pathogen, 86, 210, 219
pathological: forgetting, 206; self, 40, 43
peace, 27, 36, 61, 67, 102, 106–7, 149, 172, 178, 197, 201, 205, 218, 230
periaqueductal gray, 34, 50
peripheral nervous system (PNS), 10, 130
pleasure-reward, 157, 187, 190, 226
polyvagal theory, 14
positron emission tomography (PET), 207
posterity, 12, 35, 42–43, 67, 84, 106, 122, 237, 239
post-traumatic: growth, 9–10, 235–37, 240; slave syndrome, 103
power: healing, 40, 208, 215–17, 219; *See also* brain, power
predation, 28, 100, 111, 146
prefrontal cortex. *See* cortex, prefrontal
prejudice, 37, 47, 59, 153, 156
premature: death, 8, 27, 43, 48, 82, 100, 110, 115, 145, 155, 172–73, 180, 202; separation, 110, 117, 173
prenatal nervous system, 94
preservation of life, 9, 41, 127, 225
pride, 52, 64–65, 139
privation, 68, 155, 172, 199, 203
prosocial: behaviour, 50, 52, 69, 132–33; emotion, 175, 194; neurochemistry, 51, 131, 170, 179, 228
psoas nerve, 133, 214
psycho-emotional, 52, 68, 119

psychological: dis-ease, 92, 98, 206–7, 209, 213; health, 114, 152, 201, 207; integrity, 22, 25–26, 41, 52, 54, 61, 88, 118, 198–99, 200–201, 236

psychosocial: deficit, 62, 93, 231; development, 4–7, 18–20, 22, 27, 30, 35, 51–52, 66, 69–70, 173, 188; distress, 100, 104–5; legacies, 19, 37, 65, 75, 109; needs, 14, 28, 201; resources, 14, 19–20, 25, 29, 56, 70, 89, 128, 134, 145, 151, 163, 175, 195, 215, 228, 235; stress, 89, 93–95, 97–104, 106–7, 109, 117, 128–30, 133–35, 139, 156, 193, 210, 236

psychosocial trauma: across the generations, 14, 76, 93, 109–110, 127, 147; adaptations to, 13, 21, 71–72, 87–88, 100, 115, 134, 160, 175, 193, 197, 212; chaotic energy of, 149, 159, 225, 193, 232; conceptualisation of, 12, 120, 143; depleted or lost due to, 178, 189; discharge of 153, 161; in early life, 194, 198, 206; features of, 37, 59, 131, 140, 155, 174, 187, 203–4, 214, 218, 226; as legacy, 91, 94, 107; nature of, 82, 86, 89, 146, 182, 196, 213; therapy for, 220, 228; vector of, 94, 110, 113–14, 116; vulnerability to, 23, 78, 198, 200, 203, 215

psychosomatic maladies/diseases, 40, 49, 61, 71, 75, 87, 89, 91, 93, 116, 118–119, 121–22, 127, 129, 143, 172

psychosomatic vulnerabilities, 47

purposefulness, 199, 201–2, 226, 236

purposelessness, 51, 199

quiver of spears, 23, 26–27, 98, 160

racism, 122, 195

rationalisation, 135, 197–98

recovery, 21, 109, 116–17, 123, 129, 164–65, 172, 204, 231, 234, 239–40

regeneration, 177, 219

regression, 60, 66–67, 151, 235

relational: boundaries, 13, 176; competencies, 104, 112, 120, 170–71; distress, 112, 183; fulfilment, 52, 176; injuries, 172, 174; insecurity, 160, 173; integrity, 178; intimacy, 20, 28; needs, 64, 70, 173–74, 183, 200; resiliency, 169; resources, 173, 179; satisfaction, 22, 25–26, 41, 56, 61, 88, 118, 152, 180, 236; security, 7, 14, 22, 39, 52, 102, 109, 111, 118, 143, 160, 173, 182; therapy, 164, 174, 181–83; trauma, 36, 40, 170–71, 173, 177–78, 181–83

religion, 56, 121, 137–38, 173, 203

religiosity, 109, 113–14, 116, 178, 220

REM. *See* eyes, rapid eye movement

resilience: collective, 239; neural, 197; transgenerational, 237, 240

resonant relationship, 19, 140, 170, 180–82, 231, 235

resourcefulness, 13, 18–20, 23, 50, 70–71, 92, 128, 138, 162, 201, 204, 236–37, 239

restfulness, 49, 51, 211, 218–20, 236

restlessness, 65, 100, 143, 209, 211, 215–16, 218–19, 229

rhythm: of the breath, 216; circadian, 218; of our heart, 4, 32; in our voice, 143. *See also* bodily, rhythm

righteousness, 199, 205–6

sadness, 4, 43, 64, 115, 128, 152, 179, 185

schadenfreude, 42

schizophrenia, 49, 78–79, 82, 87–88, 93, 110, 115, 159

self: abandonment, 35, 65–67, 105, 116, 154, 176; actualisation, 29, 175, 204; alienation, 112, 187–89; authenticity, 22, 25–26, 52, 61, 70, 118, 233; awareness, 44, 55, 205, 231; care, 105, 131, 154; compassion, 13, 157, 175–76, 178, 181–82, 194, 213, 220, 227; concept, 66, 69, 153; destruction, 22, 28, 41, 66, 105,

172, 175, 189, 193; development, 159, 205; discovery, 21, 27, 123, 159, 204, 232, 238; esteem, 21, 42, 64, 102, 173, 195, 199–201; harm, 115–16, 146, 196; heal, 17, 40, 134, 156, 163, 205; image, 66, 120, 172; inauthentic, 30, 35, 37, 39, 67, 116, 151, 173; loath, 66, 105, 116, 172, 183; medicate, 18, 67, 105, 206, 238; possession, 30, 119; preservation, 29–30, 55, 62, 64, 170, 175, 195, 200, 204; protection, 32, 36, 44, 146; regulate, 7–8, 29, 115, 135, 153, 187, 189, 193; rescue, 30, 97, 203, 234; sacrifice, 34–37, 42, 63, 67, 114, 172, 176, 200, 211–12. *See also* acceptance, self

serotonin, 42, 45–46, 51, 69, 87, 103, 131, 133, 171, 193, 218

settler, 99, 102, 104–7, 111, 116, 147, 203, 213

sexual: abuse, 8, 64, 89, 92, 98, 101, 114–15, 135, 144–45, 154, 165, 173, 186, 194, 214, 230; predation, 111, 146; violence, 147, 181–83, 197, 206, 227, 230

shame, 20, 34, 36, 43–44, 63–66, 112–13, 128, 152, 155, 162, 176, 180, 183, 185–86, 189, 192, 194, 202, 206, 213, 231

slavery, 120–22, 127, 140, 160, 195, 239

sleep, 12, 49, 117, 144, 185, 218–21, 229

social-emotional: brain, 29, 45, 69, 87, 95, 105, 170, 186, 191, 210, 221, 227–8, 238; deprivation, 64, 140; injuries, 69, 194; self, 41, 43, 51–52, 56–57, 69, 150. *See also* memories

socialisation, 51–52, 56, 109, 111, 115, 128, 139, 195–96

somatic: anchorage, 227; death, 172; disease, 61, 135, 147; harmony, 52–54, 88, 118; narrative, 213, 216; safety, 22, 25–26, 41, 61, 210, 236;

states, 11, 215, 217, 219. *See also* memories, somatic

soul, 104, 113, 135–39, 141, 153, 161, 163, 180, 206, 222

spears: intelligence spears, 50, 66, 71, 75, 88, 92, 115, 127, 150, 203; native spears, 14, 20, 22, 109, 111, 139; neuro-emotional spear, 136, 187–88, 190, 193; neuro-relational spears, 174, 182; neuro-somatic spear, 210–11, 229; resilience spears, 25–27, 37, 41, 50, 61, 88, 119, 139–40, 149, 178, 183, 200, 228–29, 232, 237. *See also* psychological

spine, 10, 32–33, 25, 59–61, 94–95, 99, 103, 130–31, 133, 177, 197

spirituality, 97, 110, 141, 150, 153, 160, 205, 217–18

stereotypes; 47, 63, 180, 183

stress: disorder, 174, 197, 219; response, 7, 46, 50, 57, 62, 67, 86, 95, 97–98, 109, 122, 131, 146, 221

subconscious process, 106, 141, 156, 222

subconsciousness, 57, 60, 66, 71

suffer, 7, 9, 19, 22, 88, 97, 110, 117, 136, 165, 175–76, 178, 200, 225, 230–31, 234

suicidality, 22, 43, 110, 115, 155, 212, 220

supraconscious, 153–54

survival: demands, 86, 94; needs, 44, 66; neurochemicals, 49–50, 62; states, 156, 218, 239; strategy, 69. *See also* instincts

sustenance, 3, 13, 44, 72, 82–83, 112, 211–12, 236

sympathetic: activation, 96, 103, 131, 146, 155, 157; chain, 95–97, 99, 134, 147, 154; nerve, 48, 60, 216

synaptic cleft, 31–32, 42, 46, 79, 78–79, 88, 133, 187, 193, 207

synchroneity, 61, 129, 150–51, 186, 191–92, 216, 232

synchronies, 3, 12, 22, 151, 190, 208

tai chi, 57, 215
temporal lobe, 66, 145, 165
thalamus, 34, 131, 141–42, 145, 228
thorax, 95–96
thymus, 46, 131
toxic levels of stress, 49, 94, 97, 197
transcendence, 161, 237
transgenerational: trauma, 71, 76, 84, 91, 93, 119, 221. *See also* resilience
transpersonal, 153–54, 161, 163
transposons, 84
trauma-based: adaptation, 76, 87, 89, 92–93, 95, 112, 115, 122, 151–52, 213, 240; responses, 13, 162, 217
traumatic: memories, 12, 40, 62, 72, 133, 165, 186, 197–98, 216, 221; stress, 9, 47, 49, 60, 70, 82, 85, 89, 97, 151, 163, 172, 174, 182, 186–87, 197, 214–15, 219–20, 231; wound, 13, 36, 58, 61, 70, 89, 151, 162–63, 196, 216, 226, 230
tribe, 3, 63, 68, 91, 106, 215, 221

unconscious, 57–58, 66, 88, 98, 138, 150, 201, 219
unregulated: grief, 64; growth in cells, 229
unsafe feeling, 34, 26, 97, 147, 189, 205
unworthiness, 27, 189, 213
uterine: life, 87, 94–95, 97–98, 101–2, 107, 111, 161, 185. *See also* environment, uterine

vagal: breaks, 153, 190; dysregulation, 131, 147; fibres, 131, 153, 171, 186, 192; flexibility, 147, 153; state, 153, 183

vagus. *See* cranial nerve, vagus
ventral-tegmental area, 118, 157, 227
ventromedial: hypothalamus, 29. *See also* cortex, prefrontal
violence: acts of, 64, 103; domestic, 4, 75, 143, 229; intimate partner, 173, 181; physical, 194, 104, 115
virtues, 5, 25, 42, 52, 63–64, 93, 200, 205, 231, 236
visceral: experience, 144; structures, 210; tissue, 132
voluntary movement. *See* movement, voluntary
vulnerabilities. *See* biological, vulnerabilities; native, vulnerability; psychosocial trauma, vulnerability to; psychosomatic vulnerabilities

wakefulness, 32, 218
warrior, 4, 98–99, 105–7, 111, 135, 147, 205, 213
wisdom: ancient, 170, 220; body as source of, 54, 209, 212, 216, 220, 229; intergenerational transmission of, 109. *See also* ancestral, wisdom; biological, wisdom
worthiness, 64–65, 104, 200
worthlessness, 49, 155, 231
wound. *See* traumatic, wound
woundedness 9, 17, 72, 75, 112, 123, 139, 177, 196, 209, 230, 236

yearning, 9, 21, 25, 36, 39, 45, 63, 122, 136, 214, 232

Zygote, 3, 78, 170

Name Index

Almaas, A. H., 97

Birnholz, Jason, 97
Bleuler, Eugen, 87
Bowlby, John, 170, 172, 194
Bronfenbrenner, Urie, 8
Brown, Brené, 237

Campbell, Joseph, 232
Clarke, Arthur, 117
Crick, Francis, 77

Dalton-Smith, Saundra, 219
Damasio, Antonio, 53, 144
Dana, Deb, 153, 155, 217
Darwin, Charles, 77
Davidson, Richard, 231
De Bono, Edward, 226
De Boulogne, Duchenne, 222
DeGruy, Joy, 103, 195
Dempsey, Peter, 203

Ekman, Paul, 41
Erikson, Erik, 5, 18, 35, 134, 138

Felitti, Vincent, 8, 173, 230
Fernández-Armesto, Felipe, 75
Festinger, Leon, 139
Fisher, Janina, 112
Francis, Emily, 133, 214

Frankl, Victor, 202
Freud, Sigmund, 11, 40, 41, 150, 219

Hanson, Rick, 136
Harvey, Thomas, 120
Hebb, Donald, 187
Holme, Jeremy, 6, 67
Hübl, Thomas, 59

Jablonka, Eva, 79
James, William, 200
Jirtle, Randy, 83, 146
Jung, Carl, 21, 60, 68

Kernis, Michael, 21

Lamarck, Jean-Baptiste, 83, 193
Lamb, Marion, 79
Ledoux, Joseph, 69, 95
Lemaître, Georges, 76
Levine, Peter, 50
Lipton, Bruce, 139, 154
Loewi, Otto, 130

Maslow, Abraham, 27, 28, 70, 203
Maté, Gabor, 7
McEwen, Bruce, 86
Miller, Alice, 25, 72

Nietzsche, Friedrich, 202

Nowak, Martin, 65

Ornish, Dean, 211, 212

Patel, Vinay, 43
Porges, Stephen, 141, 153
Prescott, James, 4

Raskind, Murray, 219
Rogers, Carl, 27, 70, 149, 151
Rose, Brian, 7
Rosenberg, Marshall, 200, 201
Rothschild, Babette, 26, 153, 209
Rousseau, Jean-Jacques, 7

Schore, Allan, 69, 170, 185
Selye, Hans, 47

Siegel, Dan, 130, 135, 153
Spearman, Charles, 49, 54
Steele, Claude, 63
Sturge, Joseph, 120

Templeton, John, 201
Terkeurst, Lysa, 234
Thomas, Lennox, 62

Vajda, Peter, 178
Vygotsky, Lev, 7, 8, 159

Walker, Matthew, 219
Watson, James, 77
Watts, Terrance, 27, 99–102, 104, 106
Winnicott, Donald, 30, 71
Wolynn, Mark, 76

About the Author

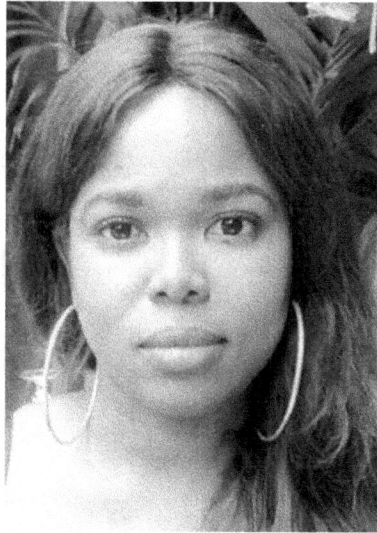

Dr. Winniey E. Maduro is a research psychologist and lecturer in the neurobiology of the psychosocial. Her research focuses on neuropsychosocial adaptations to adverse lived experiences (ALEs) and post-traumatic growth (PTG) across generations. Dr. Maduro lectures internationally on psychosocial trauma and resources, teaches and supervises integrative psychotherapy and research methods at the University of South Wales, and is a specialist examiner for child's health and well-being at the University of Cambridge. Her educational background includes a PhD in social-educational-developmental psychology from the University of Manchester and a master's degree in education psychology and social change from the Linköping University.